Handbook of Bioterrorism and Disaster Medicine

Handbook of Bioterrorism and Disaster Medicine

Edited by

Robert E. Antosia
Harvard Medical School
and
Department of Emergency Medicine
Beth Israel Deaconess Medical Center
Boston, Massachusetts, USA

John D. Cahill
Department of Emergency Medicine and
Division of Infectious Diseases
St. Luke's/Roosevelt Hospital Center
New York, New York, USA

Springer

Robert E. Antosia
Harvard Medical School
and
Department of Emergency Medicine
Beth Israel Deaconess Medical Center
Boston, MA 02215
USA

John D. Cahill
Department of Emergency Medicine and
Division of Infectious Diseases
St. Luke's/Roosevelt Hospital Center
New York, NY 10019
USA

Cover illustration: Cover design "Tribute in Light" courtesy of Charles Nesbit and Richard Nash Gould. A project of John Bennett, Gustavo Bonevardi, Richard Nash Gould, Julian Laverdiere, Paul Marantz, Paul Myoda, The Municipal Art Society, Creative Time.

Library of Congress Control Number: 2006922412

ISBN-10: 0-387-24369-0 e-ISBN-10: 0-387-32804-1
ISBN-13: 978-0387-24369-6 e-ISBN-13: 978-0387-32804-1

Printed on acid-free paper.

9 8 7 6 5 4 3 2 1

springer.com

To all victims of terrorism or disaster
throughout the world

Acknowledgments

I am indebted to Andrea Macaluso from Springer for her patience and faith in this book. A special thanks to Aaron Johnson for helping to get this project off the ground, to Tim Oliver for his expertise in copyediting and typesetting, and to Mara Aloi MD for all her efforts and help. Thank you to all the contributing authors, for this book would not have been possible without them.

Finally, thanks to my wife Rachel for her endless support and help with this project.

—John D. Cahill

Numerous people have helped and supported me in my endeavors. Most especially, I thank my mother and father for showing me the right path and for their endless love and support.

I would also like to acknowledge Dr. Bert Woolard for introducing me the specialty of Emergency Medicine; Drs. Dave Wagner, Jim Roberts, Bob McNamara, and Thomas Alessi for showing me what an emergency physician is and for being such great role models; Dr. Jennifer Leaning for both helping me and inspiring me to understand the need to enhance disaster medical care throughout the world—and the passion for making a difference; and Dr. Troy Brennan for his mentoring and unwavering support.

Finally, I wish to thank my wife Janelle; she gives me the love and strength to follow on the path.

—Robert E. Antosia

PREFACE

The *Handbook of Bioterrorism and Disaster Medicine* was created because we felt there was no effective handbook that covered the breadth and scope of this field. Our book incorporates concise chapters, on topics and diseases with abundant web-based references, and careful organization. We hope that all healthcare providers interested or involved with the care of victims of bioterrorism or disaster — including prehospital care providers, medical students, nurses, physicians, and those involved with public health or humanitarian aide — find it indispensable.

We wish to thank the numerous authors who contributed to this handbook. Throughout the book, consistency of style and depth provide the reader with easy and reliable access to the vast amount of information needed to understand, prepare for, and deal with a bioterrorist attack or disaster. The chapters in this book have been based on scientific studies and data when available. However, more research is needed to more fully understand these complex events.

These events often occur with little or no warning, and they typically disproportionately harm the very young, the very old, and the impoverished.

Contents

CONTRIBUTORS

Amesh Adalja, M.D., Department of Emergency Medicine, Allegheny General Hospital, Drexel University College of Medicine, Pittsburgh, Pennsylvania, USA

Mara Aloi, M.D., Department of Emergency Medicine, Allegheny General Hospital, Drexel University College of Medicine, Pittsburgh, Pennsylvania, USA

Phillip Anderson, M.D., Harvard Medical School, Beth Israel Deaconess Medical Center, Boston, Massachusetts, USA

Robert Antosia, M.D., M.P.H., Harvard Medical School, and Department of Emergency Medicine, Beth Israel Deaconess Medical Center, Boston, Massachusetts, USA

Robert Buckner II, M.D., Department of Emergency Medicine, Allegheny General Hospital, Drexel University College of Medicine, Pittsburgh, Pennsylvania, USA

Frederick Burkle, M.D., M.P.H., The Center for International Emergency, Disaster and Refugee Studies, The John Hopkins University Medical Institutions, Baltimore, Maryland, USA

Michelle Burns, M.D., Children's Hospital, Harvard Medical School, Boston, Massachusetts, USA

John D. Cahill, M.D., Department of Emergency Medicine and Division of Infectious Diseases, St. Luke's/Roosevelt Hospital Center, Columbia College of Physicians and Surgeons, New York, New York, USA

Christopher Cammarata, M.D., Department of Emergency Medicine, Allegheny General Hospital, Drexel University College of Medicine, Pittsburgh, Pennsylvania, USA

Anna Chen, M.D., Harvard Medical School, Beth Israel Deaconess Medical Center, Boston, Massachusetts, USA

Scott Cohen, M.D., Global Pediatric Alliance, Oakland, California, USA

Manuel Colon, M.D., Department of Emergency Medicine, St. Luke's/Roosevelt Hospital Center, Columbia College of Physicians and Surgeons, New York, New York, USA

Marina Del Rios, M.D., Department of Emergency Medicine, St. Luke's/Roosevelt Hospital Center, Columbia College of Physicians and Surgeons, New York, New York, USA

Alexandra Epee-Bounya, M.D., Children's Hospital Boston, Harvard Medical School, Boston, Massachusetts, USA

Stephen Epstein, M.D., M.P.P., Harvard Medical School, Beth Israel Deaconess Medical Center, Boston, Massachusetts, USA

Megan Fix, M.D., Brigham and Women's Hospital, Harvard Medical School, Boston, Massachusetts, USA

Medley Gatewood, M.D., Brigham and Women's Hospital, Harvard Medical School, Boston, Massachusetts, USA

Ann-Jeannette Geib, M.D., Children's Hospital, Harvard Medical School, Boston, Massachusetts, USA

Frank Guyette, M.D., Department of Emergency Medicine, University of Pittsburgh Medical Center, University of Pittsburgh, Pittsburgh, Pennsylvania, USA

Dennis Hanlon, M.D., Department of Emergency Medicine, Allegheny General Hospital, Drexel University College of Medicine, Pittsburgh, Pennsylvania, USA

Fred M. Harchelroad, M.D., Department of Emergency Medicine, Allegheny General Hospital, Drexel University College of Medicine, Pittsburgh, Pennsylvania, USA

Richard V. Hausrod, M.D., Department of Emergency Medicine, Allegheny General Hospital, Drexel University College of Medicine, Pittsburgh, Pennsylvania, USA

Michael Hoffman, Office of International Humanitarian Affairs, American Red Cross, Washington, D.C., USA

Liudvikas Jagminas, M.D., Department of Emergency Medicine, Memorial Hospital, Pawtucket, Rhode Island, USA

Catherine James, M.D., Children's Hospital, Harvard Medical School, Boston, Massachusetts, USA

Sarah M. Kelmenson, M.D., Department of Emergency Medicine, Rhode Island Hospital, Brown University, Providence, Rhode Island, USA

Kristin Kent, M.D., Department of Emergency Medicine, St. Luke's/Roosevelt Hospital Center, Columbia College of Physicians and Surgeons, New York, New York, USA

Barbara Kilian, M.D., Department of Emergency Medicine, St. Luke's/Roosevelt Hospital Center, Columbia College of Physicians and Surgeons, New York, New York, USA

Kevin King, M.D., Department of Emergency Medicine, Boston University, Boston, Massachusetts, USA

Atul Kukar, M.D., Division of Cardiology, St. Luke's/Roosevelt Hospital Center, Columbia College of Physicians and Surgeons, New York, New York, USA

Rashid Kysia, M.D., M.P.H., Brigham and Women's Hospital, Harvard Medical School, Boston, Massachusetts, USA

Jerry Lambert, M.D., Department of Emergency Medicine, Allegheny General Hospital, Drexel University College of Medicine, Pittsburgh, Pennsylvania, USA

Michael Levine, M.D., Brigham and Women's Hospital, Harvard Medical School, Boston, Massachusetts, USA

Lawrence Lo, M.D., Department of Emergency Medicine, St. Luke's/Roosevelt Hospital Center, Columbia College of Physicians and Surgeons, New York, New York, USA

Rishi Malholtra, M.D., Department of Medicine, St. Luke's/Roosevelt Hospital Center, Columbia College of Physicians and Surgeons, New York, New York, USA

Shannon Manzi, Pharm.D., Children's Hospital Boston, Boston, Massachusetts, USA

Peter S. Martin, M.D., Department of Emergency Medicine, Allegheny General Hospital, Drexel University College of Medicine, Pittsburgh, Pennsylvania, USA

George F. McKinley, M.D., Division of Infectious Diseases, St. Luke's/Roosevelt Hospital Center, Columbia College of Physicians and Surgeons, New York, New York, USA

Roland Merchant, M.D., Department of Emergency Medicine, Rhode Island Hospital, Brown University, Providence, Rhode Island, USA

Maria Mileno, M.D., Division of Infectious Diseases, The Miriam Hospital, Brown University, Providence, Rhode Island, USA

Matt Miles, M.D., Department of Emergency Medicine, Albany Medical Center, Albany, New York, USA

Mischa Mirin, M.D., Department of Emergency Medicine, Allegheny General Hospital, Drexel University College of Medicine, Pittsburgh, Pennsylvania, USA

Joshua Nagler, M.D., Brigham and Women's Hospital, Harvard Medical School, Boston, Massachusetts, USA

Lise Nigrovic, M.D., Children's Hospital, Harvard Medical School, Boston, Massachusetts, USA

Neha Parikh, M.D., Department of Emergency Medicine, Allegheny General Hospital, Drexel University College of Medicine, Pittsburgh, Pennsylvania, USA

William Porcaro, M.D., Harvard Medical School, Beth Israel Deaconess Medical Center, Boston, Massachusetts, USA

Charles Pozner, M.D., Brigham and Women's Hospital, Harvard Medical School, Boston, Massachusetts, USA

David J. Prezant, M.D., Pulmonary Division, Montefiore Medical Center, Albert Einstein College of Medicine, Bronx, New York, USA

Arathi Rao, M.D., Division of Infectious Diseases, The Miriam Hospital, Brown University, Providence, Rhode Island, USA

George J. Raukar, M.D., Department of Orthopedics, West Virginia University, Morgantown, West Virginia, USA

David Riley, M.D., Department of Emergency Medicine, St. Luke's/Roosevelt Hospital Center, Columbia College of Physicians and Surgeons, New York, New York, USA

Kaushal Shah, M.D., Department of Emergency Medicine, St. Luke's/Roosevelt Hospital Center, Columbia College of Physicians and Surgeons, New York, New York, USA

Michael Shannon, M.D., Children's Hospital, Harvard Medical School, Boston, Massachusetts, USA

Sam Shen, M.D., M.B.A., Harvard Medical School, Beth Israel Deaconess Medical Center, Boston, Massachusetts, USA

Sophie Skarbek-Borowska, Verso Publishing, London, UK

George W. Skarbek-Borowski, M.D., Department of Emergency Medicine, Memorial Hospital, Brown University, Pawtucket, Rhode Island, USA

Dorsett D. Smith, M.D., Division of Pulmonary Disease and Critical Care, Department of Medicine, University of Washington, Seattle, Washington, USA

Ramona Sunderwirth, M.D., Department of Emergency Medicine, St. Luke's/Roosevelt Hospital Center, Columbia College of Physicians and Surgeons, New York, New York, USA

Stephen Traub, M.D., Harvard Medical School, Beth Israel Deaconess Medical Center, Boston, Massachusetts, USA

Deborah Weiner, M.D., Ph.D., Children's Hospital, Harvard Medical School, Boston, Massachusetts, USA

Dan Wiener, M.D., Department of Emergency Medicine, St. Luke's/Roosevelt Hospital Center, Columbia College of Physicians and Surgeons, New York, New York, USA

Tommy Wong, M.D., Department of Emergency Medicine, St. Luke's/Roosevelt Hospital Center, Columbia College of Physicians and Surgeons, New York, New York, USA

Tracy H. Zivin-Tutela, M.D., Division of Infectious Diseases, St. Luke's/Roosevelt Hospital Center, Columbia College of Physicians and Surgeons, New York, New York, USA

PART I

GENERAL CONCEPTS

1

DEFINING A DISASTER

Robert E. Antosia, MD, MPH*

Disasters are highly complex events resulting in immediate medical problems, as well as longer-term public health consequences. They are generally considered "low probability–high impact" events. As such they are not defined by a specific number of casualties but rather by the event itself and the venue in which it occurs.

The definition of disaster is variable and usually reflects the nature and focus of the organization or individuals defining it. The World Health Organization (WHO) defines a disaster as a sudden ecological phenomenon of sufficient magnitude to require external assistance. This broad definition may exclude some events that result in mass casualties. A more focused definition generally accepted by the specialty of emergency medicine is: *when the number of patients presenting within a given time period are such that the emergency department cannot provide care for them without assistance*. This definition excludes events that result in mass death but place little or no stress on the medical system. At the community level, disasters can be defined operationally as any emergency that seriously affects people's lives and property and exceeds the capacity of the community to respond effectively to that emergency.

Disasters affect a community in numerous ways. Roads, telephone lines, and other transportation and communication lines are often destroyed; public utilities and energy supplies are often disrupted. Many victims are often rendered homeless. The community's industrial or economic base may be damaged or destroyed. Casualties may require urgent or emergent medical care. Damage to water and sanitation systems, food sources and utilities may create public health threats.

All disasters are unique because each affected region of the world has different social, economic, and baseline health conditions. However, some similarities exist and each disaster follows a general pattern in its development. This pattern is often repeated and is illustrated in Figure 1. While the divisions are artificial as one phase merges with another, this simplified disaster cycle model is useful to help understand and plan for these complex events.

Initially, a quiescent level or interdisaster period is seen during which the combination of events that will lead to a disaster are occurring but not readily apparent. A

*Department of Emergency Medicine, Beth Israel Deaconess Medical Center, Harvard Medical School, Boston

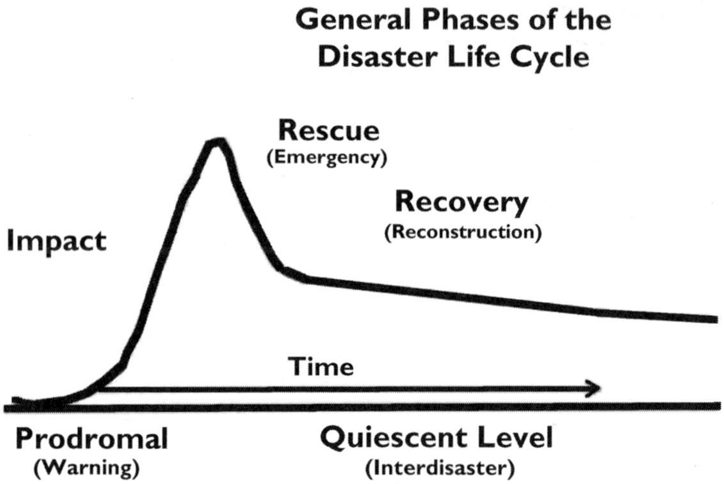

Figure 1. General phases of the disaster life cycle. Reprinted with permission from Hogan and Burstein (2002).

prodrome or warning phase develops next and lasts a variable length of time. The warning period represents a time during which a particular event (e.g. a hurricane, volcanic eruption, military conflict) is likely to occur. However, some disasters occur with little or no warning. The impact phase coincides with the occurrence of the event and may be short or protracted depending upon the particular event. The rescue phase (also known as the emergency, relief, or isolation phase) represents a time when immediate assistance can save lives. During this time, first responders' actions, basic and advanced life support, as well as search and rescue, are critical but often overwhelmed or incapacitated. The recovery or reconstruction phase constitutes all of the actions and elements needed to return the population back to a functional society. It involves the coordinated efforts of emergency medical services, public health agencies, government and social services as well as other agencies and can last months or years.

REFERENCES

Hogan DE, Burstein JL. 2002. *Disaster medicine*. Philadelphia: Lippincott, Williams, and Wilkins.

Noji EK. 1997. *The public health consequences of disasters*. New York: Oxford University Press.

Waeckerle JF. 1991, Disaster Planning and Response. *N Engl J Med* **324**:815–821.

2

EARLY WARNING SYSTEMS

Robert E. Antosia, MD, MPH*

Early warning systems rely on both intelligence information and surveillance data for mitigation and response to a disaster. They have been developed to help predict many types of disasters: natural, manmade, war/conflict, and humanitarian crises. Such systems may include: seismic monitors, weather forecasts, satellite images, food stores and agriculture, economic activity, political situations, infant/child mortality rates, and disease-surveillance systems. Additionally, there must be a routine flow of information so that people are both disaster-aware and mitigation-aware. Evacuation can be considered a step in mitigation, by removing people from an area of potential harm. There are several threats that can result in evacuation, including natural disasters (flood, tsunami, volcano, etc.) and some manmade disasters. This chapter will focus on early warning systems for natural disasters and bioterror (BT) events.

While some natural disasters such as hurricanes may be predicted with some advanced warning, we remain unable to predict earthquakes with any degree of reliability. However, after the occurrence of large-scale undersea earthquakes, which can be recorded on seismic monitoring networks worldwide, preliminary warnings can be raised for coastal regions at risk for tsunamis. These warnings are circulated via established communication systems. In the US, for example, a national warning system is in place that is used to contact emergency personnel, as well as the use of radio, television, and the internet. The US National Tsunami Hazard Mitigation Program highlights the key principles of Tsunami hazard planning, including hazard assessment, mitigation, and warning guidance. Early warning systems for tsunamis exist for the Pacific Rim, Japan, the west coast of the US (including Alaska and Hawaii), and South America. The effectiveness of these systems is proven, and could have prevented tens of thousands of deaths on December 26, 2004 if an early warning system was present in the Indian Ocean. The tsunami that struck 11 countries in South Asia that day resulted in a disaster of apocalyptic proportions. Had alerts from existing networks reached the stricken countries, the impact could have been mitigated further with improved communication systems and education regarding awareness of the true danger.

*Department of Emergency Medicine, Beth Israel Deaconess Medical Center, Harvard Medical School, Boston

Unfortunately, most terrorist attacks occur with little or no warning. In response to the terrorist attacks in the US on September 11, 2001, the United States created the Department of Homeland Security. This entity has nine components: border and transportation security, emergency preparedness and response, information analysis and infrastructure protection, science and technology, management, coast guard, secret service, citizenship and immigration services, and the inspector general. The department overlooking emergency preparedness and response established a five-tiered, color-coded security advisory system based on the perceived threat level of a terrorist attack. The highest risk level is termed "severe" and is coded red; a "high" level of risk is coded orange; an "elevated" or significant risk is coded yellow; a "guarded" or general level of risk is coded blue; and a "low" risk of terrorist attacks is coded green. This serves to notify the media, general public, police and military officers, and public health agencies in an attempt to improve awareness and readiness should an attack occur.

European governments and most other countries have avoided the drastic organizational changes for disaster planning and management that have recently occurred in the US. In many countries, the preparation and response to bioterrorism and other public health problems are led by applied epidemiology and training programs (AETPs), which are part of, or closely affiliated with, the host country's ministry of health. AETPs cover approximately 45 countries, and most are strengthened by support from various partners, including representatives from the Centers for Disease Control (CDC) and the World Health Organization (WHO).

Improved global surveillance efforts should be instituted with as close to real-time data gathering as possible. All facets of surveillance should be used and should include emergency department visits, laboratory data, pharmacy use, school absenteeism, and any other data that may correlate with an outbreak of infectious disease. Robust surveillance systems are essential in detecting any emerging or reemerging diseases that may represent a possible BT attack. Quick recognition of any change in disease patterns will facilitate determination of the source and help limit further exposure. With applied epidemiology and training programs, close attention to disease patterns, and a basic knowledge and understanding of the threat of BT, actions can be taken to decrease the impact of disease and disasters, regardless of their etiology.

RESOURCES

http://www.hewsweb.org/home_page/default.asp
http://www.reliefweb.int/resources/ewarn.html

REFERENCES

Department of Homeland Security. 2004. www.dhs.gov/dhspublic

Perry RW, Lindell MK. 2003. Preparedness for emergency response: guidelines for the emergency planning process. *Disasters* **27**(4):336–350

Sandhu HS, Thomas C, Nsubuga P, et al. 2003. A global network for early warning and response to infectious diseases and bioterrorism: applied epidemiology and training programs. *Am J Pub Health* **93**:10.

Zygmunt-Lubkowski JB. 2005. Managing tsunami risk. *Lancet* **365**:271–273.

3 EPIDEMIOLOGY OF DISASTERS

Robert E. Antosia, MD, MPH*

Epidemiology is based on two fundamental assumptions; first, that human disease does not occur at random, and second, that human disease has causal and preventable factors that can be identified through systematic investigation. It is the study of the distribution, determinants, and frequency of disease in human populations. Epidemiology is also concerned with the broader causes of disease. Note that the term "disease" refers to a broad array of health-related states and events, including diseases, injuries, disabilities, and death.

Disasters are predictable—not in time or place, but in their inevitability. A major disaster occurs almost daily, and a natural disaster that requires international assistance for affected populations occurs weekly. The rate of occurrence of such events may be increasing; this is possibly due to regular variation in natural cycles such as solar flares, earthquakes, and volcanic activity. Also, global warming is projected to increase storm activity in some areas and to cause drought in others.

Although the likelihood of natural disasters is relatively high, the chance of a bioterrorist (BT) attack or other manmade disaster is both unknown and unpredictable. In contrast to nuclear and chemical weapons, for which both short- and long-term consequences can be rather well established, the consequences of the use of biological weapons are hardly foreseeable. The spread of BT agents, unlike other weapons, can go undetected, and when noticed they may have already infected a major portion of the population.

Despite advances in preparedness, nations remain vulnerable. This is especially true of civilian populations, who often do no have readily available protective equipment or vaccines. Unlike natural disasters, the unfortunate fact remains that humans are often the most sensitive, or the only, detector of a biological attack. Without prior knowledge of an attack, an increased number of patients presenting with signs and symptoms caused by the disseminated disease agent is most likely the first indicator that a BT attack has occurred.

A comprehensive epidemiologic investigation of a disease outbreak, whether natural or manmade, will assist medical personnel in identifying the pathogen as well as

*Department of Emergency Medicine, Beth Israel Deaconess Medical Center, Harvard Medical School, Boston

Table 1. Phases of a Complex Emergency

Parameter	Acute emergency	Late emergency	Post-emergency
Timeframe	0–1 mo.	1–6+ mo	>6 mo
Health profile	High CMR High CFR Outbreaks of communicable disease Malnutrition	Declining CMR	Stable CMR "Village" profile
Priority needs	Food Water/sanitation Shelter	Security Fuel Improve basic needs	Expand self-sufficiency
Public health interventions	General ration, possible elective feeding Measles immunization HIS Primary care clinics and outreach and ORT centers	Train community health workers Standardize treatment protocols Expand HIS Develop rational drug supply Begin MHC and STD programs	Develop tuberculosis and mental health programs Expand MHC and STD programs

United Nations Office of the Coordinator of Human Affairs (OCHA) organized to coordinate large-scale humanitarian emergencies
Abbreviations: CFR = case fatality rate; CMR = crude mortality rate; HIS = health information system; MCH = maternal and child health; ORT = oral rehydration therapy; STD = sexually transmitted disease.
Reprinted with permission from Burkholder and Toole (1995).

the appropriate medical interventions. Documenting who is affected, the possible routes of exposure, the signs and symptoms of disease, and rapid identification of the causative agents will enhance the ability to plan an effective and comprehensive public response. This includes establishing priorities for action and is essential to determine appropriate relief supplies, equipment, and personnel needed to respond effectiv ely to such situations. Additionally, such information will allow appropriate follow-up of those potentially exposed as well as help determine public information guidelines and response to the media.

Unfortunately, most diseases caused by BT agents present with nonspecific signs and symptoms that could be misinterpreted as natural occurrences. The developing disease pattern, including measures of disease frequency, is an important factor in differentiating between a natural event and a BT attack. In most naturally occurring epidemics, there is a gradual rise in disease incidence as people are progressively exposed to an increasing number of patients, formites, or vectors that spread the pathogen. In contrast, all those exposed to a BT attack would come into contact with the agent at approximately the same time. This results in a compressed epidemic curve with a peak attack rate within a matter of days or even hours after a specific exposure. Most point-source exposures will present in this fashion with a large difference in attack rates for exposed and unexposed individuals. Such outbreaks may be naturally occurring, such as food-borne outbreaks, or possibly intentionally induced. Further information should be obtained to help establish the causal agent.

Since a disease outbreak can be the result of intentional contamination, the differential diagnosis of an outbreak should first be considered. The possibilities include a spontaneous outbreak of a known epidemic disease, a spontaneous outbreak of a new or reemerging disease, a laboratory accident, or an intentional attack with a BT agent.

The basic epidemiologic approach in the evaluation of a potential attack is not different from any standard epidemiologic investigation. The first step is to use laboratory and clinical findings to confirm that a disease outbreak has occurred. A case definition should be constituted to determine the number of cases and the attack rate. The use of specific objective criteria in the development of a case definition is very important in determining the attack rate, as steep epidemic curves can be seen in natural point-source exposures. Additional characteristics of the outbreak should be investigated in determining whether it is the result of a BT attack. Possible clues to a terrorist attack include: the presence of a large epidemic, especially in a discrete population; more severe disease than expected for a given pathogen, as well as unusual routes of exposure, such as a preponderance of inhalation disease (as seen in the US with the intentional release of Anthrax spores), a disease unusual for given geographical areas, one focused outside its normal transmission season, or a disease impossible to transmit naturally in the absence of the normal vector for transmission; multiple simultaneous epidemics of different diseases; unusual strains or variants of organisms with unusually high antimicrobial resistance; higher attack rates in those exposed within certain areas, such as inside a building if the agent was released indoors; claims by terrorist of the release of a BT agent; and direct evidence of the release of an agent, with findings of equipment or tampering. If an attack with BT agents is suspected, the proper authorities, either military or civilian, should be notified immediately.

Burkholder and Toole (1995) described complex emergencies or disasters as having acute, late, and post-emergency phases, each of which is characterized by predictable patterns of health indicators and expected public health responses. If these patterns are addressed with appropriate management responses, a decline in mortality and morbidity and a shortening of the duration of each epidemiologic phase will result.

REFERENCES

Aschengrau A, Seage GR. 2003. *Essentials of epidemiology in public health.* Boston: Jones and Barlett.

Buckholder BT, Toole MJ. 1995. Evolution of complex emergencies. *Lancet* **346**:1012–1015.

Henderson DA, Inglesby TV, O'Toole TJ. 2002. *Bioterrorism: guidelines for medical and public health management*. American Medical Association Press, pp. 1-12, 54-68.

Hennekens CH, Buring JE. 1987. *Epidemiology in medicine.* Philadelphia: Lippincott, Williams, and Wilkins.

Hogan DE, Burstein JL. 2002. *Disaster medicine.* Philadelphia: Lippincott, Williams, and Wilkins, pp. 3-9.

Noji EK. 1996. *Disaster epidemiology*. Philadelphia: W.B. Saunders, pp. 289–300.

4

TRIAGE

Frederick M. Burkle Jr., MD, MPH*

DEFINITION

Triage occurs when clinicians sort, screen, and prioritize victims in a resource-constrained environment.

Operational Characteristics

- In preparing and planning for a disaster, it is a legal expectation that a triage plan exist.
- Legally, ethically, and morally, under a triage plan there is an obligation to treat as many victims as possible who have a chance of survival.
- The methodology by which this plan occurs is called the triage process.
- Recognizing the limiting circumstances of any disaster event, international law requires that the best "opportunity" for survival be provided to all victims. This "opportunity," in fact, translates operationally into a well thought out and designed triage plan and process that ensures resources be used appropriately and fairly.
- When performed in accordance with accepted medical practice, triage is recognized and sanctioned by law in most countries.
- Providers of care are held accountable for the triage process, but the process itself cannot ensure either treatment or survival.

Triage Decision Criteria

Disaster medicine recognizes guidelines that emphasize decisions for populations, not necessarily individuals. Triage exists to provide the greatest good to the

*The Center for International Emergency, Disaster and Refugee Studies, The Johns Hopkins University Medical Institutions, Baltimore, Maryland

greatest number. The decision criteria for triage is that victims who receive care have a likelihood of success, and that scarce resources, the driving force of triage decisions, are appropriately conserved and utilized through the triage decision-making process.

Exclusion Criteria

Western industrialized countries pride themselves on a robust health system that has rarely been forced to engage a triage process during disasters. Hospitals enjoy almost limitless resources (referred to as inclusion criteria) for natural disasters and trauma care. However, if a large-scale communicable disease disaster would occur today, over half of US hospitals lack enough antibiotics to treat more than 50 victims. Studies suggest that triage of resources would be required for up to 72 hours (based on surge capacity expectations in the US). During that time some victims would be triaged to obtain full treatment based on inclusion criteria, whereas other medical and surgical conditions might not receive the resources normally expected (referred to as utilizing exclusion criteria). Healthcare providers who have worked in complex humanitarian emergencies—such as the wars and conflict events in Somalia, Rwanda, the Sudan, the former Yugoslavia, and Liberia—recognize that triage based on exclusionary criteria is commonplace and prolonged.

Minimal Qualification for Survival (MQS)

An MQS is a predetermined and agreed-upon criterion, based on available resource constraints, that determines what conditions/cases will not receive curative care (e.g., cardiac arrests, severe trauma, lethal radiation dose, advanced respiratory failure from pneumonic plague or inhalational Ebola, or severe burns) but will receive pain relief and emotional and spiritual support, if available. Without resources, the hopelessly injured and ill die. Unrealistic triage results in unacceptable deaths rates among those who should survive.

Disaster Triage Nomenclature

The Potential Injury/Illness Creating Event (PICE) disaster nomenclature is a helpful management tool in large-scale disasters where triage occurs. PICE provides a method for consistency in disaster classification, based on the likelihood that outside medical assistance will be needed. Stage 0 means little or no chance, stage I means there is a small chance, stage II means there is a moderate chance, and stage III means local resources are clearly overwhelmed. This nomenclature emphasizes critical decisions concerning resources and extent of geographic involvement (from local to international). PICE is applicable to triage in large-scale events such as internal conflicts and war, accidental or bioterrorism induced epidemics, or to radiation/nuclear tragedies.

TRIAGE PROCESS

Simple Triage

Simple triage is defined and used at the scene of a mass casualty incident to choose patients who require immediate transport to a hospital to save their lives as opposed to patients who can wait for help. First-aid resources are triaged for patient transport. START (Simple Triage and Rapid Treatment) is a process that is readily performed by pre-hospital and inexperienced volunteer personnel in the field in trauma-related disasters such as earthquakes and accidents. Triage separates victims into four groups: DECEASED, those who require IMMEDIATE transportation, those who would not be compromised by DELAYED transport, and those "walking wounded" with MINOR injuries.

Advanced Triage

Advanced triage refers to the process used in disasters where severely injured should not receive care because they are unlikely to survive, and the available care must be rationed to those patients who have some hope of survival. In advanced triage a more skilled personnel will sort the injured into five categories that are also identified by color coded triage tags:

- EXPECTANT/BLACK colored tag: those who will die from their injuries or illness.
- IMMEDIATE/RED colored tag: those who require immediate surgery or advanced care.
- OBSERVATION/YELLOW colored tag: condition is currently stable but requires close observation by trained healthcare providers. May be re-triaged to immediate category.
- WAIT/GREEN colored tag: would tolerate delay in treatment for hours or days. Many minor fractures and soft tissue injuries fall into this group. Require designated follow-up arrangements.
- DISMISS/WHITE colored tag: minor injuries or illnesses. First aid and/or home treatments are appropriate, with early follow up.

LESSONS LEARNED

Military Triage in Conventional Warfare

Traditional battlefield model for triage is defined as a procedure whereby the wounded are classified, to type and urgency, and then routed under assigned priorities to echelons of advanced care. Conventional warfare focuses on retaining the fighting force. By western military standards support to the military is robust with equipment, supplies, and personnel, with readily available urgent care, forward surgical teams, and rapid evacuation to specialized surgical care, within or without the theater of war. These criteria are expected and required for morale.

Triage categories vary. Conventional military schemes commonly utilize a MEDIC-type approach to classification. Likely percentages of victim categories found apply to conventional war and large-scale trauma-related disasters. Major variations would suggest unique nonconventional characteristics exist—for example, high-velocity blast weaponry or the presence of a large-scale accidental or deliberate (bioagent) contagious disease:

- Minimal (require only limited care before return to duty; makes up about 40% of those triaged).
- Expectant (the dead or nearly dead; constitutes about 20% of those triaged).
- Delayed (delay in treatment will not compromise survival; comprises about 20% of those triaged).
- Immediate (requires acute care management and/or surgery to survive; constitutes 20% of those triaged).
- Contaminated: Chemical, biological, or radiation/nuclear contamination, with or without primary trauma.

Reverse triage is practiced when the less wounded or ill may are treated first, thereby delaying those patients who are severe. This may be deemed necessary in war to rapidly return soldiers to combat.

Triage in Complex Emergencies

Up to 90% of victims in complex emergencies (CEs), from both trauma and illness, are civilians. Access and availability of health care and basic public health resources are scarce. Nongovernmental organization (NGOs), the International Committee of the Red Cross (ICRC)/International Federation of Red Cross and Red Crescent (IFRC) societies, United Nations (UN) Agencies, and UN and non-UN militaries often provide healthcare resources in these conflicts. Nongovernmental agencies (NGOs) and the ICRC are often the only providers of emergency medical assistance in long-term CEs such as the Sudan and Liberia, who have both suffered totally collapsed health systems as the result of decades of war.

A major characteristic of CEs is that resources for health are scarce or nonexistent. Basic medical care, public health infrastructure, and essential resources are lacking. Relief equipment and supplies are imported by relief agencies through a complicated and often looted logistics system. Healthcare professionals are mostly expatriates. These countries are usually in a constant state of triaging all essential services, not just health. As such, the triage process must take into account multisectoral (i.e., water, food, sanitation, shelter, fuel, security) factors in making triage decisions.

In Kigali, Rwanda, where over 20,000 trauma casualties occurred in April 1994, scant resources required the rapid development of a triage system that could only provide minimal operative treatment for those victims "left standing." The triage objective was limited to prevention of secondary wound infections and mitigation of further morbidity and disability in victims who had the likelihood of survival. Any more serious victims did not receive treatment other than pain medication and comfort. In refugee camps in the former Zaire, there were limited rehydration salts and liquids to adequately treat epidemics of cholera and dysentery. Minimal qualification for survival criteria (MQS) constituted an essential part of the camp triage process. All triage criteria were resource driven but could change on an hourly or daily basis depending on the ability of camp managers and logisticians to obtain outside resources by whatever means possible.

Large-Scale Bioterrorism Events

The goal of triage in a noncommunicable disease disaster is to successfully treat primary infections. In the example of an inhalational anthrax event, the major triaged resources would be available: organism-sensitive antibiotics, ventilators, and intensive-care beds and staff. However, in the post-9/11 anthrax terrorist event, only 20 primary cases were treated (half pulmonary, half cutaneous), but up to 35,000 people were treated with outpatient antibiotics.

If triage of antibiotics or vaccines becomes a priority, it will require resources to ensure more stringent history-taking to better identify those exposed from those potentially exposed but psychologically traumatized or impaired, individuals with multiple unexplained physical symptoms (MUPS), and those simply susceptible but concerned they might have been exposed. This subgroup may make up most of those seeking immediate care. A triage process that does not recognize and plan for these victims will certainly fail. A rapidly fielded Health Information System (HIS) is required to first clarify and mitigate risk and vulnerability, and to then stovepipe timely and accurate information to those in need. It is the major resource tool in triage management. Triage planning must provide predesignated programs for evaluation, education, reassurance, and emotional support separate from but close to any health facility, to ensure ready access, availability, and compliance.

In communicable disease disasters such as smallpox and inhalational plague, the goal of triage is to successfully identify and treat primary infections and to prevent secondary infections. Public health measures such as surveillance, disease containment strategies (i.e., isolation, quarantine), immunization, and prophylactic antibiotics are the major management tools to prevent secondary infections. The Centers for Disease Control and Prevention (CDC) in Atlanta was overwhelmed with testing of bogus anthrax samples, as were several other remote state laboratories. In the SARS epidemic in Toronto, the laboratory resources were quickly compromised. The triage plan and process must be broad based to include laboratory, pharmaceutical, hospital, and outpatient care center resources, to name but a few. The CDC/Homeland Security facilitated Strategic National Stockpile (SNS) will provide pharmaceutical resources within 12 to 72 hours, thereby decreasing significantly the triage time.

Large-scale communicable disease events will challenge any conventional trauma related triage system. The PICE categorization scheme is adaptable to illness and would set the stage for understanding triage and management requirements. There are five triage groups (SEIRV) for communicable disease outbreaks, both accidental (i.e., SARS) and deliberate bioagents:

- SUSCEPTIBLE individuals make up the majority of victims and require robust health information and education resources; includes those with incomplete or unsuccessful vaccination.
- EXPOSED individuals: those who are infected but not yet symptomatic or contagious.
- INFECTIOUS individuals symptomatic and contagious; includes remains of those who died but are still contagious (i.e., Ebola).
- REMOVED individuals, who are no longer sources of infection, who either survived or died from the illness, including remains no longer contagious.
- VACCINATED successfully, or those who completed a course of immunity.

Triage tags, signifying one of the SEIRV triage groups, can serve as temporary medical records.

Large-Scale Radiation Disasters

The Cold War produced medical modeling for potential low- and high-yield nuclear explosion scenarios. Studies then suggested that mass casualty consequences would be dire, and a 1977 casualty policy warned not to waste medical staff/resources on "organized life saving operations." The goal of triage would be to save the maximum number of lives by refusing medical care to those unlikely to recover. Triage groups, which can be used even today, are either "survival possible" or "survival impossible." In a mass casualty event, reverse triage would be standard practice.

If victims are transported to a radiation-free area, contaminated injured patients will not be a radiation hazard to healthcare providers. Life-supporting measures and emergency treatment take precedence over specific treatment for radiation injury. Triage-management will be:

- Confirm radiation contamination with a radiation detector.
- Decontaminate with 0.5% hypochlorite solution.
- Confirm removal of 95% of radiation with detector.
- If life-threatening injuries from blast or flying objects require surgery, it must be performed within 48 hours or immune system compromise will delay healing.

The severity of symptoms of acute radiation syndrome depends on radiation dose, type, and individual sensitivity. Severity is marked by rapid onset of nausea, vomiting and malaise. The clinical triage markers of individual radiation dose are:

- time to onset of symptoms (nausea and vomiting)
- severity of nausea and vomiting
- decrease in absolute lymphocyte count for hours or days after exposure
- peripheral blood lymphocytes evidencing dicentric and ring forms, indicating chromosomal aberrations

Based on the above, triage decisions would depend on the availability and access to the following resources:

- antimicrobial, antiviral, and antifungal therapies
- antiemetics
- analgesics
- potassium iodide to reduce thyroid uptake

Triage will require observation, over time, of signs and symptoms involving the hematopoietic, gastrointestinal, cerebrovascular, and cutaneous systems. The resources for more advanced treatment options of a hematopoietic syndrome, in select cases, include hematopoietic cytokines, blood transfusions, and stem-cell transplantation.

Triage in a "dirty bomb" event would deal with concerns over potential exposures. An example of what to expect occurred in Brazil in 1987, where a disassembled medical radiation device found in a city dump and passed around to unsuspecting individuals measurably contaminated 249 people, causing 30 to suffer radiation sickness and 4 to die; however, over 112,000 requested radiation screening. Whereas potassium iodide might be useful in a thermonuclear disaster event, it may be of little value in a dirty bomb event.

REFERENCES

Barclay L, Lie D. 2004. New guidelines address radiation syndrome. Medscape Medical News, June 14. http://www.medscape.com/viewarticle/480890. Accessed 1 July 2004.

Burkle FM. 1999. Lessons learnt and future expectations of complex emergencies. *BMJ* **319**:422–426.

Burkle FM. 2002. Mass casualty management of a large-scale bioterrorist event: An epidemiological approach that shapes triage decisions. *Emerg Med Clin North Am* **20**:409–436.

Burkle FM, Orebaugh S, Barendse BR. 1994. Emergency medicine in the Persian Gulf War, part 1: preparations for triage and combat casualty care. *Ann Emerg Med* **23**(4):742–747.Burkle FM, Newland C, Orebaugh S, Blood CG. 1994. Emergency medicine in the Persian Gulf War, part 2: triage methodology and lessons learned. *Ann Emerg Med* **23**(4):748–754.

Campbell D. 1982. *War plan UK: the truth about civil defence in Britian*. London: Burnett Books, pp. 112–413.

Coupland RM. 1994. Epidemiological approach to surgical management of the casualties of war. *BMJ* **308**:1693–1697.

Information headquarters: Triage. http://www.informationheadquarters.com/health_science/triage.shtml. Accessed 7 April, 2004.

Koenig KL, Dinerman N, Kuehl AE. 1996. Disaster nomenclature—a functional impact approach: the PICE system. *Acad Emerg Med* **3**:723–727.

Neal CJ, Moores LKE. 2002. Weapons of mass destruction: radiation. *Neurosurg Focus* **12**(3), http://www.medscape.com/viewarticle/43113. Accessed 1 July 2004.

Ring JP. 2004. Radiation risks and dirty bombs. *Health Phys* **86**(suppl 1):S42–S47.

Vastag B. 2003. Experts advise on potassium iodide use: no protection against "dirty bombs." *JAMA* **289**(16):2058.

Winslow GR. 1982. *Triage and justice*. Berkeley: University of California Press, pp. 1–23.

5 DISASTER LOGISTICS

Robert E. Antosia, MD, MPH*

Logistics generally refers to the method of procuring, distributing, maintaining, and replacing goods, equipment, and personnel. The basic task of a logistics system is to provide essential operations support by delivering the appropriate supplies, in the quantities required, at the places and times they are needed. In reality, disaster logistics is a systems exercise involving integrated and coordinated performance from a diverse group of skilled specialists and support staff. It is both the largest and most complex element of disaster operations, and overcoming logistical obstacles is often much more difficult than characterizing the health priorities.

The critical components of logistics include medical supply, communications, facilities, and security (see Figure 1). Supplies are those materials and medications that are consumed and cannot be reused. Supplies are listed in several categories, and detailed lists are found in various other areas of the text. A disaster area is supplied using the "push-pull" method. In a pull supply system, field units order supplies as needed. This system has several disadvantages, including the need for an effective communications system and the inherent lag time from order to arrival. In a push supply system, predetermined supplies are forwarded to the disaster scene. The push system is a military logistics concept that has also been adopted by EMS and fire department operations. In this system, supply needs are anticipated and stored in caches in forward areas at key locations throughout a city, county, or region. In disasters, these caches are designed to be easily mobilized and to be used by regional or national disaster teams. In a best-case disaster scenario, the pushed supplies account for 95% of logistical needs. The additional supplies are pulled to ensure that adequate needs are met.

Communications is a key support unit in logistics. Effective communications may involve handheld radio transmissions, telephones (landline and cellular), computers, or portable fax machines. The specific information that must be communicated includes vehicle status, unit assignments, resource consumption, and emergency traffic. These transmissions should include only relevant information, and the messages should be clear and concise. In addition, feedback is a critical loop to ensure that the

*Department of Emergency Medicine, Beth Israel Deaconess Medical Center, Harvard Medical School, Boston

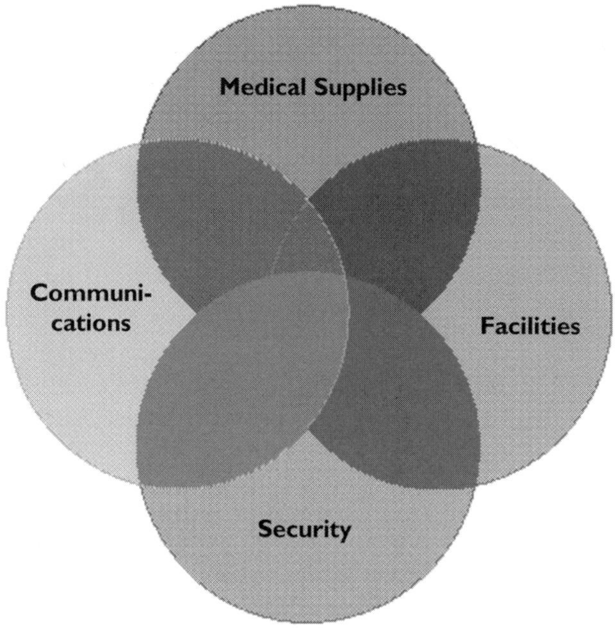

Figure 1. Logistic components.

message is received and understood. Finally, in a large-scale mass casualty incident or disaster, Medical Control serves as a gatekeeper and is responsible for maintaining the patient receiving status for all medical facilities in the area. Medical Control is usually located at the dispatch center or hospital command post. Medical Control contacts all appropriate medical facilities to determine patient availability and maintain the status of specialized facilities, such as burn units, pediatric hospitals, etc.

The facilities unit provides food, water, and living facilities for on-scene personnel. Such units are usually only required for large-scale mass casualty incidents or disasters. Adequate site facilities also function as a rest and rehabilitation area for working personnel. Facilities support is often provided by local public health agencies or ministries of health as well as various Intergovernmental Organizations and Nongovernmental Organizations.

Security is an essential component of logistics. It may require the appointment of an incident manager and involvement of police, fire, or military personnel. The key role of the security unit is to provide protection to medical personnel and first responders. In addition to controlling civil order, the security unit is responsible for traffic control, treatment area security, and security against secondary terrorist attacks.

Planning and anticipation form the cornerstone of a good logistics program, which usually involves a central coordination body. The preparedness plan requires a thorough knowledge of the operating environment as well as an appropriate implementation and operations plan. All plans must allow for potential breakdowns in the system and contingencies with redundancy, extra capacity, and alternative procedures to provide flexibility as needed. This is critical since a mass casualty incident will consume the supplies of responding units; a medical disaster will deplete regional supplies.

Logistical activities should be coordinated with other components of a comprehensive disaster plan and be based at the command post. For example, information, communication, and control systems are vital to monitor the performance of ongoing operations and to optimize support. This is especially important since personnel support is closely related to supply support.

A challenge of logistics is the prompt and reliable delivery of supplies when infrastructure is damaged or nonexistent. Different means of delivery may include aircraft if an appropriate and accessible landing strip exists; trains, boats, and trucks may also provide the necessary means depending on the situation. In large-scale disasters, consumption of supplies may occur rapidly and deplete regional supplies. While distribution-related activities will usually be improvised at the local level, there may be a need for very rapid and very specific deliveries from outside the area. This can include supply of critical medical items, delivery of communications equipment, or provision of relief food, water, shelter, sanitation, and electrical power, as well as other basic items. Medical and public health care, as well as provisions for civic order and security, must also be provided. No one agency or organization has control of such resources. The major participants, all of which have vital roles to play, include local and national government organizations, the United Nations (UN) and UN agencies, other nongovernmental organizations (NGOs), international organizations such as the International Committee of the Red Cross (ICRC), and military forces can play important supporting roles.

REFERENCES

Chrisen HT, Maniscalo PM. 2002. *Mass casualty and high-impact incidents—an operations guide.* Englewood Cliffs, NJ: Prentice-Hall.

Stephenson RS. 1993. *Logistics: disaster management training program.* New York: United Nations Development Program.

6 PUBLIC HEALTH PREPAREDNESS

Robert E. Antosia, MD, MPH*

The most common approach is to describe disaster preparedness and response as a series of stages in which the reaction to the disaster ends in a return to normalcy. The various stages are concomitant and overlapping, but are nonetheless useful to better understand the process. While the historical origin of these cycles is in natural disasters, they can be adapted to other types of disasters. The public health model for disasters highlights a cycle of preparedness, mitigation, response, and recovery. This is used by the US Federal Emergency Management Agency (FEMA) in its instructional materials and courses.

Risk Assessment: Basic surveys of a given area are conducted to locate potential disaster hazards. Accurate knowledge of the threat comes from thorough hazard assessment and vulnerability analysis and is a sustained and ongoing process. This includes identification of the risk, an estimation of the probability of occurrence, and an estimation of the possible damage.

Mitigation: This includes contingency plans that are drawn up to "mitigate" or limit the effects of a disaster. This may include evacuation of patients away from an imminent threat or movement from a disaster site to unaffected areas.

Response: As a disaster strikes, response agencies are activated to help support coordinated relief efforts. This often involves EMS providers, police, firefighters, local and regional Emergency Departments, as well as governmental and public health officials and agencies. In large-scale disasters, the response may require regional, national, or international humanitarian aide agencies depending on the number of victims and the severity of injuries. Both initial and definitive medical care as well as psychological support and crisis counseling are provided. Temporary housing, financial contributions, and donations of goods and services help to support relief efforts.

Recovery: After the immediate response is completed, long-term recovery begins. Depending on the severity, this process may take months to years to complete. The goals are to promote the recovery of individuals as well as the restoration of the economic and civil life of the community. Victims remain at risk for depression, guilt, and posttraumatic stress disorder. Displaced populations are particularly vulnerable. The

*Department of Emergency Medicine, Beth Israel Deaconess Medical Center, Harvard Medical School, Boston

needs of affected individuals and families should be identified and met, including access to vital services and assistance from available disaster programs. The process of recovery is integrated with starting the disaster cycle with renewed risk assessment.

In large-scale mass casualty events, physicians and other healthcare workers must be knowledgeable of the need for efficient coordination among local, state, and federal response efforts; how to protect themselves and others from further harm; how to communicate effectively with other emergency personnel and the media; and how to address the unique psychological impacts and related social chaos that may ensue. The National Disaster Life Support (NDLS) training program serves to better prepare healthcare professionals and emergency response personnel and to help standardize emergency response nationwide and strengthen the nation's public health system.

REFERENCES

National Disaster Life Support. American Medical Association. www.ama-assn.org/ama/pub/category/print/12606.html. Accessed 3 April 2005.

Levinson J, Granot H, eds. 2002. *Transportation disaster response handbook*, pp. 27–33. San Diego: Academic Press.

7 INTERGOVERNMENTAL AND GOVERNMENTAL ORGANIZATIONS

Robert E. Antosia, MD, MPH*

INTRODUCTION

Humanitarian organizations are vital to help mobilize resources and activities to address the consequences of any major disaster that overwhelms the capabilities of state and local governments. By convention, humanitarian aid agencies are divided into three groups: Intergovernmental Organizations (IGOs); Governmental or International Organizations (GOs); and Nongovernmental Organizations (NGOs). The first two types will be discussed in this section, and the latter, NGOs, will be discussed in a separate chapter.

INTERGOVERNMENTAL ORGANIZATIONS (IGOs)

IGOs are organizations or institutions created and joined by governments. Their members are states that give them the authority to make collective decisions to manage particular problems on the global agenda. They may be universal, such as the United Nations, or regional as in the case of the European Union. The purpose of these organizations may vary from a military alliance (NATO) to health care (United Nations agencies). Other organizations have multiple purposes and areas of interest with specialized agencies and autonomous organizations.

United Nations

The United Nations (UN) is the best-known international organization. This world assembly of sovereign states was founded in October 24, 1945, when 51 member states ratified the Charter. By 1994 the United Nations had grown to 185 members.

*Department of Emergency Medicine, Beth Israel Deaconess Medical Center, Harvard Medical School, Boston

When states become members of the UN they must agree to its goals and accept the obligations of the UN Charter. Its goals are to promote world peace and security and to develop international cooperation in economic, social, cultural, and humanitarian problems. The Charter expresses the fundamental purpose of the UN and sets out a basic framework for international relations. The member states of the UN Charter agree to:

- Maintain peace and security
- Develop friendly relations between nations
- Cooperate in solving international problems
- Promote respect for human rights

The UN is composed of five main bodies, which are based at UN Headquarters in New York.

- The General Assembly
- The Security Council
- The Economic and Social Council
- The Trusteeship Council
- The Secretariat

The judicial arm of the UN, the International Court of Justice, is located in The Hague, The Netherlands.

Specialized agencies—including The International Monetary Fund, the World Bank, the World Health Organization (WHO), the International Civil Aviation Organization, and ten other independent organizations—are linked to the UN through cooperative agreements. These organizations are autonomous bodies created by intergovernmental agreements.

Within the UN system there also exist a number of offices and funds, including the Office of the UN Commissioner for Refugees (UNHCR) and the UN Children's Fund (UNICEF). These important agencies work to improve economic and social conditions around the world, and report to the General Assembly or the Economic and Social Council. The Office for the Coordination of Humanitarian Affairs was established in 1998 to coordinate humanitarian response, policy development, and humanitarian advocacy. OCHA works in hand with the Emergency Relief Coordinator.

GOVERNMENTAL OR NATIONAL ORGANIZATIONS

A number of countries, in addition to belonging to and participating in IGO and NGO activities, have developed their own national aid agencies. While the goals and objectives of these agencies are similar to those of many IGOs and NGOs, governmental agencies also help promote the advancement of particular national interests. Two such agencies are the US Agency for International Development (USAID) and the United Kingdom's Department for International Development (DFID). Both agencies receive direction and foreign policy guidance from their respective national governments. USAID is an independent federal government body that conducts foreign assistance and humanitarian aid to advance the political and economic interests of the United States. The DFID is charged with carrying out the British government's aid and development efforts. These goals are achieved by its own personnel or by funding specialist agencies within the NGO network.

RESOURCES

http://www.un.org/
http://ochaonline.un.org/
http://www.unhcr.ch/cgi-bin/texis/vtx/home
http://www.usaid.gov/

8 NONGOVERNMENTAL ORGANIZATIONS

Jerry Lambert, MD*

DEFINITION

Although many disagree as to how to define a nongovernmental organization, the World Bank recognizes these private entities as groups that "pursue activities to relieve suffering, promote the interest of the poor, protect the environment, provide basic social services, or undertake community development." An NGO must be independent of governmental control, and receive its support through charitable donations and voluntary services.

HISTORY

During the eighteenth and nineteenth centuries, NGOs developed to meet community needs, defend interests, and promote new policies for the increasing number of citizens who were gaining extended civil rights within Europe and the Americas. The antislavery movement, the International Committee of the Red Cross, and trade unions represented some of the first precursors for NGOs. Over the last fifty years NGOs have become a major force worldwide and now address almost every conceivable issue. They are most effective when they work in coalitions, pooling their resources and coordinating their lobbying efforts. There are more than 30,000 NGOs, most of which operate within a single country, from where they disburse millions of dollars in aid to developing countries.

NGO STRENGTHS

*Drexel University College of Medicine, Department of Emergency Medicine, Allegheny General Hospital, Pittsburgh

- Strong grassroots links
- Innovative
- Acts as conscience of humanity
- Cost-effectiveness
- Common ideology among members
- Long-term commitment and emphasis on sustainability

NGO WEAKNESSES

- Limited financial and management expertise
- Limited institutional capacity.
- Lack of understanding of broader social or economic context
- Lack of interorganizational communication/coordination.
- Small-scale intervention

SUMMARY

NGOs and their networks provide accountability to the global civil society. They always carry out an important advocacy mission. As globalization increasingly creates both cross-border issues and communities, NGOs will play a vital role in relief and development within these dynamic processes.

9 COMPLEX HUMANITARIAN EMERGENCIES

Frederick M. Burkle Jr., MD, MPH, FAAP, FACEP*

DEFINITION

Complex emergencies (CEs)—as seen in Angola, Liberia, Somalia, the Former Yugoslavia, Kosovo, and East Timor—can be defined as nation-state internal conflicts in which the capacity to sustain livelihood and life is threatened primarily by political factors, and, in particular, by high levels of violence.

CHARACTERISTICS

CEs have existed for many years; however, they have become the most common human-generated disasters during the last two decades. Currently, there remain 35 countries at risk of serious conflict, 11 of which are near collapse.

The large majority of victims are civilians, with mortality and morbidity primarily among vulnerable and unprotected children, women, the elderly, and the handicapped.

CEs may also exacerbate social, economic, and gender inequalities, poverty, injustices, cultural and religious persecution, ignorance, racism, oppression, religious fundamentalism, and other lethal factors that contribute to internal strife among varied ethnic, tribal, and religious groups.

CEs must be understood and managed in the context of politics. The success and failure of intervention and relief during CEs are dependent on the politics of the situation and outside military actions to cease or at least contain the violence. The world community has, with varying success, responded to the more publicized CEs in the decade of the 1990s (the Kurds in Northern Iraq, Somalia, the Balkans, East Timor), but with other conflicts (Rwanda, Democratic Republic of the Congo, the Sudan) outside assistance has been limited or avoided. Primarily because of unresolved war and conflict, hunger has climbed 18%, representing more than 850 million people without

*The Center for International Emergency, Disaster and Refugee Studies, The Johns Hopkins University Medical Institutions, Baltimore

food sufficient for basic health. Conflict has also degraded agricultural and public health infrastructure over the past decade, directly increasing the toll in terms of civilian morbidity and mortality.

Outmoded international laws and treaties favor the primacy of a given nation's sovereignty over any international legal mandate and prevent intervention to protect victims who remain within the nation in conflict. These victims are referred to as *internally displaced populations* (IDPs), and they suffer the highest mortality and morbidity rates. Once fleeing populations cross the border of the country in conflict they become *refugees* and benefit from the protections mandated under UN Agencies, specifically the UN High Commissioner for Refugees (UNHCR).

EPIDEMIOLOGICAL MODELS

Populations suffer both the direct and indirect effects of a conflict. Direct effects include injuries, deaths, disabilities, human rights and international humanitarian law abuses, and psychological stress. Indirect effects actually contribute to the majority of mortality and morbidity due to population displacement, disruption of food supplies, and destroyed health facilities and public health infrastructure. At least three epidemiological models exist that may guide the current practice of the humanitarian response effort.

Developing Country Model

The health profile for countries in Africa and Asia during the acute phase of a conflict or war is usually identified by moderate or severe malnutrition, outbreaks of communicable diseases, and often both. Three-fourths of all epidemics of the last decade took place in the context of a CE. Epidemiological indicators show high crude mortality rates and, if disaggregated, expose the vulnerability among the populations as to age (children under 5 years and the elderly) and gender (women and female-headed households). There is a linear relationship between under age 5 childhood mortality (per 1000) and the percentage of nations engaged in armed conflict. The worst conditions and highest mortality rates are recorded among orphaned and unaccompanied children. High case fatality rates were common among malnourished children in Somalia, with measles contributing to between 50 and 81% of deaths. As such, all children in developing countries in conflict should receive measles vaccine and vitamin A supplementation to mitigate the complication rate of measles and other infectious diseases, such as diarrheal and respiratory diseases. Malaria, HIV, and STDs also take a severe toll. Once humanitarian assistance reaches these populations the mortality rates should decline, and the priorities in camps should become ensuring security and fuel and rebuilding the basic public health infrastructure. Abuses against women and failures in reproductive health have led to high rates of STDs and pregnancy in refugee camps. Immediate assistance in CEs comes in the form of WHO Emergency Health, Surgical, and Safe Birthing Kits, which provide care for a 10,000 population for 3 months, and safe birthing and surgical kits. Medical and nursing assets more often needed under this model include public health, preventive medicine and infectious disease specialists, primary care, obstetrics and gynecology, and family practice and emergency medicine personnel.

Developed Country Model

Countries such as Iraq, the former Yugoslavia, Macedonia, and Kosovo had relatively healthy populations with demographic profiles similar to Western countries. The few epidemics and low prevalence of malnutrition among children and infants were superseded by undernutrition and chronic diseases among the elderly, who could not flee the conflict or were unable to access health care. In these settings war-related trauma from advanced weaponry contributed to the primary mortality. Rape and traumatic exposures commonly contributed to psychological morbidity. For such models the desired expatriate medical and nursing care includes surgery, anesthesia, and emergency medicine.

Smoldering Country Model

Both Haiti and the Sudan have unique problems relating to long-standing conflict and unrest that prevent progress in health, healthcare delivery and access, disease prevention, and education. Except for high rates of HIV/AIDS, Haiti represents a health profile in disease last seen in the United States in the early 1900s. Massive deforestation has led to severe environmental collapse, which contributes inextricably to chronic health and infrastructure loss. Haiti represents a developmental as well as an emergency situation. The Sudan has experienced war since 1955 and as such its children grow up chronically malnourished and know only a culture of violence, with little access to health care and education. Reproductive health is an unknown luxury, and most health care must be imported.

Whatever the epidemiological model, the larger humanitarian community has found itself often unprepared and at times overwhelmed with the demands for assistance.

CURRENT PRACTICE

Training for work in a complex emergency environment is essential before deployment.

Rapid assessments provide for quick identification and analysis of vulnerable populations, setting priorities requiring immediate aid, which is then followed by more detailed surveys and ongoing surveillance and monitoring of the populations at risk. Research suggests that certain health-related issues should be the focus of assistance to minimize mortality and morbidity. Endemic disease control is always a priority. Surveillance, outbreak investigation, and preventive control measures—such as ensuring adequate quantity and quality of water and sanitation facilities, food and shelter, and immunizations for measles, tetanus, diphtheria, and polio, as well as vector control for malaria—are priority measures, especially in the developing and smoldering country models. Food programs must ensure proper nutrition for the general displaced population as well as therapeutic or supplemental feedings for the acutely malnourished; they should address micronutrient deficiencies as well as give special attention to nutrition for those with HIV/AIDS and TB. Emphasis must be placed on maternal and child health, reproductive health, and protection of those with disabilities and injuries. Healthcare providers have been instrumental in developing unique solutions through negotiating "immunization days" with rebel groups and delineating "tranquility zones," whereby vulnerable groups are isolated from the surrounding fighting.

CEs may require the immediate response of healthcare personnel who serve with a wide range of international and national relief agencies or with international military forces called in to quell the conflict. In the mid-1990s concerns over inconsistencies in humanitarian assistance led to the development of field standards in a multi-agency collaborative known as SPHERE, a series of qualitative and quantitative minimum standards that guide relief efforts in health services, food and nutrition, water and sanitation, and shelter.

MULTINATIONAL MODEL

The traditional humanitarian response model follows a UN Security Council Resolution that spells out the terms of intervention. The UN Office of the Coordinator for Humanitarian Assistance (OCHA) is the lead agency that coordinates international relief agencies. These include the such UN agencies as the World Food Program (WFP), the World Health Organization (WHO), and the UN Children's Fund (UNICEF); the Red Cross Movement, including the International Committee of the Red Cross (ICRC) and the Federation of Red Cross and Red Crescent Societies (FRC/RC); Nongovernmental Organizations (NGOs); UN Peace Keepers or Peace Enforcement troops sanctioned by a UN Security Council Resolution; and donor agencies representing national governments such as the US Agency for International Development (USAID), the Canadian International Development Agency (CIDA), and Japan's International Cooperation Agency (JICA), among others.

International relief organizations are protected under international humanitarian laws and treaties, such as the Geneva Conventions. Wanton violations of the Geneva Conventions and international humanitarian law make it increasingly difficult for relief workers to maintain security for their programs and projects. The recent trend since the Balkan wars—to militarize and politicize humanitarian assistance—has made it increasingly difficult for international relief organizations to maintain neutrality and impartiality. The urbanization of populations in warfare has caused humanitarian assistance to move from rural to urban settings. Almost two-thirds of African populations are now living in urban settings with tenuous social and physical protections, and 95% of the Iraqi population is urbanized in areas where the public health infrastructure is in disrepair and there is an extreme lack of security—major impediments to recovery and reconstruction.

UNILATERAL MODEL

In the 2003 Iraq war, the United States and Coalition Forces chose a *unilateral* route of response rather than the traditional *multinational* and multi-agency response. The unilateral approach requires military and private sector contractors to lead humanitarian, recovery, and reconstruction efforts, while specifically avoiding dependency on UN and NGO resources. Whether this unilateral approach to conflict and war will represent a new model for dealing with CEs has yet to be determined.

REFERENCES

Burkle FM. 1999. Lessons learnt and future expectations of complex emergencies. *BMJ* **319**:422–426.

Crisis Watch. 2004. International Crisis Group, May 01, 2004. Available at www.crisisweb.org. Accessed 14 May, 2004.

Sphere Project. 2003. *Humanitarian charter and minimum standards in disaster response*, 2nd ed. Geneva: Sphere Project. www.sphereproject.org.

Toole MJ, Waldman RJ. 1993. Refugees and displaced persons: war, hunger and public health. *JAMA* **270**:600–605.

Van Rooyen MJ, Eliades MJ, Grabowski JG, Stress ME, Juric J, Burkle, FM. 2001. Medical relief personnel in complex emergencies: perceptions of effectiveness in the former Yugoslavia. *Prehospital Disaster Med* **16**(3):145–149.

Zwi A, Uglade A. 1991. Political violence in the third world: a public health issue. *Health Policy Planning* **6**:203–217.

PART II

Natural Disasters

10 EARTHQUAKES

Kevin King, MD*

OVERVIEW

Earthquakes are one of the most destructive natural disasters. At least 1.3 million deaths occurred during the previous century from earthquakes. On average 16 earthquakes resulting in significant loss of life occur every year. Earthquakes are produced by the movement of the plates that form the earth's crust. The boundaries where the plates meet and slide across each other are called faults. If movement of plates becomes arrested, energy can accumulate along the fault line. When the accumulated energy exceeds the strength of the rocks along the plate boundary, the rock may fracture and the plates can move suddenly up to a few meters. This sudden movement produces vibrations or seismic waves that radiate outward from the focus of the quake. Surface waves that travel along the earth's crust have the strongest vibrations and thus produce the greatest damage. Earthquakes tend to recur along fault lines but may also occur in the middle of a plate.

The intensity of an earthquake is based on the magnitude of the vibrations produced. Seismographs are used to measure these vibrations, whose increasing wave amplitude is associated with a correspondingly stronger earthquake. The Richter Scale is used to further qualify the strength of an earthquake. For every increase of 1 on the Richter scale a quake is 10 times stronger. Earthquakes over a magnitude 7.0 have the potential to cause thousands of deaths and significant structural damage.

RISK FACTORS FOR INJURY

Ground movement during an earthquake is seldom the direct cause of death or injury. Most injuries result from collapsing structures, falling masonry, flying glass, and falling objects, or when people attempt to move during a quake. Structural failure

*Department of Emergency Medicine, Boston University, Boston

of a building is generally recognized as the most common cause of death in large earthquakes. There is generally a higher risk of fatal injury associated with multilevel commercial and residential buildings, though this is dependent on the construction of the building. The peak in deaths and injuries occurs during the 24-hour period after an earthquake, with the highest number of fatalities recorded within minutes after the quake. Hospitalization for nonfatal injuries also peaks on the day of an earthquake, but may also have subsequent peaks depending on the presence of secondary disasters and the strength of aftershocks.

The most common causes of injury and death may vary depending on the earthquake and the construction of local buildings. Analysis of injury patterns during the Northridge earthquake in 1994 found that falling building masonry was the most common cause of injury, followed by being pinned between furniture and objects. Investigation of the 1988 Armenian earthquake identified building collapse as the most common cause of injury and death. Data from multiple earthquakes has shown that exiting from a building is both a risk factor and protective against death.

Earthquake lethality can be magnified by promulgation of secondary disasters. Ground vibrations can collapse buildings and bridges, disrupt gas and electric service, and trigger landslides, avalanches, flash floods, fires, and sometimes huge tsunamis. Tsunamis are a particular risk when earthquakes occur near or beneath the ocean floor. Immense waves that may reach greater than 15 meters in height and travel at speeds greater than 960 kilometers per hour can be generated. These waves may cause significant damage and loss of life in communities near the ocean.

Care should also be taken to avoid injuries from aftershocks. These are smaller quakes that follow the main seismic event and may cause collapse of previously weakened or damaged structures. Aftershocks may occur within minutes to weeks after the main earthquake. Motor vehicle accidents are also a source of earthquake-related injury and death.

PREVENTION OF INJURIES

The best method of injury prevention during an earthquake is adequate warning. Unfortunately, earthquakes are not predictable in their magnitude or time of occurrence. This places a premium on preventative strategies to limit loss of life and damage to property. The first line of public protection is the institution of building codes that ensure construction will withstand potential earthquake strengths expected for the region. Local governments should ensure that the local population is educated through media campaigns to identify earthquake hazards within the home. The local government, emergency services, and public utility companies should have disaster plans in place to mitigate fires, gas explosions, aftershocks, and other secondary earthquake effects.

During the earthquake those who are in buildings constructed to withstand earthquakes should not attempt to move and should find cover under sturdy furniture for protection from falling objects. They should avoid going outside during the quake unless the building is in danger of collapse. Drivers of motor vehicles should make their best attempt to come to a safe stop during the earthquake and remain in their cars with seatbelts fastened. They should not attempt to drive until all ground vibrations have subsided and should proceed cautiously, avoiding damaged road, ramp, and bridge structures.

After the earthquake has abated, people should survey their surroundings for signs of potential danger. People should leave buildings in danger of collapse. Gas or other utilities should not be used since there may be damage to lines resulting in increased risk of fire and explosion. Buildings that appear structurally unsound or are partially collapsed should not be entered because subsequent aftershocks might cause their collapse.

INJURIES

Injuries during earthquakes are primarily from blunt trauma. In the 1988 Armenian earthquake there were 831 fatalities, 533 fractures, 397 crush injuries, and 646 minor injuries, with greater injury rates noted in females. During the 1994 Northridge earthquake in California there were 33 related fatalities and 138 hospitalizations. Analysis of the injury pattern for the Northridge earthquake found specific injury patterns for fatalities and hospitalized cases. Among fatalities, the head was the most commonly injured body region, followed by thoracic, abdominal, and lower extremity injuries. The most common causes of death were asphyxia and body compression from building collapse. Orthopedic injuries were the most common cause of hospitalization.

EMERGENCY DEPARTMENT TREATMENT

As previously described, most injuries and fatalities occur within the first 24 hours after the initial shock. The majority of injuries seen will be blunt trauma, crush injuries, fractures, lacerations, abrasions, burns, and penetrating injuries in varying numbers. Since the occurrence of earthquakes is unpredictable, it is important to have a previously prepared and rehearsed disaster plan that can be rapidly activated. An emergency department should be prepared to treat an anticipated post-event surge in multi-trauma patients. In situations where local resources are overwhelmed, all efforts should be made to stabilize critical patients and expeditiously transfer stabilized individuals to other medical facilities outside the disaster zone. In situations where the patient surge completely overwhelms the emergency department, it may be necessary to implement a mass casualty triage approach to maximize the number of lives saved. It is also important to ensure that the hospitals and emergency rooms are structurally sound and in no potential danger from secondary earthquake effects.

RESOURCES

http://www.fema.gov/hazards/earthquakes
http://www.fema.gov/hazards/earthquakes/quake.shtm
http://www.seismo.unr.edu/ftp/pub/louie/class/100/plate-tectonics.html

REFERENCES

Armenian HK, Melkonian A, Noji EK, Hovanesian AP. 1997. Deaths and injuries due to the earthquake in Armenia: a cohort approach. *Int J Epidemiol* **26**:806–813.

Peek-Asa C, Kraus JF, Bourque LB, Vimalchandra D, Yu J, Abrams J. 1998. Fatal and hospitalized injuries resulting from the 1994 northridge earthquake. *Int J Epidemiol* **27**:459–465.

Peek-Asa C, Ramirez M, Seligson H, Shoaf K. 2003. Seismic, structural, and individual factors associated with earthquake related injury. *Inj Prev* **9**:62–66.

11

VOLCANOES

William Porcaro, MD*

OVERVIEW

Volcanoes are one of the more prominent natural creative and destructive forces. Over 80% of the earth's surface is known to be volcanic in origin. The gases emitted from volcanoes throughout the history of the planet have played a vital role in the creation of its atmosphere, oceans, and life itself. While relatively rare, modern-day volcanic eruptions have great potential to cause serious human and property disasters.

HISTORY

Many classic eruptions have been noted throughout human history. On August 24, AD 79, Mount Vesuvius erupted in southern Italy. Although the volcano had been classified as extinct by contemporaries, a massive eruption literally buried two cities "alive" under ash fall within a period of several hours. In modern times, the May 1980 eruption of Mt. St. Helens is one of the more notable events in US history. This eruption also boasts the largest landslide in recorded history, as the volcano's bulge and summit slid away. In 1985, ineffectual planning and evacuation contributed to more than 22,000 deaths related to the predicted eruption of Mount Nevado del Ruiz in Colombia. In 1995, the Soufriere Hills Volcano on the island of Montserrat in the Caribbean underwent a massive eruption that buried a great portion of the island in ash and caused two-thirds of the population to flee the island. Hawaiian volcanic activity continues to be on the forefront of news with ongoing eruptions, most notably on Mauna Loa, which exhibits more gradual lava flows rather than cataclysmic eruptions.

*Beth Israel Deaconess Medical Center, Harvard Medical School, Boston

INCIDENCE/FREQUENCY

Roughly 600 volcanos are currently considered active, meaning that they have erupted during recorded history. Thousands of other volcanos are classified as dormant, acknowledging that they have the potential for future activity. While the exact time and place of volcanic eruptions cannot be predicted, research at specific volcanic observatories and the historical behavior of a volcano can provide some guidance to the local population. Some volcanos demonstrate gradual activity through multiple minor recurrent events that eventually culminate in a larger episode. However, history teaches us that extended periods of dormancy offer no guarantee for paucity of future activity. On average there are about 50 volcanic eruptions per year contributing to various degrees of human impact depending, in part, on the local resources available to monitor them.

PREVALENCE: AREAS AT RISK

The peoples and areas at most risk for volcanic eruptions are, obviously, those in the vicinity of mountains. Some of the more notorious regions worldwide include the Hawaiian Islands, the Cascade Range in the western United States, Iceland, the Pacific Rim, Southeast Asia, western South America, and the Middle East/Western Africa.

RISK FACTORS

While everyone is at risk for the various dangers posed by volcanic activity, certain groups are more susceptible. Infants and the elderly as well as people with cardiac or respiratory conditions such as asthma and COPD may have an increased vulnerability to volcanic gases and ash.

PRESENTATION

As alluded to above, there are many possible scenarios for volcanic eruptions that vary by time course, severity, and type of eruption. Depending on the type of eruption, different hazards may be encountered, ranging from lava to debris to gas and ash clouds to landslides.

TYPES OF ERUPTIONS

The types of volcanic eruptions are named for the sites/volcanos that exhibited such characteristics in history. The main classes of eruptions are listed below in relative order of decreasing intensity or potential for destruction.

Pelean — Volcanic blast mainly though the side of the mountain of great intensity, causing a high degree of destruction. Avalanches of dust, ash, and lava move down slopes at speeds in excess of 100 mph.

Plinean — Violent upward blast expanding into atmosphere.

Vesuvian — Infrequent, intense eruption with large cauliflower-shaped ash cloud spreading over a wide area.

Vulcanian — Repeat eruptions in which lava crusts over vents, enlarging the volcano cone. Recurrent eruptions displace more material and gradually increase in intensity.

Strombolian — Relatively continuous series of eruptions with occasional "clots" or chucks of lava being ejected into the sky.

Hawaiian — Freely flowing lava, usually originating from liver fissures or fractures in the volcano.

HEALTHCARE CONCERNS

Volcanic eruptions pose numerous dangers that vary based on the type of event. Listed below are some of the common volcanic hazards and their potential health risks.

Gas

Volcanic eruptions liberate large quantities of gas mixtures. Plumes contain water vapor, carbon dioxide, carbon monoxide, sulfur dioxide, hydrogen compounds, and acids, including Hydrogen Chloride (HCl) and Hydrogen Fluoride (HF). Sulfur dioxide gas and the acid rain it produces may manifest clinically through skin and mucous membrane irritation and upper respiratory tract symptoms. Such acid rain may contaminate surrounding agricultural lands, resulting in long-term crop failure. Gas reactions with dust, sunlight, and oxygen may produce volcanic smog, which can exacerbate symptoms in patients with lung disease. In addition, the combination of acid rain and volcanic smog can lead to local famine conditions and also have substantial effects on worldwide climate. Hydrogen sulfide, a flammable gas, can cause effects ranging from headache, dizziness, upper airway irritation, and bronchitis to depressed mental status and pulmonary edema. Carbon dioxide is liberated in large amounts from volcanos. However, it usually poses little threat to people as it rapidly disperses. In some cases it may concentrate in low-lying areas (it is heavier than air) and cause unconsciousness and death. Volcanic chlorine gas combines with water to form acid that, depending on concentration, may cause effects ranging from membrane irritation to pulmonary edema and laryngeal spasm. Hydrogen fluoride can trigger mucous membrane irritation as well as bone and teeth degeneration.

Pyroclastic Flows

Bursts of high pressure/velocity blasts of gas and rock explode from eruption vents. Virtually everything in the path of this phenomenon is destroyed. Asphyxiation and major trauma are the foremost concerns in management.

Lahars

The combination of volcanic eruption and melting snow and ice or subsequent heavy rainfalls may generate these hot or cold mixtures of water, rock fragments, and other debris. Lahars expand as byproducts from their path of destruction are incorporated. The obvious effects of such events cause trauma, property destruction, and drowning.

Landslides

These entities consist of large amounts of rock and soil, and may be wet or dry. They are triggered during eruptions from the steep and unstable slopes of volcanic cones that tend to have cleavage planes secondary to lava layering and the gases and acidic fluids that are byproducts of eruptions. Landslides can reach speeds over 100 km/hr and can cause wreck through a number of mechanisms, including direct destruction, triggering further explosions, creating lahars, and initiating tsunamis.

Lava Flows

As implied, lava flows consist of streams of molten rock emanating from volcanic vents. The largest threats from this phenomenon occur when gases are liberated from combustion of materials or lava is splattered when reacting with water. As the flow rate is often quite slow, people are generally injured when they are too close to the flow and suffer burns or the escape route is cut off from further flow.

Ash/Tephra

Volcanic eruptions spew forth a great magnitude of rock fragments. *Tephra* is a general term for this material, while *ash* describes fragments less than 2 millimeters in diameter. Large fragments, sometimes called "bombs," may travel great distances and cause destruction and fires at remote sites. Ash flow may obscure sunlight and markedly decrease visibility in surrounding areas. Ash also infiltrates into virtually all crevices, creating mechanical and biological disfunction such as respiratory symptoms and auto/jet engine malfunction. Wet ash can become slippery, triggering further incidents. Ash is also quite abrasive to substances that it contacts and may simply destroy structures under its sheer weight. Deposition of volcanic material into water supplies can also cause particulate and chemical contamination, making the supply non-potable.

Volcanic activity also has the potential to trigger earthquakes and tsunamis before, during, and after the actual eruption. These natural disasters pose obvious threats that are discussed elsewhere in this volume.

TREATMENT

During or following a volcanic eruption, a wide range and degree of medical care may be required. Baseline medical instructions should include a direction to remain indoors while sealing windows and doors, and wearing masks or damp cloths over the nose and mouth if outside.

Acutely, large volumes of traumatic injury may be encountered, necessitating the use of the mass casualty principle in conjunction with conventional trauma management. Special attention may be required in the areas of chemical and thermal burn management. Acute and later chronic upper and lower respiratory pathology will occur, requiring treatments ranging from oxygen and bronchodilators to intubation. In the subacute and chronic phases following a volcanic incident, large numbers of people may be displaced from their homes, triggering numerous public health concerns from ensuing infections and disease.

PREVENTION

While no one can predict the exact time and nature of a volcanic eruption, most events are heralded by observable geophysical and geochemical changes. In "hot spots" of volcanic activity, people and governments need to have disaster and evacuation plans in place to avert enormous human tragedy.

If an eruption occurs, escape via automobile should be avoided due to the risk of engine failure, fire-extinguishing material should be at hand, and ash should be promptly removed from buildings to avert structural compromise.

RESOURCES

CDC Volcanoes Emergency Preparedness and Response: http://www.bt.cdc.gov/disasters/volcanos

U.S. Geological Survey Volcano Hazards Program: http://volcanoes.usgs.gov

REFERENCES

Auerbach PS, ed. 2001. *Field guide to wilderness medicine*, 4th ed. St. Louis: Mosby.

Baskett P, Weller R. 1988. *Medicine for disasters*. London: Wright-Butterfield.

Global Volcanism Program: Smithsonian Institute http://www.volcano.si.edu

Tilling RI. Volcanos: On-line edition, United States Geological Survey website.

Volcanic Hazards Program: http://volcanoes.usgs.gov.

12

FLOODS

Kevin King, MD*

OVERVIEW

Floods are a chronic and costly hazard to life and property. In the United States alone, an average of 140 fatalities and 5 billion dollars of damage are caused by floods each year. Flooding is defined as excess water overflow onto normally dry land. The most important factor that determines if a flood will occur is the absorptive capacity of the soil. If water influx exceeds the capacity for soil absorption then flooding may occur. Rivers swollen by excess runoff can overflow their banks, surmount or breach dikes, and flood adjacent low lying areas.

Flash floods are of particular concern where soil has low absorptive capacity and severe storms are common. Flash floods happen within 6 hours of a rain event or when there is sudden release of water, as occurs with dam or levee failure. They may develop anywhere—including dry streambeds, flood plains, and low-lying areas. Normal urbanization and development can potentiate the risk of severe flooding. Paving and cementing inhibit normal water absorption by soil, while settlement on flood plains increases the size of the population at risk for exposure to floods.

RISK FACTORS FOR INJURY

Floods pose a risk of injury during and after the disaster. An analysis of flood-related injuries in Oklahoma determined that location was the major factor in injury occurrence. Creeks accounted for over half of submersion injuries. Key human factors were: a lack of knowledge regarding the risks and hazards for flooding, ignorance of proper actions to take in a flood situation, and limited time to seek safety. Flooding may last for weeks and thus increase the risk for waterborne communicable diseases.

*Department of Emergency Medicine, Boston University

During flood cleanup there is a risk of electrocution from water-damaged electrical circuits as well as damaged equipment.

PREVENTION OF INJURIES

Practicing good flood safety techniques is the best method for reducing flood-related injuries. It is important to stay out of areas subject to flooding. If outdoors when flooding occurs, climb to higher ground and stay there until rescued or the waters have receded. If water in a stream is above your ankles, turn around and do not enter the stream. Attempting to drive through water and playing in higher water are the most frequent causes of flood mortality. When traveling in or along stream channels, be aware of distant events that may cause flash floods in the area. Camp or park away from all streams and washes, particularly during threatening conditions. Evacuate immediately through recommended evacuation routes when advised.

After a flood or flash flood, measures can be taken to reduce the risk of further injury and death: avoid all disaster areas, stay out of any buildings if floodwaters remain around the base, do not enter any building unless deemed safe, wear sturdy shoes to limit the chance of foot and ankle injuries, avoid smoking because of possible explosion risks from damaged to gas lines, and do not drink tap water unless authorities have advised it is safe to do so. Epidemiological surveillance for waterborne and communicable diseases should continue until flood cleanup has been completed.

INJURIES

Submersion injuries are the most common injury in flooding, with the majority of deaths occurring from drowning. Other injuries commonly seen include: sprains, strains, lacerations, abrasions, and contusions. Common related illnesses include: gastrointestinal problems, rashes, and heat related illness.

MEDICAL TREATMENT

If a medical facility is located in an area at risk for flooding, a disaster and evacuation plan should be in place. Ensuring appropriate tetanus prophylaxis and disease surveillance are both of primary importance. Heightened surveillance for communicable diseases should continue until all floodwaters have receded and public health authorities have determined that risks have returned to pre-disaster levels.

RESOURCES

http://www.stillwaterredcross.org/floodsafe.htm.
http://www.cdc.gov/niosh/flood.html.

REFERENCES

Azeredo R. 2001. Hazards related to nature, environment, and human behavior leading to flood-related submersion injuries in Oklahoma. Injury Update. May 30. www.health.state.ok.us/program/injury/updates.

Jonkman SN, Kelman I. 2005. An analysis of the causes and circumstances of flood disaster deaths. *Disasters* **29**(1):75–97.

Morbidity surveillance following the Midwest flood—Missouri. 1993. *MMWR* **42**(41):797–798.

O'Connor JE, Costa JE. 2003. *Large floods in the united states: where they happen and why*. US Geological Survey Circular 1245. Washington, DC: US Government Printing Office.

13 TSUNAMIS

Robert E. Antosia, MD, MPH*

Tsunamis, commonly but incorrectly called tidal waves, have inspired both awe and fear among coastal peoples for millennia. Although today we have a more scientific understanding of the phenomenon, tsunamis remain an awesome and deadly natural disaster. On December 26, 2004, an earthquake triggered a devastating tsunami that struck 11 countries on two continents in South Asia. The devastation caused by this tsunami was catastrophic—more than 200,000 people dead, tens of thousands of people missing or injured, thousands of miles of coastline destroyed, and loss of livelihood for millions of the survivors. With coastal populations that are continuing to increase, especially in the tsunami-prone Pacific region, more tsunami disasters are inevitable. Minimizing the potential morbidity and mortality requires: assessment of potential tsunami hazards; public education and awareness; early warnings and effective communication; and prompt evacuation of threatened areas. Emergency care providers in tsunami-prone areas should be familiar with this particular type of natural disaster as well the public health model for disasters that highlights preparedness, mitigation, response, and recovery.

THE PHYSICS OF TSUNAMIS

A tsunami is a series of waves generated by an undersea disturbance. Approximately 90 to 95% are the result of earthquakes; the devastating December 2004 tsunami in the Indian Ocean was caused by the second-largest earthquake in recorded history. Other tsunamis may be caused by volcanic eruptions or massive landslides. Although tsunamis are often (incorrectly) called tidal waves, they have nothing to do with tides. They are, rather, very long waves that race along the ocean at speeds that can reach 500 miles an hour. Tsunami waves are remarkable for their destructiveness, speed of propagation, and ability to cross thousands of miles of ocean with little or no diminution in strength, thus causing destruction in areas far distant

*Department of Emergency Medicine, Beth Israel Deaconess Medical Center, Harvard Medical School, Boston

from their origin. Large tsunamis are not that rare, especially in the Pacific, where the vast majority (90–95%) occur within the so-called hyperactive "Ring of Fire" in the Pacific Ocean.

Historic evidence for massive tsunamis exists in many locations around the world. Almost everyone is familiar with the recent massive 2004 tsunami in South Asia, which resulted in more deaths than all other tsunamis combined. However, the coast of New South Wales in Australia has suffered the impact of six large tsunamis over the past few centuries. In addition, large tsunamis have affected Japan, Hawaii, New Guinea, and other areas of the globe. In the US tsunami danger is not confined to those generated in the Pacific: in the Canary Islands, the Cumbre Vieja volcano poses a threat to Atlantic coastlines.

The tsunami phenomenon is divided into the following three phases: (1) generation, (2) propagation, and (3) inundation. The generation phase is the production of tsunami waves caused by a large vertical displacement of ocean floor; the propagation phase is the spread of the tsunami away from the disturbance; the inundation phase is the interaction of the tsunami with the affected coastal areas—as a massive breaking wave, a wall of water, or a tide-like flood.

TSUNAMI EFFECTS

Due to the tremendous amount of mass and energy contained in a tsunami, damage to structures and the affected areas is universal and devastation near total. Most coastal buildings are likely to be obliterated, and many utilities—such as water, sewage, power lines, and gas lines—may be damaged, leading to such hazards as electrical fires, gas explosions, and septic contamination of water supplies. In a large tsunami, fatalities are high in relation to injuries as a result of the relatively short warning time, lack of protective structures, and difficulty of timely rescue. Average death rates are approximately 50% for the population caught by the tsunami, though rates up to 80% have been reported. The major causes of death are drowning and blunt trauma. Survivable but serious injuries primarily result from complications of near-drowning and aspiration pneumonia. Orthopedic and soft tissue injuries are the most common conditions among survivors. They may also suffer from associated dehydration, hypothermia, and sunburn.

The short-term public health needs of the surviving population are similar to those in other disasters and include: water, sanitation, food, shelter, and appropriate medical care administered to persons remaining in place and those who are living in self-settled displaced communities. As with many disasters, the medical infrastructure of the community impacted by the tsunami may be destroyed, leaving no source for even routine medical care of the victims. Initial medical aid efforts should focus on search and rescue and pre-hospital care. The latter should focus on ensuring adequate oxygenation since ear drowning and aspiration are common. Intravenous fluids should be administered to correct dehydration, injured extremities should be splinted, and open wounds need to be covered to prevent further contamination. Emergency department and hospital care will include definitive care for traumatic injuries and respiratory support for patients with severe aspiration pneumonia, and provisions for psychological support should be continued or initiated. Relief work, including medical and public health response, ideally represents the collaboration of affected communities with global partners in government, nongovernmental organizations, and humanitarian aid organizations.

The intermediate-term public health needs in the affected areas are less certain, and the threat of an epidemic looms. Damage to sewer systems and contamination of drinking water supplies poses the gravest threat and can lead to a multitude of common water- and food-borne diseases: cholera and shigella dysentery, hepatitis A, and rotavirus. Pools of standing water increase the risk of mosquito-borne diseases such as malaria and dengue fever. Overcrowding in large camps can also lead to the spread of such communicable diseases as pneumonia and measles. Preventive measures and interventions should focus on ensuring the health of survivors: adequate supplies of clean water and sanitation facilities; appropriate medications as indicated and distribution of health kits; targeted measles vaccination; treatment and control of vector-borne illnesses including mosquito-control measures; and careful epidemic surveillance to detect and treat the early appearance of communicable diseases.

The longer-term recovery and rehabilitation needs in the affected areas are more poorly understood. This includes the loss of livelihood for distraught survivors. In addition, the psychological trauma of the tsunami will lead survivors to experience grief, loss, and guilt, and impair individual and community coping abilities for a long time to come. The incidence of posttraumatic stress disorder and depression is expected to be high. Disasters that ravage economies can also elevate infant mortality and disease transmission rates for years. As a result, the devastated communities will often take many years to return to some sense of normalcy, and public health efforts should also be directed at rehabilitation and reconstruction efforts.

TSUNAMI PLANNING

A tsunami is an extremely powerful natural phenomenon that cannot be prevented or modified by any method that is known at this time. Seawalls and engineering provide minimal protection. Early warning systems and timely evacuation of coastal communities at risk provide the most effective response. At present, the Tsunami Warning System is made up of 26 participating member states throughout the Pacific basin. The system has the capacity to provide up to several hours of early warning of tsunamigenic activity in the Pacific (though not for the Atlantic or Indian Ocean). As presently configured, the detection system produces a 75% rate of false alarms. However, the US National Oceanic and Atmospheric Administration (NOAA) plans in the next two years to deploy 32 new advanced-technology Deep-ocean Assessment and Reporting of Tsunami (DART) buoys for a fully operational enhanced tsunami warning system by mid-2007. This new system will cover the US coast to include the Pacific, Atlantic, Caribbean basin, and the Gulf of Mexico and should considerably lower the number of false alarms. The United States also supports an international effort to build a global tsunami warning system that would include coverage of the Indian Ocean. In addition, minimizing tsunami risk must also focus on improved communication systems, local public education, and low-technology solutions related to design, planning, and protection.

REFERENCES

Hogan DE, Burstein JL, eds. 2002. *Disaster preparedness*. Philadelphia: Lippincott, Williams and Wilkins.

Van Rooyen M, Leaning J. 2005. After the tsunami: facing the public health challenges. *N Engl J Med* **352**:435–438.

Wattanawaitunechai C, Peacock SJ, Jipratoom P. 2005. Tsunami in Thailand: disaster management in a district hospital. *New Engl J Med* **352**:962–964.

US plan for an improved tsunami detection and warning system. Global Earth Observation System of Systems, Office of Science and Technology Policy, Executive Office of the President of the United States. http://www.ostp.gov/html/TsunamiFactSheet.pdf.

14 HURRICANES AND TYPHOONS

Manuel Colon MD* and John D. Cahill MD**

OVERVIEW

Hurricanes and typhoons have been responsible for the loss of millions of lives around the world. Even with the more sophisticated and faster weather tracking and communications systems now available, hurricanes continue to be responsible for the loss of many human lives and the loss of billions of dollars in property.

New technology and a detailed historical analysis of previous hurricanes have helped keep death tolls to a minimum. It is estimated that 1 of every 3 people affected by a hurricane in South America would have died in 1930, compared to 1 of every 100,000 in 1989. However, the potential for a major catastrophe has increased exponentially, as more people continue to move into low-lying areas close to the shore.

In contrast to other natural disasters such as earthquakes, tsunamis, and tornadoes, hurricanes are predictable. People who experience a hurricane have the distinct advantage of knowing about the threat days, even weeks, in advance. A thorough understanding of the events surrounding the hurricane, such as expected rainfall and wind speed, help the population prepare for the disaster and government agencies coordinate relief efforts.

DEFINITIONS

The term "tropical cyclone" is a generic name used to refer to all organized, circulating weather systems of low pressure that develop over tropical waters. The center axis of this system is known as the eye of the system. The direction of the winds is

*Department of Emergency Medicine, St. Luke's/Roosevelt Hospital Center, New York

**Department of Emergency Medicine and Division of Infectious Diseases, St. Luke's-Roosevelt Hospital Center, New York

clockwise in the Southern Hemisphere and counterclockwise in the Northern Hemisphere.

Tropical cyclones are classified into three groups:

- **Tropical Depression**: organized system of clouds and thunderstorms with a well defined circulation and maximum sustained winds of 38 mph (62 km/hr)
- **Tropical Storm**: organized system of clouds and thunderstorms with a well-defined circulation and maximum sustained winds of 39 to 73 mph (62 to 118 km/hr)
- **Hurricanes**: organized system of clouds and thunderstorms with a well-defined circulation and maximum sustained winds of more than 74 mph (118 km/hr). The terms typhoon, severe tropical cyclone, and cyclonic storm are also used in different regions of the world and are all synonymous with the term hurricane. For easy identification and tracking, the storms are generally given alternating masculine and feminine names or numbers that identify the year and annual sequence.

CLASSIFICATION OF HURRICANES

In 1969 Herbert Saffir and Bob Simpson developed a standardized system to categorize hurricanes. This allows researchers and meteorologists to better compare hurricanes and to predict potential damage for future hurricanes. The Saffir-Simpson Hurricane Scale, as it is known, categorizes hurricanes by the intensity of their sustained winds (wind speed average over one minute). There are five categories:

- **Category 1 Hurricane**: wind speeds of 74 to 95 mph (119 to 151 km/hr). Minimal damage is expected. Most damage is to unanchored mobile homes, trees, and shrubs. Tide level rises 4 to 5 feet over normal levels.
- **Category 2 Hurricane**: wind speeds of 96 to 110 mph (152 to 176 km/hr). Moderate damage is expected. Some damage will occur to roofs, windows, and doors. Significant damage to road signs, trees, shrubs. Tide level rises 6 to 8 feet over normal levels.
- **Category 3 Hurricane**: wind speeds of 111 to 130 mph (177 to 209 km/hr). Severe damage expected. Mobile homes will be destroyed. Some damage to small buildings and residences. Floating debris will damage structures near shores. Tide level rises 9 to 12 feet over normal levels.
- **Category 4 Hurricane**: wind speeds of 131 to 155 mph (210 to 248 km/hr). Extreme damage expected. Trees and shrubs are destroyed. Collapse of roof and walls of small buildings and residences. Tide level rises 13 to 18 feet above normal levels.
- **Category 5 Hurricane**: wind speeds > 155 mph (248 km/hr). Catastrophic damage expected. Complete failure of roof and walls of small buildings and some large or industrial buildings. Tide level rises >18 feet over normal levels.

It is important to recognize that the Saffir-Simpson Hurricane Scale only uses wind speed to classify hurricane severity. This scale can be deceiving at times, since the actual damage caused by the hurricane might be more or less than expected based on this scale alone. Factors such as timing of the event, sea surge, and expected rainfall must also be taken into consideration. A category 1 hurricane, for example, can cause devastating damage if it is accompanied by severe rainfall or if it occurs after a tropical storm has struck and saturated soil and rivers with water.

INJURIES

Most injuries can be associated with: flying debris during the hurricane, debris lying on the ground after the hurricane and during cleanup, and structural collapse. Soft-tissue injuries are most common: lacerations, abrasions, contusions, and crush injuries. These wounds are at risk for tetanus and need proper wound management and identified vaccination status. Orthopedic injuries of the extremities are not uncommon as well: sprains and fractures. Significant blunt trauma, penetrating trauma, and head injuries are less common but may also occur. With flooding comes the risk of drowning, water-borne illnesses, electrical injuries, and potentially mosquito-borne illness. Damage to the local infrastructure can lead to increased frequency of motor vehicle accidents, electrical injuries, and food/water-borne illness. It should also be remembered that everyday medical emergencies do occur and treatment may be difficult secondary to lack of access to medical care or medications.

SPECIAL CONSIDERATIONS

As stated earlier, prevention is the best means for avoiding injury and death. Whenever possible, individuals should heed the advice of local authorities in regards to evacuation plans and relocation details.

Special considerations include:

- Remain indoors until it has been confirmed that the hurricane has passed.
- During the eye of the hurricane, winds may significantly diminish.
- Shelter should be sought in the most solid structure possible.
- Avoid staying in higher floors.
- Windows and doors should ideally be boarded.
- Prior to the hurricane, free-standing outside objects should be secured: bicycles, barbecues, etc.
- Do not rely on the usual water supply.
- Have water-purifying kits available.
- Fill tub and containers with water prior to the hurricane.
- Hand-washing decreases food- and waterborne illness.
- Do not rely on electricity.
- Have batteries and flashlights available.
- Do not rely on refrigeration for foodstuffs.
- Carbon monoxide poisoning can occur with improper indoor cooking techniques and during attempts to heat or dry articles/rooms.
- Assume downed electrical wires are live and be aware that electricity can travel through water.

— Be prepared for fires: fire extinguishers.
— Have a form of communication that does not rely on telephone landlines or electricity.
— Be prepared for hypothermia- or hyperthermia-related problems.
— Beware of structural collapse or instability.
— Wear proper protective wear during cleanup: eye protection, ear protection, hard hats, gloves, pants, long sleeves, and watertight steel boots.

RESOURCES

National Hurricane Center: http://www.nhc.noaa.gov/aboutsshs.shtml
Atlantic Oceanographic and Meteorological Laboratory: http://www.aoml.noaa.gov/general/lib/laescae.html

REFERENCES

Cardona Arboleda, OD. 1993. *Guías para la mitigación de riesgos naturales en las instalaciones de la salud de los países de América Latina*. Washington, DC: Panamerican Health Organization.

CDC. 2000. Morbidity and mortality associated with Hurricane Floyd, North Carolina, September–October 1999. *MMWR* **49**:369–372.

CDC. 1998. Deaths associated with Hurricane Georges, Puerto Rico. *MMWR* **47**:897–898.

CDC. 1989. Deaths associated with Hurricane Hugo, Puerto Rico. *MMWR* **38**:718–725.

CDC. 1995. Deaths associated with Hurricanes Marilyn and Opal, United States, September–October 1995. *MMWR* **45**:32–38.

CDC. 1986. Epidemiologic notes and reports: hurricanes and hospital emergency-room visits, Mississippi, Rhode Island, Connecticut. *MMWR* **34**:765–770.

CDC. 1994. Flood-related mortality, Georgia, July 4–14, 1994. *MMWR* **43**:526–530.

CDC. 2001. Tropical storm Allison, rapid needs assessment, Houston, Texas, June 2001. *MMWR* **51**:365–369.

Diaz JH. 2004. The public health impact of hurricanes and major flooding. *J La State Med Soc* **156**:145–150.

Jarrell JD, Mayfield M, Rappaport EN, Landsea CW. 2001. *Deadliest, costliest, and most intense United States hurricanes from 1900 to 2000 (and other frequently requested hurricane facts), updated October 2001*. NOAA Technical Memorandum, NOAA-TM-NWS-TPC-3 (PB2002-100134).

Holland GJ. 1993. Ready reckoner. In *Global guide to tropical cyclone forecasting*, chap. 9. WMO/TC-No. 560, Report No. TCP-31. Geneva: World Meteorological Organization.

Pielke RA, Landsea CW. 1998. Normalized hurricane damages in the United States: 1925–1995. *Weather Forecasting* **13**(3):621–631.

Sheets RC. 1994. *The United States hurricane problem: an assessment for the 1990s*. Miami: National Hurricane Center.

15 TORNADOES

Sarah M. Kelmenson, MD*

OVERVIEW

Tornadoes are one of the most violent and lethal wind-related natural disasters in the world. They appear as funnel-shaped clouds that rotate at high velocity. Severe tornadoes can have wind speeds up to 310 mph and travel as far as 185 miles. There were 3653 fatalities caused by tornadoes in the US between 1953 and 1992, and over 70,000 injuries from tornadoes between 1950 and 1994. There are approximately 800 tornadoes each year in the United States, and they occur in all 50 states as well as in most of Canada. However, most tornadoes occur in "Tornado Alley," which is comprised of Texas, Oklahoma, Kansas, and Nebraska.

RISK FACTORS FOR INJURY

Mobile homes are one of the greatest risk factors for injury during a tornado. The rate of serious injury for mobile home occupants is 85.1 per 1000, compared to 3 per 1000 for occupants of standard homes. Although mobile home parks have tie-downs, they are only effective for wind speeds up to 50 mph, which is well below that of most tornadoes.

People who are outdoors during a tornado are also at increased risk for morbidity and mortality compared with people who are sheltered. Injuries from wind-accelerated projectiles cause a significant number of tornado-related injuries.

The elderly population also has an increased risk of morbidity and mortality, with people older than 60 being seven times more likely to sustain an injury than people younger than 20. The reasons for this fact include the decreased mobility of the elderly, a greater number of comorbid diseases, and increased susceptibility to trauma.

*Department of Emergency Medicine, Brown University, Rhode Island Hospital, Providence

PREVENTION OF INJURIES

The best means of prevention for tornado-related injuries is adequate warning. A tornado watch is issued when weather conditions favor storm formation. A tornado warning in issued when a funnel cloud is detected, either visually or by radar. In the United States, all watches and warnings are issued from the Storm Prediction Center (SPC). Since 1950, the number of tornado-related fatalities has been steadily declining, mostly as a result of improvements in warning systems. People should be encouraged to watch alerts on local radio and television stations. In addition, alert sirens can warn a greater number of people than media bulletins alone.

People should seek shelter indoors, in the basement or lowest floor, and away from windows. Rooms in the center of a structure are more secure than rooms around the perimeter. Furthermore, lying under a blanket, mattress, sleeping bag, or other such object can provide additional protection to tornado victims.

However, mobile home residents should not remain inside during a tornado. Some mobile home parks have tornado shelters that can be used by residents. If there is no such shelter, people in mobile homes should find an alternative structure, ideally one with a basement. If there is no such shelter nearby, the mobile home resident should go outdoors and lie in a ditch, ravine, or culvert.

Drivers should not try to outrun a tornado, an action which is a risk factor for increased morbidity and mortality. If there is no shelter readily available, drivers should get out of the vehicle, find a low-lying area such as a ditch, gully, or culvert, and lie down flat, covering their heads with their hands. Drivers should not lie down underneath the vehicle, and they should try to avoid an area with numerous trees.

Tornado victims who are outdoors at the time of a tornado should find nearby shelter if possible. If not, they should follow the above instructions for drivers who are forced to leave their vehicles.

Finally, people in public buildings such as offices, schools, and shopping malls should congregate on the lowest, most centrally located area, avoid windows, and find shelter under secure objects (doorframes, counters). Elevators should be avoided to prevent a power failure trapping victims inside.

INJURIES

The leading cause of death in tornadoes is severe head injury, followed by cervical spinal injury and crush injuries to the chest. Most of these serious injuries result in death at the scene. Soft-tissue injuries, including lacerations, contusions, abrasions, and musculoskeletal strain, are the most common reported nonfatal injuries resulting from tornadoes, and make up more than 50% of the injuries seen in emergency rooms after a tornado. These injuries are also usually highly contaminated with foreign material. Fractures, the most common cause of admission, are seen in approximately 30% of injuries after a tornado. Electrical injuries can occur due to damage to utility lines, and flooding, hail, or lightning during a tornado or afterwards can cause injuries to tornado victims as well as to rescuers.

EMERGENCY DEPARTMENT TREATMENT

As previously mentioned, most fatalities after a tornado occur on the scene. However, there will be serious injuries that arrive in the emergency department (ED). Most severe injuries arrive within 1–4 hours. These patients should be cared for like other trauma patients.

Since over 50% of injuries consist of soft-tissue wounds, wound care after a tornado is a most important topic. Many wounds will be heavily contaminated with dirt, glass, wood, grass, and other foreign matter. As a result, there is a significant concern with infection. Copious irrigation and removal of foreign bodies should be performed. Studies have shown that wound infections in tornado victims are polymicrobial, with the most common organisms including *Escherichia coli*, *Klebsiella*, *Serratia*, *Proteus*, and *Pseudomonas* species. *Staphylococcus aureus*, *Bacteroides*, and fungi also occur, but less frequently. In addition, there has been one documented case of tetanus and two cases of gas gangrene from *Clostridium perfringens* in tornado victims.

It has been shown that wounds in tornado victims that are closed primarily, even with the use of antibiotics, have a high rate of infection. Although no formal studies have been conducted, delayed primary closure for heavily contaminated post-tornado wounds with broad-spectrum antibiotic coverage is likely the best course of treatment. In addition, patients with any skin break should receive a tetanus shot unless they have received a booster shot within the previous five years.

REFERENCES

Brenner SA, Noji EK. 1992. Head injuries and mortality in tornado disasters. *Am J Public Health* **82**:1296.

Bohonos JJ, Hogan DE. 1999. The medical impact of tornadoes in North America. *J Emerg Med* **17**:67–73.

Carter AO, Millson ME, Allen DE. 1989. Epidemiologic study of deaths and injuries due to tornadoes. *Am J Epidemiol* **130**:1209–1218.

CDC. 1991. Tornado disaster—Illinois, 1990. *MMWR* **40**:33–36.

CDC. 1994. Tornado disaster—Alabama, March 27 1994. *MMWR* **1**:339–343.

CDC. 1997. Tornado disaster—Texas, May 1997. *MMWR* **14**:1069–1073.

Eidson M, Lybarger JA, Parsons JE, MacCormack JN, Freeman JI. 1990. Risk factors for tornado injuries. *Int J Epidemiol* **19**:1051–1056.

Liu S, Quenemoen LE, Malilay J, Noji EK, Sinks T, Mendlein J. 1994. Assessment of a severe-weather system and disaster preparedness, Calhoun County, Alabama, 1994. *Am J Public Health* **86**:87–89.

Mandelbaum I, Nahrwold D, Boyer DW. 1966. Management of tornado casualties. *J Trauma* **6**:353–361

Saunderson LM. 1989. Tornadoes. In *The public health consequences of disaster, 1989*, vol. 127, pp. 39–49. Ed MB Gregg. Atlanta: Centers for Disease Control.

16 DROUGHT

Robert E. Antosia, MD, MPH*

Drought may be defined as a period of abnormally dry weather that is sufficiently prolonged so that the lack of water causes a serious climate imbalance in the affected areas. Drought is a natural disaster that is found at some time in every region of the world. It can induce famine, malnutrition, diseases, and significant morbidity and mortality.

Throughout history, the most dreaded consequence of drought is famine. As water tables drop, a corresponding decline in amount of vegetation is observed. The reduction in crop productivity increases the morbidity and mortality of livestock, fish, and wildlife. While the immediate effect is a significant increase in food prices, the most serious economic burden is borne by farmers and ranchers. Drought-related farm industry losses often run into billions of dollars and can have catastrophic effects on the regional or national economy, as well as the individual consumer.

The environmental effects of drought force local wildlife into human-occupied areas in search of food and water. Under such circumstances, the invasion of neighborhoods and homes by rodents, deer, and coyotes is very common.

The medical consequences of drought include an increased incidence of malnutrition and infectious diseases. The resultant lack of nutrition can ultimately lead to the classic conditions of marasmus (the lack of caloric intake) and kwashiorkor (lack of protein intake). Collectively, the states of inanition are referred to as protein-energy malnutrition (PEM). PEM results in impaired immune system function and increased mortality.

The other direct consequence of drought is contamination of the existing water supply with waterborne pathogens. As the surface water level recedes, reservoirs become stationary and stagnant and serve as a medium for unusual parasites and opportunistic bacteria. Under these circumstances, an increase in the incidence of zoonotic and parasitic infections in man is seen. Primary amebic meningoencephalitis is caused by the facultative parasite *Naegleria fowleri*. Infection often results from inhaling contaminated water while swimming. The signs and symptoms are similar to those for bacterial meningitis. Leptospirosis is a febrile bacterial illness acquired by

*Department of Emergency Medicine, Beth Israel Deaconess Medical Center, Harvard Medical School, Boston

contact with water contaminated by infected rat urine. The diagnosis should be suspected in those who participate in recreational water sports and subsequently develop an acute febrile illness complicated by jaundice and renal failure. Enterotoxigenic *E. coli* has a worldwide distribution and transmission, and spreads by the fecal-oral route via contaminated food or water sources. It is a major cause of gastroenteritis and traveler's diarrhea.

The drought-induced migration of wildlife to areas inhabited by man can also result in exposure to a number of diseases. In this case, either the animal is a vector, or parasites on the host animal serve as a vector for the illness. Tick-borne diseases such as Rocky Mountain Spotted Fever, Tularemia, and Lyme Disease are common examples. Flea-borne diseases include the Plague and Hantavirus Pulmonary Syndrome.

Droughts are important natural disasters that have far-reaching effects on society. Because of increasing population and the ever-changing climate of the world, droughts remain inevitable. They are also the result of highly complex meteorological phenomena, which makes forecasting them accurately extremely difficult.

REFERENCES

Barwick RS, Levy DA, Craun GF, Beach MJ, Calderon RL. 2000. Surveillance for waterborne disease outbreaks, United States, 1997–1998. *MMWR CDC Surveill Summ* **49**(4):1–21.

Hogan DE, Burstein JL. 2002. *Disaster medicine*, pp. 212–221. Philadelphia: Lippincott, Williams, and Wilkins.

17

FIRESTORMS AND WILDFIRES

Medley O'Keefe Gatewood, MD*

OVERVIEW

The urban/wildland interface is the area where the private citizen meets wildland, and it is the zone of greatest concern for contemporary firefighters. Attendance at US parks and recreational areas has been steadily increasing for many years. Wilderness areas lack highly developed urban emergency medical services. In attempting to escape the dangers and troubles of an urban lifestyle, many place themselves at greater risk for loss of life and property through wildland fire.

In the United States, about 70,000 wildland fires per year burn almost 2 million acres and require the efforts of approximately 80,000 firefighters. Nearly every state has experienced fires in the urban/wildland interface that have resulted in significant losses. The National Fire Protection Agency (NFPA) estimated that, from 1985 to 1995, wildfires destroyed more than 9,000 homes and resulted in many deaths of firefighters, as well as civilians, with untold numbers of injuries. From 1990 to 1998, 133 fatalities were associated with wildland fire activities. While California had the highest number of fatalities, wildland fire fatalities occurred in 33 different states spanning every region of the country.

The most common cause of death from fighting wildland fires from 1990 to 1998 was burnover. This occurs when a firestorm burns over an individual in the path of the advancing front. Other causes include aircraft accidents, followed by heart attack and vehicle accidents. Lastly, falling snags, which refer to dead trees that have begun to burn, account for 5% of reported fatalities.

*Harvard-Affiliated Emergency Residency Program, Brigham and Women's Hospital/Massachusetts General Hospital, Boston

Physical Principles of Heat Transfer

Heat energy is transferred by conduction, convection, radiation, and spotting, but generally only the latter three processes are significant in a wildland setting. Convection, or the movement of hot masses of air, accounts for most of the heat transfer outward from the fire. Convective currents usually move vertically unless a wind or slope generates lateral movement. Convection preheats fuels upslope and in shrub and tree canopies, further contributing to a fire's spread and the onset of crown fires. Radiant energy is emitted in direct lines or rays and decreases inversely in proportion to the square of the distance from the source. Radiant heat does not penetrate solid objects and is easily reflected. Spotting is a mass transfer mechanism by which wind currents carry burning or glowing embers beyond the main fire to start new, often unpredictable and unexpected, fires.

FIRE-RELATED INJURIES AND FATALITIES

While no comprehensive data are available concerning wildfire injury, clearly, many more injuries than fatalities are seen in each event. Those with underlying medical conditions and poor physical conditioning are at higher risk of death or disability while fighting or escaping from a wildland fire. All the potentially injurious events that one normally associates with the outdoors are magnified for those closely associated with wildland fires. The most serious injuries from wildland fires are smoke exposure, respiratory problems, heat illness, burns, and thermal injury. Wildland firefighters generally do not wear the same level of protective equipment as their urban counterparts. It is rarely feasible for a wildland firefighter to wear a self-contained breathing apparatus or fireproof clothing. The risks of burning and smoke inhalation are magnified for those fighting wildfires. However, due to the nature of the open environment, the risk of injury from heat stress is decreased.

Thermal Injury

The most common cause of thermal injury is direct contact with flames. While the temperatures created by a forest fire can be extreme, they are often of short duration. The most severe burns typically involve civilians who are inexperienced with wildland fire behavior or with rapid, unanticipated changes in fire behavior. Burns can be partial thickness or full thickness. Immediate death is due primarily to hypovolemia or frank incineration.

Airway Injury

Contact with superheated air brings the risk of respiratory tract injury. Respiratory tract injury should be suspected with burns around the face, neck, or upper body, and with nasal hair singing, facial edema, stridor, and early respiratory distress. The level of injury is directly correlated with the amount of time spent in the burning area and the actual temperature of the air breathed. Air is a poor conductor of heat, and the upper airway is very efficient in thermal exchange. Thermal injuries to the respiratory tract can be insidious, with respiratory distress presenting as late as 24 hours after exposure to superheated air.

Heat Stress

All persons involved with a wildland fire are at increased risk for heat-related illness. Wildland fire suppression is usually prolonged and extremely strenuous. Individuals working in the heat rarely replace fluids at the same level of that lost through exertion. For more information on heat-related disorders, see chapter 18 on Hyperthermia.

Smoke Inhalation

Asphyxia is always a risk when an individual is exposed to smoke. While many wildland firefighters use particulate masks, private citizens may be unprepared and have no form of airway protection. Wildland firefighters are not as likely to experience the extreme, acute exposures that structural firefighters encounter. However, they are more likely to have prolonged exposure to smoke. Common compounds found in the air of wildland fires include carbon monoxide, sulfur dioxide, particulate carbon and silica, polyaromatic hydrocarbons, aldehydes, and benzene. Of greatest concern are aldehydes and carbon monoxide. Aldehyde exposure results in local irritation, while carbon monoxide exposure is associated with nonspecific warning signs such as headache, and high levels can be potential fatal. While the long-term effects of respiratory contaminants are not fully known, studies have shown decreased short-term pulmonary function in wildland firefighters. Also of concern are exacerbations of underlying pulmonary conditions, like asthma, emphysema, and COPD.

SYSTEMS PLANNING: FIRE SAFETY AND EMERGENCY MEDICAL SERVICES

For wildland fires, as in almost all disasters, planning is essential for reducing loss of life and property. Proper planning begins and ends with education. The National Fire Protection Association has produced a wildfire training course that helps both volunteer and professional fire departments plan for and safely fight wildland fires. Instruction in entrapment procedures, wildfire behavior, communications, and escape protocols should be given. Minimum safety equipment for the wildland firefighter should include a hard hat, safety goggles, brightly colored clothing, long sleeves and pants, boots, and gloves. A personal fire shelter should also be carried to deploy in the event of imminent burnover.

Collaborative Planning

As almost all wildland fires are fought with the help of several municipal, state, and federal agencies, mutual aid agreements are vital in combating wilderness fires. Planning should take into account the expected extended nature of wildland fire suppression efforts. Communication and chain of command should be addressed in advance. Rescue protocols, equipment needs, personnel needs, and evacuation procedures must be addressed as well.

EMS

A wildland fire is an ongoing disaster that may last for days to weeks. Emergency Medical Services can play a critical role in wildland fire safety. Typically at or near the fire front, EMS can play a critical role in triage and field treatment of those injured in these events. A mobile command post with the capabilities to treat several patients simultaneously for heat-related illness, trivial trauma, and respiratory complaints is able to reduce morbidity and the emergency department visits for fire personnel. Triage and treatment may occur simultaneously with stabilization, and the units must have the capacity to move from the area rapidly if this is required by the changing fire environment.

Emergency Department Preparedness

During a wildland fire, the emergency departments should maintain close contact with medical support at the scene of the fire. This will help assess civilian risk and guide resource utilization. The most common injuries seen are respiratory complaints, heat stress, burns, and minor trauma. However, serious trauma associated with involvement or responses to these events, as well as heart attack and stroke, are also seen. Emergency visits increase during these events, but hospitalization rates do not appear to be significantly increased.

PUBLIC EDUCATION

The general public tends to underestimate existing fire hazards and is usually not experienced in avoiding fire threats. Civilians entering the wilderness or building homes in the wilderness must be educated and informed about fire safety. Individuals should carry personal safety equipment and be familiar with safety and suppression procedures. Structures should be erected with attention to adequate ingress and egress routes, preferably multiple. Structures should be constructed with cognizance of possible fire hazard, built accordingly, and have a safe perimeter. Adequate resources for personal suppression efforts should be available. Such education and preparation is essential prior to entering the wilderness or building in the wilderness or urban/wildland interface. The general public must share responsibility with suppression organizations to minimize fire hazards created by humans. Care with fire, proper cleanup of debris, fuel reduction efforts on wildland property, fire-safe construction guidelines, and the application of survival skills will minimize fire threats.

RESOURCES

www.fs.fes.us
www.firepreventionteams.us
www.nifc.gov
www.nwcg.gov
www.firewise.org

REFERENCES

Davis KM, Mutch RW. 2001. Wildland fires: dangers and survival. In *Wilderness medicine: management of wilderness and environment emergencies*, 4th ed., pp. 318–341. Ed PS Auerbach. St. Louis: Mosby.

Frantz RR. 2002. Firestorms and wildfires. In *Disaster medicine*, pp. 194–201. Ed DE Hogan, JL Burstein. Hogan DE, Burstein JL, eds. Philadelphia: Lippincott, Williams and Wilkins.

Mangan R. 1999. *Wildland fire fatalities in the United States 1990 to 1998*. Missoula, MT: USDA Forest Service.

Rothermel RC. 1991. *Predicting behavior and size of crown fires in the northern Rocky Mountains*. USDA Forest Service Research Paper INT-438.

Rothman N, Ford DP, Baser ME, Hansen JA, O'Toole T, Tockman MS, Strickland PT. 1991. Pulmonary function and respiratory symptoms in wildland firefighters. *J Occup Med* **33**(11):1163–1167.

US Department of the Interior and USDA. 1995. *Federal wildland fire management policy and program review: final report*. Boise: National Interagency Fire Center http://www.fs.fed.us/fire/management/policy.html.

18 HEATWAVE/ HYPERTHERMIA

Stephen Epstein, MD,* and Atul Kukar, DO*

OVERVIEW

Historical Significance

Heat waves have caused large-scale human deaths throughout history. The effects of heat on military campaigns have been described in the Bible, as well as in recorded history from Alexander the Greek to the Crusades. Battles have been won and lost in part as a result of superior or inferior heat management. However, heat waves are not only an ancient phenomenon, and technological advances have not prevented catastrophic heat waves from occurring as recently as the past decade. In July 1995, 739 deaths were ascribed to a heat wave in Chicago over a 5-day period—more than the number of deaths from floods, hurricanes, and tornadoes combined for an average year. In 2003, 35,000 deaths were tallied during an August heatwave in Europe.

Etiology

Extensive analysis of the Chicago heat wave of 1995 revealed that most of the victims were elderly urban dwellers, without air conditioning, and hesitant to open doors and windows due the threat of crime. Appropriate warnings (which did not come until the last day of the heatwave), use of air conditioning and ventilation, as well as appropriate clothing and hydration might have prevented many deaths.

Urban dwellers are at particular risk, as cities tend to be warmer than surrounding suburbs. This is due to the concentration of manmade materials that tend to absorb more heat during the day and release heat into the environment at night. Power failures can also affect cooling equipment, which is more critical in urban areas.

*Beth Israel Deaconess Medical Center, Harvard Medical School, Boston
**Division of Cardiology, St. Luke's-Roosevelt Hospital Center, New York

Other risk factors include medications that inhibit the body's cooling mechanisms: anticholinergic medications can inhibit sweating and evaporative cooling while sympathomimetics can increase heat production. Beta blockers and other cardiac medications can limit the heart's ability to increase cardiac output in response to heat stress and circulate a larger blood volume to the peripheral tissues where cooling might occur. Diuretics lead to hypovolemia and limit the ability of the body to shunt blood to the periphery for cooling.

Finally, many elderly are without access to free water on their own are subject to dehydration. The elderly are therefore at particularly high risk of heat illness.

PRESENTATION

Heat-related illnesses are a continuum from the minor heat illnesses and dehydration to heat stroke. Generally, patients who succumb to heat stroke during a heat wave have gone through the other stages of heat illness first, particularly volume-depletion heat exhaustion. That said, classic heat stroke can strike suddenly, the hallmark being a markedly elevated core temperature and altered mental status

Heat Rash

Heat rash usually consists of a maculopapular, pruritic, erythematous rash over cloth-covered areas of body. It has been noted to be due to acute blockage of sweat glands. If in the acute phase, antihistamines can be used to manage the rash. More severe cases require vigilance, as the level of damage may predispose the patient to *Staphylococcus aureus* skin infections.

Heat Cramp

Heat cramp consists of painful, involuntary muscle spasms that usually occur after vigorous exercise and, surprisingly, during a rest period that includes showering. This condition is usually self-limited, but may be a harbinger of a more serious condition. Although caused by excess heat, the core body temperature may be normal. It is usually managed with salt tablets and water.

Heat Exhaustion

Heat exhaustion is a condition of both salt and water depletion that usually strikes people in a hot environment who are without adequate water repletion. Salt losses are expected with heavy sweating and hypotonic replacement. This condition is sometimes difficult to diagnose, as it presents with myriad nonspecific symptoms, including: headache, fatigue, nausea, vomiting, diaphoresis, weakness, irritability, and muscle cramps. The rectal temperature will be less than 40°C, and mental status should be normal. This is important in distinguishing this state from that of heat stroke, which will usually have a temperature above 40°C (unless treated prior to arrival) and mental status changes.

Heat Stroke

This is classically seen in debilitated patients during disaster conditions, such as heat waves. The signs and symptoms of heat exhaustion are unfortunately nonspecific, and include weakness, fatigue, nausea and vomiting, headache, and orthostatic syncope. By comparison, key features of heat stroke include the following:

- Exposure to heat stress
- CNS dysfunction, with delirium and coma most common
- Elevated core temperature (usually >40.5°C)
- Dry, hot skin; sweating in exertional heat stroke
- Elevation of liver transaminases

Patients with heat stroke will often appear similar to patients in septic shock, with tachycardia and low peripheral vascular resistance, as the body attempts to shunt blood to the periphery.

DIAGNOSIS

Hyperthermia leads to a number of biochemical changes that can alter key bodily functions. Coagulopathies are common, as liver damage depletes stores of clotting factors, and clotting factors are activated by heat leading to disseminated intravascular coagulation (DIC).

Marked elevations of transaminases are seen and are a consistent feature of heat stroke.

Renal damage is also common due to hypovolemia and shock.

Laboratories should include a CBC, electrolytes, BUN and creatinine, ABG, lactate, CPK, hepatic enzymes, coagulation studies and DIC screen.

DIFFERENTIAL DIAGNOSIS

In the appropriate circumstances of heat stress, heat-related illness is at the top of the differential diagnosis when the patient responds appropriately to cooling with improvement in mental status and hemodynamic stability. However, should the patient not respond, the following diagnoses should be considered:

- Meningitis/encephalitis
- Septic shock
- Thyroid storm
- Drug-induced
    - Anticholinergics
    - Sympathomimetics
- Delirium tremens

TREATMENT

Treatment involves removal of the offending agent, namely the hot environment. Once the patient has been stabilized, the next step is rapid cooling to a temperature lower than 39.5°C (103°F). This may be accomplished by cold-water immersion or evaporative cooling, which involves spraying lukewarm water over the patient's skin via air circulated by fans. Evaporative cooling is the most effective and practical method, as immersion makes monitoring difficult. The use of ice packs is not recommended, as there is no reduction in cooling time and it is often poorly tolerated by the patient. Cold peritoneal lavage is effective, but is a surgical procedure contraindicated in patients with prior abdominal surgery.

Adjunctive therapies including cold gastric lavage, cooling blankets, and cold intravenous fluid may help, but alcohol sponge baths should be avoided, as they may cause toxicity due to greater absorption with dilated cutaneous circulation. In addition, antipyretics are of no benefit because the underlying mechanism is not one of cytokine-induced inflammation.

Rectal or esophageal (in intubated patients) probes are the best means by which to monitor temperature. If this is not available, tympanic temperatures are taken every 5 minutes. In addition to monitoring the cooling process, it helps prevent iatrogenic hypothermia. Of note, shivering usually requires treatment with sedatives, as it will increase heat production. Intravenous fluids are only necessary if the patient is unable to tolerate oral solutions (secondary to severe gastrointestinal upset), is hemodynamically unstable, or has severe electrolyte disturbances. If patients are quickly treated with cooling and management of laboratory abnormalities, they usually recover without sequelae.

PREVENTION

The mainstay of hyperthermia management is prevention. All types of people—including workers, athletes, and the general population—need to be wary of certain dangerous situations and take proper preventative measures. These include frequent breaks, wearing lightweight, light-colored, loose-fitting clothing, properly functioning air-conditioning, increased heat loss with fan evaporation, appropriate isotonic fluid repletion (excess fluid repletion has led to hyponatremia), and avoiding activity during maximum temperatures (noon to 4:00 pm). Air conditioning is helpful, but it places strains on electrical power grids, and backup plans to maintain power are essential.

RESOURCES

www.bordeninstitute.army.mil/medaspofharshenvrnmnts/Ch1-IntroductiontoHeat-RelatedProblemsinMilitaryOpera.pdf

REFERENCES

Bross MH, Nash BT, Carlton FB. 1994. Heat emergencies. *Am Fam Physician* **50**:389–396.

Dematte JE, O'Mara K, Buescher J, Whitney CG, Forsythe S, McNamee T, Adiga RB, Ndukwu IM. 1998. Near-fatal heat stroke during the 1995 heat wave in Chicago. *Ann Intern Med* **129**(3):173–181.

Kaiser R, Rubin CH, Henderson AK, Wolfe MI, Kieszak S, Parrott CL, Adcock M. 2001. Heat-related death and mental illness during the 1999 Cincinnati heat wave. *Am J Forensic Med Pathol* **3**:303–307.

Khosla, R, Guntapalli, KK. 1999. Heat-related illness. *Crit Care Clin* **15**:251–263.

Lu KC, Wang TL. 2004. Heat stroke. *Ann Disaster Med* **2**(suppl 2):S97–S109.

Seraj MA, Channa AB, Al-Harthi SS, Khan FM, Zafrullah A, Samarkandi AH. 1991. Are heat stroke patients fluid depleted? Importance of monitoring central venous pressure as a simple guideline for fluid therapy. *Resuscitation* **21**:33–39.

19 WINTER STORM DISASTERS AND HYPOTHERMIA

Matt Miles, MD, and Robert E. Antosia, MD, MPH*

OVERVIEW

A specific combination of weather conditions must be present to trigger a winter storm. Typically, such storms develop along the boundary between two air masses: warmer moist air overrides denser, cold air. This results in condensation, cloud formation, and precipitation. Depending on what the surface conditions are, precipitation may fall as snow, ice, or rain. Such storm systems may extend over a wide area, and may result in large amounts of snow in a relatively short period of time.

COMMUNITY PREPARATION AND PUBLIC EDUCATION

The National Weather Service (NWS) in the United States issues winter storm warnings. Both historical and current data are used in computer models to create long-range weather forecasts. Short-range predictions are made by coupling these models with real-time data from surface and air measurements, as well as with radar and various types of satellite imaging.

Various weather advisories and warnings may be issued by the NWS. A frost or freeze warning means that temperatures below freezing are expected for some defined period of time. A winter storm advisory implies that winter weather conditions can be expected to cause inconveniences and delays, especially for motorists. A winter storm watch implies that a winter storm is likely. Protective action by the public should be taken when a winter storm warning is issued. A blizzard warning refers to a severe winter storm with significant snow and high winds that will lead to deep snow drifts,

*Department of Emergency Medicine, Albany Medical Center, Albany, New York

**Department of Emergency Medicine, Beth Israel Deaconess Medical Center, Harvard Medical School, Boston

poor visibility, and life-threatening cold. The public should seek protection immediately.

Specific measures should be emphasized before the arrival of a winter storm. These measures include the following: monitoring of a National Oceanic Atmospheric Administration (NOAA) weather radio, local radio, or TV station for forecast updates and information including emergency instructions; avoid going outdoors unless absolutely necessary; dress appropriately when going outside, including multiple layers of loose-fitting, lightweight dry clothing, a hat to minimize heat loss through the head, as well as gloves or mittens, and a scarf; beware of overexertion and recognize that shoveling snow can induce a heart attack; be cautious of structural damage to homes due to snow and ice buildup; have an adequate supply of home staples, including bottled water and canned foods; and develop an emergency survival kit for the home and car.

PATHOPHYSIOLOGY OF COLD INJURIES

Heat is lost through the following four mechanisms: radiation, convection, conduction, and evaporation. Radiation, in which heat is transferred by electromagnetic waves, accounts for almost two-thirds of heat loss in a cold environment. Radiant heat loss can be minimized by wearing appropriate warm clothing and minimizing the body surface area exposed to the cold environment. Conduction refers to the transfer of heat from warmer to cooler objects by direct contact. Heat loss through this mechanism is usually minimal, but it becomes a major source of heat loss in wet clothes or with cold-water immersion. Convection is the loss of heat to surrounding air and water vapor. Heat loss by convection is dependent on a combination of environmental factors, including wind velocity and temperature. The wind chill index, which estimates the equivalent temperature effect on exposed skin, is a combination of the ambient temperature and the wind velocity. It is a more important consideration than the actual temperature. This index and the time required to cause skin damage are demonstrated in Figure 1. Evaporation is the heat lost when a liquid is converted to gas. Sweating and an increased respiratory rate with physical exertion increase heat loss in the cold.

COLD INJURIES

Cold injuries can be divided into local cold injuries and the systemic state of hypothermia. Local cold injuries are further subdivided into the freezing injuries of frostbite and frostnip and the nonfreezing injuries of chilblains and trench foot. In general, the prognosis is better for nonfreezing injuries. Trench foot is seen when wet feet are exposed continuously to cold temperatures and develops over hours to days. Chilblains refer to localized skin lesions seen in the hands, feet, ears, and lower legs. It is caused by chronic, intermittent exposure to damp, nonfreezing cold conditions. Frostnip is an early stage in the continuum of frostbite, and is a superficial cold injury without tissue damage. Clinically, the involved area appears pale and is associated with a mild burning or stinging sensation. Symptoms improve with rewarming and no permanent injury occurs. Frostbite is a more serious condition, and is most commonly seen on the nose, ears, face, hands, and feet. It can be subdivided into superfi-

APPARENT WIND CHILL

	45	40	35	30	25	20	15	10	5	0	-5	-10	-15	-20	-25	-30	-35	-40
4mph	45	40	35	30	25	20	15	10	5	0	-5	-10	-15	-20	-25	-30	-35	-40
5mph	43	37	32	27	22	16	11	6	0	-5	-10	-15	-21	-26	-31	-36	-42	-47
10mph	34	28	22	16	10	3	-3	-9	-15	-22	-27	-34	-40	-46	-52	-58	-64	-71
15mph	29	23	16	9	2	-5	-11	-18	-25	-31	-38	-45	-51	-58	-65	-72	-78	-85
20mph	26	19	12	4	-3	-10	-17	-24	-31	-39	-46	-53	-60	-67	-74	-81	-88	-95
25mph	23	16.	8	1	-7	-15	-22	-29	-36	-44	-51	-59	-66	-74	-81	-88	-96	-103
30mph	21	13	6	-2	-10	-18	-25	-33	-41	-49	-56	-64	-71	-79	-86	-93	-101	-109
35mph	20	12	4	-4	-12	-20	-27	-35	-43	-52	-58	-67	-74	-82	-89	-97	-105	-113
40mph	19	11	3	-5	-13	-21	-29	-37	-45	-53	-60	-69	-76	-84	-92	-100	-107	-115
45mph	18	10	2	-6	-14	-22	-30	-38	-45	-54	-62	-70	-78	-85	-93	-102	-109	-117

Unpleasant

Frostbite likely. Outdoor activity dangerous.

Exposed flesh will freeze within half a minute for the average person

Figure 1. Wind chill index and time to skin damage. Adapted from a chart provided by the National Weather Service.

cial and deep injuries. First-degree frostbite is characterized by erythema, mild edema, and no blisters. This is also accompanied by mild stinging or burning. Second-degree frostbite is characterized by initial erythema, followed by clear blisters in 6 to 12 hours. Clinically, the patient will also have initial numbness, followed by a deep throbbing. The blisters may desquamate into black eschars over several days. Deep frostbite injuries extend beyond the epidermis and portend a worse prognosis. Third-degree frostbite results in dark hemorrhagic blisters and skin necrosis. Fourth-degree frostbite is characterized by extension into the muscle, tendons, or bone. The skin is mottled and cyanotic and will transform over time to a dry black eschar. Definitive treatment for fourth-degree frostbite frequently requires debridement and amputation.

HYPOTHERMIA

Hypothermia is defined as a core temperature of less than 35°C (95°F). While hypothermia can affect virtually any organ system in the body, the most prominent effects are on the neurologic and cardiovascular systems. Further classification of severity is also based on core temperature:

- Mild: 32–35°C
- Moderate: 29–31°C
- Severe: 26–28°C

Etiology

Virtually any disaster situation can produce conditions that result in hypothermia. While primary hypothermia may result from prolonged exposure to a cold environment, the loss of normal regulatory functions may cause secondary hypothermia.

Therefore, while it is associated with cold weather, cases also occur during summer months in warm climates. It is also commonly associated with water-related accidents.

Diagnosis

A measured core temperature (esophageal or rectal) below 35°C is sufficient for confirming the diagnosis. Most standard thermometers do not provide readings below 31°C, so an accurate measure requires a temperature probe with an adequate range. The diagnosis is typically supported by physical signs and symptoms (see Table 1), but those signs may be paradoxical (e.g., vasodilation and flushing) and misleading unless the diagnosis is considered. In addition, mild and even moderate cases may not be readily apparent in the unconscious disaster victim or those with significant comorbid conditions. Specific organ system effects include myocardial depression, renal hypoperfusion, acute tubular necrosis, bronchorrhea and pulmonary edema, GI ileus, pancreatitis, hepatic failure, cerebral hypoperfusion, and altered mental status. In the setting of delirium, the phenomenon of paradoxical undressing may occur in which the victim sheds their protective clothing while still in the cold environment.

Initial Evaluation, Triage, and Prognosis

Survival from mild hypothermia without other comorbid conditions is essentially 100%. Therefore, triage of such patients should be based on the presence of other worrying conditions.

The prognosis of moderate and severe cases are much more difficult to establish, particularly in the pre-hospital setting. There is a trend toward decreased survival at lower core temperatures, but presenting core temperature is not a clear predictor of mortality. Therefore, triage decisions must consider other factors, including duration of hypothermia, preexisting medical conditions, and concurrent insults.

Thrombosis (fibrinogen <50 mg/dl), severe acidosis, hyperkalemia (>10 mEq/L), and hyperammonemia (>250 μmol/L) are markers of cell death and are grave prognostic indicators, but no clear upper limits that define survival have been established. Shock is an independent risk factor for mortality.

An ECG finding of Osborn J waves is pathognomonic for hypothermia but is not always present and does not correlate with outcome. The presence of ventricular fibrillation or asystole indicates a poor prognosis. The survival rate is much lower if asystole occurs prior to arrival at a hospital.

Management

The patient should be moved carefully and quickly to a safe environment. If unresponsive and not shivering, the hypothermia should be presumed severe and the myocardium considered irritable, so that excessive manipulation of the patient may induce cardiac dysrhythmia. Once in a safe environment, further cooling should be prevented by removing wet clothes, applying warm, dry garments, and warming the air. It is appropriate to spend 30–60 seconds palpating for a pulse and auscultating for breath sounds in order to avoid unnecessary CPR, which may precipitate ventricular fibrillation.

Table 1. Clinical Findings of Progressive Hypothermia

Stage	Core temp	Physiologic changes	Physical signs
Mild	33°–35°C 91°–95°F	Increased basic metabolic rate Increased sympathetic tone Peripheral vasoconstriction Shiver reflex	Increased activity, tachypnea Tachycardia Cool extremities Shivering/clumsiness
Moderate	28°–32°C 82°–90°F	Decreased basic metabolic rate Decreased renal tubular resorption Decreased cerebral blood flow Decreased ADH function Loss of shiver reflex	Bradycardia, bradypnea Confusion/delirium Atrial fibrillation Hypotension Rigidity/loss of shivering
Severe	<27°C <80°F	Loss of all thermoregulation Vasodilation Bradycardia, decreased CO Decreased nerve conduction Decreased cardiac stability	Stupor leading to coma Cutaneous erythema Absent BP/loss of DTRs Arrhythmias including VF, and asystole

Monitoring

Continuous rectal probe monitoring with esophageal confirmation provides a reliable assessment of core temperature. Vital signs should be recorded at short intervals (2–5 minutes) in moderate and severe cases. Continuous pulse oximetry and cardiac monitoring are important, but pulse oximetry may be inaccurate with the poor perfusion seen in hypothermia.

Resuscitation

The first priority is reestablishing respiration and tissue perfusion. The effectiveness of chest compressions may be reduced by 50% or more. Nevertheless, neurologically intact survival after prolonged CPR has been reported. Rapid volume expansion, with fluids heated to 40–42°C, is indicated in moderate and severe hypothermia in anticipation of rewarming shock. Normal saline is preferred to Ringer's lactate solution and can be heated by microwave (approximately 2 minutes on "high" per one-liter bag). Rapid central venous administration can precipitate dysrhythmias; therefore, this route should be avoided for large volumes of warm fluids.

Most dysrhythmias caused by hypothermia will resolve with rewarming. Asystole should be treated no differently than in the warm patient. Bretylium tosylate is the antidysrhythmic of choice for ventricular fibrillation associated with hypothermia. External pacing is preferred to transvenous pacing.

Afterdrop

Afterdrop, a fall in core body temperature after removal from a cold environment, is a common occurrence. Though the definitive cause of this phenomenon is unknown, it is presumed to be caused by improved peripheral circulation, which draws cold blood back to the core. Active external rewarming of the trunk only and inhalation rewarming may limit afterdrop, which can have significant adverse effects in moderate and severe hypothermia.

Rewarming Shock

Rewarming of moderate or severe hypothermia may cause shock. An increase in peripheral circulation in the setting of hypovolemia and a depressed myocardium can result in profound hypotension. Furthermore, the hydrostatic pressure of water may support circulation during immersion. The hydrostatic pressure support is lost when the victim is removed from water. Anticipation of rewarming shock and aggressive intravascular volume expansion are crucial.

REWARMING TECHNIQUES

The basic steps in the rewarming process are:

1. Removal from the cold environment
2. Removal of wet clothing
3. Passive and/or active rewarming
4. Monitoring for afterdrop
5. Monitoring for rewarming shock

Passive External Rewarming (PER)

Consists of insulating the patient (generally with warming, dry clothing, and blankets) to stop heat loss and is sufficient for most mild cases.

Active Rewarming

Uses an exogenous heat source to provide rewarming. Indications are:

1. Cardiovascular instability
2. Moderate or severe hypothermia (T < 32°C)
3. Failure of PER
4. Impaired endogenous heat production

Active rewarming techniques are divided into external and core rewarming techniques.

Active External Rewarming (AER)

Provides heat to the patient's skin surface, particularly the torso. Common AER methods include immersion in warm (40°C) water, and application of heating pads or warm water bottles. Forced air warmers circulate warm air through inflated tubing and are most practical in the ED.

Active Core Rewarming (ACR)

Provides heat directly to the patient's core via the airway, circulatory system, GI tract, or body cavities such as the thorax, peritoneal cavity, or bladder. Airway rewarming is relatively simple, very effective, and indicated for all cases of moderate and severe hypothermia. Humidified air heated to 42–45°C can increase core temperature at 1–2.5 °C/hr. Peritoneal lavage provides dialysate (or saline) heated to 40–45°C to the peritoneal cavity. Two liters are infused, retained for 20 minutes, then drained, and then repeated. This will typically raise core temperature by 1–3 °C/hr. Thoracic lavage provides normal saline heated to 40–42°C via an anterior chest tube and is drained continuously via a posterior chest tube. GI lavage via NG or rectal tube should use <300 ml/lavage to avoid electrolyte disturbances. Cardiopulmonary bypass and other blood rewarming techniques such as hemodialysis are indicated for severe and moderate hypothermia with an unstable cardiac rhythm.

REFERENCES

Hogan DE, Burstein JL, eds. 2002. *Disaster medicine*, pp. 202–211. Philadelphia: Lippincott Williams and Wilkins.

National Weather Service. Available at www.nws.noaa.gov.

Surviving old man winter. 1998. *Occup Health Saf* **67**(10):186–187.

PART III

Bioevents and Manmade Disasters

20

THE EPIDEMIOLOGY OF WAR AND CONFLICT

Frederick M. Burkle, Jr., MD, MPH*

In conventional wars and complex emergencies, humanitarian response must first focus on restoring public health. An epidemiological approach to determine mortality, morbidity, and vulnerable populations begins with establishment of rapid field assessments, surveys, and surveillance that will parallel any emergency response. Past epidemiological studies of war and conflict allow relief agencies and organizations to more accurately focus their emergency response priorities while monitoring ongoing evidence-based surveillance systems to ensure vulnerable populations do not go unrecognized.

The objectives of a rapid assessment in the emergency phase of a complex emergency are to:

- determine the magnitude of the emergency
- identify existing and potential public health problems
- measure present and potential impact, especially health and nutritional needs
- assess resources needed, including availability and capacity of a local response
- determine and plan an appropriate external response
- set up the basis for a health system

The five epidemiological areas that are most useful are: (1) mortality (first measure crude mortality rates, then disaggregate for age and gender), (2) incidence of the most important diseases (morbidity), (3) nutritional status, (4) "activities data," such as immunizations performed, and the "vital sectors," namely food, water, sanitation, shelter, and fuel.

*The Center for International Emergency, Disaster and Refugee Studies, The Johns Hopkins University Medical Institutions, Baltimore

Nutritional assessments measure the height, weight, and mid-upper arm circumference (MUAC) of children 65–110 cm tall (a proxy for 6–59 months of age). Severe undernutrition is defined as low weight-for-height (WFH) or wasting (WFH less than 2 standard deviations below national Center for Health Statistics/CDC/WHO reference median), or a Z-score less than –2 SD from the mean, or a low MUAC (less than 12.5 cm).

PRE-RESPONSE DATA COLLECTION

Data collection commences before the field assessment and originates from existing country profiles, maps, census data, previous demographic and health surveys, early warning system tools, and previous or ongoing in-country assessments. These are routinely performed by United Nations agencies (International Committee of the Red Cross), nongovernmental organizations (NGOs), governmental institutions (e.g., donor organizations), and academic and research centers. Additional data may come from overflights and satellite imagery, especially useful in tracking refugee migration. Background health information is gleaned from reports inherent to organizations such as the World Health Organization, the Disaster Epidemiology Research Center in Belgium, Epicentre, the Centers for Disease Control, and the Prevention Mortality and Morbidity Weekly Report (MMWR) publications, and includes baseline data on:

- endemic diseases
- baseline mortality rates
- morbidity incidence rates
- nutritional status
- sources of health care
- impact of disruption of health services

EPIDEMIOLOGY OF CONVENTIONAL WAR

Conventional cross-borders wars were the most common forms of extended violence prior to 1992. Advanced weaponry, despite claims of improved technology and targeting, respect for the Geneva Conventions, and military discipline, allow for vulnerable civilians to be killed or injured more easily. In World War I, 5% of casualties were civilian, by World War II 50% were civilian. In the Vietnam war 80% of casualties were civilian, but some would argue that this represented a civil war more similar to the complex emergencies of the last two decades.

EPIDEMIOLOGY OF COMPLEX EMERGENCIES

Since 1992 modern post–Cold War era wars have been primarily internal conflicts that target civilian populations, and are referred to as complex emergencies for the complexity of social, political, economic, religious, ethnic, and cultural issues that contribute to and maintain the violence. Inequities, torture, religious fundamentalism, poverty, and loss of sustainable public health infrastructure and development contribute to the onset and migration of populations, either across borders (as refugees) or as internally displaced populations. During the Cold War small arms and automatic weapons were easily transferred into the hands of untrained, undisciplined, or nonmilitary users, and weapon sales to nonmilitary groups increased tremendously. Landmines, always a weapon of conventional war, have proliferated in complex emergencies. An estimated 800 persons die each month from landmine-related injuries and an additional 1200 persons suffer nonfatal injuries, a third of whom require amputations.

Complex emergencies can be divided into three country models: developing, developed, and smoldering or chronic, all with differing epidemiological data presentations.

Developing Country Model

Ninety percent of all complex emergencies occur in the developing world, where basic health care is lacking, consistent nutritional health is erratic and marginalized, famine recurrent, and subsistence level poverty the norm. As such, during non-emergency situations the baseline daily crude mortality rates (CMR) in the non-famine Horn of Africa is 0.5 to 0.65 per 10,000 persons or higher. Conflict readily accelerates worsening of these numbers. Initially, mortality results from the direct effects of violence (more commonly from small arms and machetes), causing deaths, injury, and disabilities. It is the indirect effects of the conflict—the migration of populations, separation from food supplies, and destruction of the public health infrastructure—that eventually cause the greatest mortality and morbidity. A characteristic of complex emergencies is that the healthcare system with hospitals and clinics is the first to be destroyed and the often last to be rehabilitated. By fleeing the violence populations suffer almost immediate food, shelter, fuel, water, sanitation, and basic healthcare insecurities. Refugee populations, especially the most vulnerable—women, children, the elderly, and those with disabilities—suffer the most. Not uncommonly, males are either fighting competing rebel forces or have been killed.

The complexity of the environment and insecurity do not allow for accurate data collection. Aside from shifting populations, difficult terrain, and a hostile environment, the population denominators are frequently unknown and must be estimated. Mortality rates are collected from several sources: camp grave watchers, a body collection system that recovers bodies of fleeing refugees along roadsides using trucks, tallies of bodies buried in mass graves, health agency reports of deaths in camp hospitals or clinics, home-health visitor tallies who interview families of deceased persons, and by camp health units that distribute free funeral shrouds to families.

Crude mortality rates (per 10,000 population) in recent conflicts range from 4.7 (Ethiopia, 1991), 10.1 (Somalia, 1980), 10.6 (Thailand, 1979), 14 (Rwanda, 1997), 23.4 (Somalia, 1984-5), to 34–35 (Zaire, 1994), but when these figures are corrected for age, the under-age-5 mortality rates reached 69.4 in the famine-affected internally displaced and refugee populations in Somalia in 1994. The highest rates, 20 to 200 times the baseline, are seen in orphaned or parentally separated minors. In addition, 97% of all deaths occur outside health facilities

Rapid influx of persons facilitates transmission of infectious diseases and hinders establishment of emergency services. Within a week of the arrival of refugees, the Goma camp became the third largest city in Zaire, with a population of more than 300,000. Camps of over 25,000 have difficulty maintaining water, sanitation, and proper shelter. Increased incidence of infectious disease outbreaks are reflected in the daily number of camp arrivals, the total camp size and density, and the magnitude and speed of spread of the outbreaks of cholera and other transmissible diseases.

Deaths primarily result from diarrheal disease and dehydration, malaria, measles, acute lower respiratory infections, and malnutrition. Despite ongoing violence, trauma deaths usually account for only 4–11% of mortality. Under difficult and hostile circumstances, Roberts found that a uniquely modified cluster survey study was the only epidemiological tool available to estimate *excess mortality* in Eastern Congo. His data suggested that an excess mortality rate of between 2.0–4.0 million occurred over a 4-month period with the return of hostilities and the breakdown of critical infrastructure. However, only 10% of the estimated mortality was due to intentional violence. The remainder of deaths was from the preventable cases of malaria, malnutrition, and diarrheal disease. Death rates are one of the most sensitive indicators of the success of emergency relief efforts, where the goal of a successful humanitarian program would be defined as reducing the crude mortality rate to less than one death per 10,000 persons.

The most common reasons for morbidity can be found in clinic data, where diarrhea (watery, bloody, and non-bloody), malaria, lower respiratory infections, meningitis (meningococcal meningitis epidemic threshold ≥15 cases per 100,000 per week), injuries, and malnutrition, are most prevalent. Standard case definitions are critical to reduce variability in reporting. Repeated epidemiological studies confirm that control of diarrheal diseases occur through provision of clean water and sanitation systems, distribution of soap, training of clinical staff in aggressive rehydration therapy, and increased basic health services..

The severe undernutrition rates in Somalia during 1992 ranged from 50 to 75% of the population studied. However, the WFH of less than 5% suggests that chronic malnutrition was not a major factor before hostilities began. This pattern is typical of most developing country model complex emergencies.

Individual psychological trauma is often difficult to assess unless a detailed ethnographic assessment is performed. Community-focused programs must take precedence over individually oriented therapies. War trauma correlated strongly with psychosocial and somatic symptoms. The diagnoses representative of the consequences of war is found in a study of Sri Lankan families, where somatization (41%), posttraumatic stress disorder (27%), anxiety disorder (26%), major depression (25%), hostility (19%), relationship problems (13%), alcohol and drug misuse (15%), and functional disability (18%) were evident in 64% of families studied.

Smoldering/Chronic Country Model

The Sudan, Liberia, and Haiti represent countries that have suffered widespread and prolonged conflict and war, chronic decay in infrastructure, environment, and economy, food shortages, famine, crop destruction, and severe poverty. A characteristic of a chronic, smoldering country model, especially the Sudan, is a combination of severe undernutrition and prolonged wasting (low WFH rates or Z-scores). In the Sudan, up to 40–44% of children were chronically undernourished, affecting not only the very young, but also adolescents and adults. Severe undernutrition rates are associated with *excess mortality* from complications of preventable illnesses such as diarrhea, measles, malaria, and acute respiratory tract infections (ARIs). Since 1955 and the onset of internal conflict, Sudanese children have suffered acute and chronic malnutrition, received little or no education, and have grown up in an environment of continued violence. These three countries require continual expatriate assistance for basic health care. Liberia suffered three wars beginning in 1993, with extensive looting and destruction of hospitals and clinics repeated during each conflict. The international relief organizations became the proxy healthcare system for Liberia, where less than 24 physicians remained in a population of over 3 million. Environmental decay (deforestation) and high-density population growth contribute to the inability of Haiti to attain sustainable development.

Developed Country Model

Iraq, the former Yugoslavia, and Chechnya represent complex emergencies in developed countries. They differ from the previous models in that civilians caught up in the violence are more likely to be well educated and resourceful urban dwellers who maintain relatively high standards of personal hygiene and suffer little from undernutrition. Early on, acute malnutrition is usually not a major problem. Those who remain in the urban areas during and following the war suffer mostly from the trauma of advanced weaponry, and worsening of chronic diseases secondary to lack of critical medication, supplies, and equipment. Widespread destruction of public health infrastructure results in an increased incidence of enteric diseases (a 5- to 16-fold increase in the incidence rates of diarrheal disease and hepatitis in the former Yugoslavia) from cross-contamination of water supplies with sewage. High pre-war vaccination rates and overcrowded refugee camps contributed to limited occurrence of preventable diseases. Epidemics, seen in the previous models, are rare.

In Bosnia-Herzegovina the CMR from trauma increased from 0.8 to 2.9 deaths per 1000 per month. In Sarajevo, trauma casualties accounted for 57% of all reported mortality. Ninety percent of civilians displaced by the violence were able to find space in private homes, and only 10% were housed in collective centers. As the war continued, household reserves of food diminished and undernutrition was seen in the elderly, children, and pregnant women. Psychological trauma from forced displacement, ethnic targeting, rapes, torture, and abuse is commonplace.

REFERENCES

Brennan RJ, Burkle FM. 2000. Disaster assessment for the public health sector, II: risk assessment and rapid health assessment. In *Disaster preparedness in schools of public health: a curriculum for a new century*, pp. 1–20. Ed L Landesman. Atlantla: Centers for Disease Control.

Burkholder BT, Toole MJ. 1995. Evolution of complex emergencies. *Lancet* **346**:1012–1015.

Burkle FM. 1999. Lessons learnt and future expectations of complex emergencies. *BMJ* **319:** 422–426.

Burkle FM. 2003. Evidence-based health assessment process in complex emergencies. In *Emergency relief operations*, pp. 55–79. Ed KM Cahill KM. New York: Fordham University Press.

CDC. 1991. International notes: public health consequences of acute displacement of Iraqi citizens—March–May 1991. *MMWR* **40**(26):443–446.

CDC. 1992. Famine-affected, refugee and displaced populations: recommendations for public health issues. *MMWR* **41**(RR–13):1-76.

CDC. 1993. Nutrition and mortality assessment—Southern Sudan, March 1993. *MMWR* **42**(16):304–308.

CDC. 1993. Status of public health—Bosnia and Herzegovina—August–September, 1993. *MMWR* **42**(50):979–982.

CDC. 1994. International notes health status of displaced persons following civil war—Burundi, December 1993–January 1994. *MMWR* **43**(38):701–703.

CDC. 1996. Morbidity and mortality surveillance in Rwandan refugees—Burundi and Zaire, 1994. *MMWR* **45**(5):104–107.

CDC. 1997. Landmine-related injuries, 1993–1996. *MMWR* **46**(31):724–726.

Reza A, Mercy JA, Krug K. 2004. Epidemiology of violent deaths in the world. National Center for Injury Prevention and Control, CDC. http://www.cdc.gov/nicipc/pub-res/epi_of_violence.htm. Accessed 2 July 2004.

The Refugee Experience. The nature of conflict and the implications for appropriate psychosocial responses: a brief epidemiology of war. http://earlybird.qeh.ox.ac.uk/rfgexp/rsp_tre/student/natconf/nat_02.htm. Accessed 2 July 2004.

Roberts L. 2002. Mortality in eastern Democratic Republic of Congo: results from eleven mortality surveys. *MMWR* **52**(20)469–471.

Somasundaram DJ, Sivayokan S. 1994. War trauma in a civilian population. *Br J Psychiatry* **165**(4):524–527.

Spiegel PB, Salama P. 2000. War and mortality in Kosovo, 1998–99: an epidemiological testimony. *Lancet* **357**(9257):2204–2209.

Toole MJ. 199. The role of rapid assessment. In *Humanitarian crises: the medical and public health response*, pp. 15–39. Ed J Leaning, SM Briggs, LC Chen LC. Cambridge: Harvard UP.

Toole MJ, Waldman RJ. 1990. Prevention of excess mortality in refugee and displaced populations in developing countries. *JAMA* **263**:3296–3302.

Toole MJ, Waldman RJ. 1997. The public health aspects of complex emergencies and refugee situations. *Annu Rev Public Health* **18**:283–312.

21 WEAPONS OF MASS DESTRUCTION

Liudvikas Jagminas, MD,* Robert E. Antosia, MD, MPH**

The twentieth century witnessed the creation and development of Weapons of Mass Destruction (WMDs): nuclear, chemical, and biological. While such weapons have been used in major wars, regional conflicts, and terrorism, this chapter will focus on the latter. WMDs all have the potential to create mass casualties, public panic, and enormous property destruction. They represent an existing and growing security and safety risk for all the citizens of the world.

Terrorists now have an improved ability to collect information, raise money, and disseminate rhetoric. Advanced information technology available through the Internet allows extremists to communicate widely and efficiently. Additionally, publicly available databases serve as repositories for technical information relating to weapons production. Another important factor is that WMDs, together with the materials and technology used to make them, are increasingly available. Many of these materials are widely available for legitimate commercial purposes. Moreover, the disintegration of the former Soviet Union has increased concerns about the protection, control, and accountability of WMDs, related materials and technologies, and the potential unemployment and proliferation of thousands of scientists skilled in the field. A final factor is the relative ease of manufacture and delivery of WMDs. Facilities required to produce radiological, biological, and chemical weapons are small and hard to detect, compared with those associated with nuclear weapons.

While each WMD is associated with unique challenges, diverse but effective strategies are needed to counter this threat. Such strategies include: the application of new technologies for detection and prevention; preventive measures such as strict export and border control, increased emphasis on intelligence collection and analysis; the strengthening of old alliances and the establishment of new partnerships; and increased compliance with existing international agreements to both prohibit their use and proliferation.

*Department of Emergency Medicine, Memorial Hospital, Pawtucket, Rhode Island

**Department of Emergency Medicine, Beth Israel Deaconess Medical Center, Harvard Medical School, Boston

Several international agreements have been developed to achieve this goal. The Nuclear Nonproliferation Treaty is a landmark multilateral UN treaty whose objectives include: prevention of the spread of nuclear weapons and weapons technology, promotion of cooperation in the peaceful uses of nuclear energy, and furtherance of the goal of achieving nuclear disarmament. This treaty has been ratified by 188 states, including the five nuclear-weapons states. Verification of compliance is performed by the International Atomic Energy Agency. Other important agreements include: the Comprehensive Nuclear Test Ban Treaty, which bans all nuclear explosions; the Chemical Weapons Convention, which provides a framework for the elimination of this entire category of WMD under universally applied international control and includes an intrusive verification system; and the Biological Weapons Convention, which supplements the 1925 Geneva Protocol, but lacks any formal verification program. The 1925 Geneva Protocol prohibits "the use in war of asphyxiating, poisonous or other gases, and of bacteriological methods of warfare." However, it did not prohibit the manufacture and stockpiling of these weapons.

Several recent events, including the events of September 11, 2001, have caused both the United States and the international community to focus on the issues of terrorism and WMDs with renewed intensity. In the United States many new initiatives have been implemented, including the recently created Department of Homeland Security. The proposed initiatives include such measures as: improved and modernized nonproliferation laws and law enforcement cooperation; restriction of the sale and transport of nuclear technologies and equipment; expanded efforts to secure and destroy nuclear weapons and materials; and strengthening the International Atomic Energy Agency to improve the organization's ability to monitor and enforce compliance with nuclear nonproliferation obligations.

In addition, the previously mentioned public health measures of preparedness, response, mitigation, and recovery apply to WMD-related disasters. Indications of the use of a BT agent include: severe clinical presentations in healthy individuals, multiple patients from a single location with similar presentations, multiple outbreaks in different locations, rapid increase in incidence curves, an unexpected number of quickly fatal cases, or any case of a category A infection. Biological agents are more complicated and delicate to handle than nerve agents, but because they are less conspicuous and relatively easy to release into society, they are potentially more lethal. Both chemical and biological weapons cause physical harm as well as psychological consequences. It is felt by some, due to the circumstances of nonproliferation since the end of the Cold War, that the proliferation of BT agents represents more of a threat as a WMD than nuclear weapons.

BIOLOGICS

Biological agents are the oldest of the Chemical, Biological and Radiological triad, and have been used in warfare for over 2,500 years. Biologic agents occur naturally in the environment, but many have been refined and can be made more virulent and resistant to therapy in weapons laboratories. Some bacterial toxins have also been developed for use as weapons. Most notable is botulism, which can produce death after being ingested or inhaled in minute quantities. The eradication of smallpox as declared by the WHO in 1980 is threatened by the possible weaponization of stockpiled virus and use against now unvaccinated populations.

From 15 to 25 countries are currently suspected of possessing biologic weapons where political and economic instability threatens control of stockpiles. Terrorist groups have included these weapons in their armamentarium. These agents are more deadly on a compound-per-weight basis than chemical agents. They can be produced at relatively low cost and delivered surreptitiously via a building's ventilation system, aerosolized via an aircraft or rooftop dispenser, or placed into the food or water system. Biologic agent attacks have a slower course than other WMD attacks, but have the greatest potential impact for casualties by weapon size and cost.

Despite differences between the various types of biological agents, these agents, bacteria, viruses, and toxins share some common characteristics. The primary route of infection or "portal of entry" is by inhalation (pulmonary). Since biological agents are nonvolatile (do not evaporate), they must be dispersed in aerosols as 1- to 5-micron sized particles (1/30,000 of the diameter of a hair), which can remain suspended in the air for hours (depending on weather conditions). If inhaled, the particles will deposit deep into the terminal air sacs of the lungs, causing disease.

Each of these agents can be easily disseminated from a point source, such as industrial sprayers modified to generate small particle size. The aerosol can also be delivered along a line from a moving generator in an airplane or boat traveling upwind from the intended target. Military weapons have been designed to deliver biologic agents in warheads and bomblets. The ideal biological agent can be delivered as an aerosol, has a high disease/infection ratio, maintains viability/infectivity in various environments, and has a vaccine or other prophylaxis to protect the attacker. Only a few of the thousands of known microorganisms meet these requirements.

Biological agents are affected by a number of weather conditions: the ultraviolet light from sunlight helps kill many biological agents, wind can spread the biological agents and may contribute to diluting their effectiveness, biologic agents vary in their sensitivity to extremes of heat and cold (most are resistant to freezing), and, depending on the degree of desiccation, biological agents may either suffer growth inhibition or be killed.

Based on the ease of transmission, severity of morbidity and mortality, and the likelihood of use, the Center for Disease Control and Prevention (CDC) has classified biological agents into three categories, termed A, B, and C. An overview is provided here, but details on these agents are provided in disease-specific chapters, including such appropriate treatment as antidotes, antibiotics, vaccines, and decontamination methods.

- **Category A**: highest priority, easily disseminated or transmitted person to person, high mortality, potential for major health impact, causes social disruption and public panic, needs special action/intervention from public health services:

  Anthrax
  Smallpox
  Tularemia
  Plague
  Botulism
  Viral hemorrhagic fevers (e.g., Ebola virus)

- **Category B**: second highest priority, moderately easily disseminated, moderate morbidity, low mortality, needs enhanced surveillance from CDC or other public health agency:

  Q fever (*Coxiella burnetii*)
  Brucellosis
  Ricin toxin
  Epsilon toxin of *Clostridium perfringens*
  Staphylococcus enterotoxin B (SEB)
  Glanders
  Melioidosis
  Psittacosis
  Typhus fever (*Rickettsia prowazekii*)
  Viral encephalitis (Venezuelan equine encephalitis, eastern equine encephalitis, western equine encephalitis)
  Food-borne threats (*Salmonella* species, *Escherichia coli* O157:H7, *Shigella*)
  Water-borne threats (*Vibrio cholerae, Cryptosporidium parvum*)

- **Category C**: third highest priority, easy to produce and available and easy to disseminate, possible mass dissemination in future, can be high morbidity and/or mortality:

  Hantavirus
  Yellow fever
  Multidrug-resistant TB
  Tick-borne viruses (hemorrhagic, encephalitis)
  Nipah virus

CHEMICALS

Chemical warfare agents are classified as nerve agents, vesicants, pulmonary agents, and cyanides, formerly classified as "blood agents" (weapons are also addressed in specific chapters in the text). These WMDs can be made from readily available material used in various industrial operations. Delivery systems may include commercial agricultural sprayers, crop dusters, and bombs or missiles.

Nerve agents such as Sarin, Soman, Tabun, and VX—all colorless organophosphate compounds that can be vaporized and inhaled—are significantly more toxic than the more common organophosphate insecticides. These toxic substances can produce incapacitation and death within seconds to minutes and may be absorbed through any surface of the body. Theoretically, only one gram of gas can kill thousands of people. However, nerve gas must be stored in pure and stable form, including the correct temperature, density, and stability, to have optimal effects. This was demonstrated in the March 1995 Tokyo subway sarin attack, which led to 7 deaths and approximately 2000 injuries.

Vesicants include Mustard and Lewisite, so-called "blister agents," which are rapidly absorbed by the skin and mucous membranes, leading to erythroderma followed by blistering.

Pulmonary agents include phosgene and chlorine gases, which rapidly dissipate and clinically produce irritation to the skin and respiratory system, leading to pulmonary edema. Treatment includes bronchodilators, supplemental oxygen, irrigation, removal of contaminated clothing, and avoidance of secondary transmission.

Cyanides include Hydrogen Cyanide and Cyanogen Chloride, which are vaporized and inhaled, leading to severe dyspnea, confusion, and rapid cardiopulmonary arrest. Immediate lifesaving treatment is required, but decontamination is generally not required due to the extremely volatile physical properties of these agents

NUCLEAR AGENTS

There are two types of radiological weapons that may be used by a terrorist. The first would be the use of a thermonuclear device. Development of such weapons requires such technical sophistication and effort that only national military programs have constructed such weapons, meaning the terrorist would have to steal such a weapon from a national arsenal. Significantly more easy to obtain are radioactive isotopes, which are used in industrial and medical sites and are occasionally lost or mishandled. Terrorists could also cause accidents involving nuclear power plants or vehicles used in the transportation of nuclear waste.

A Radiation Dispersal Device is more commonly known as the "dirty bomb." A "dirty bomb" combines a conventional explosive, such as dynamite, with radioactive material. The conventional explosive itself would cause more casualties than the radioactive material. At the levels created by most probable sources, not enough radiation would be present in a dirty bomb to kill people or cause severe illness. However, the detection of radiation after an overt terrorist attack would lead to the development of panic and probably require decontamination or evacuation of the affected urban area with considerable disruption. A second use would be to hide a strong radiation source in a public place, exposing persons to radiation until it was detected. For further details, please chapter 40 on "Nuclear Detonation/Ionizing Radiation Exposure."

RESOURCES

National Response Center, DOJ: (800) 424-8802, or http://www.fema.gov.
CDC Bioterrorism Response Center: (770) 488-7100, or http://www.bt.cdc.gov.
Radiation Emergency Assistance Center: Training Site (REACTS) (432) 481-1000.
Homeland Security Advisory System: http://www.homelandsecurity.gov.

REFERENCES

Darling RG, Catlett CL, Huebner KD, Jarrett DG. 2002. Threats in bioterrorism. I: CDC category A agents. *Emerg Med Clin North Am* **20**:273–309.

Hogan DE, Burstein JL. 2002. *Disaster medicine*. Philadelphia: Lippincott Williams and Wilkins.

National strategies to combat weapons of mass destruction. 2002. The White House. Washington, DC: Government Printing Office.

22 ANTHRAX

John D. Cahill, MD*

Anthrax is primarily a disease of herbivorous mammals with a worldwide distribution. Humans become infected by coming into contact with infected animals and as an occupational exposure. Globally, up to 100,000 new cases occur per annum. Clinically, three forms of the disease are recognized: cutaneous, inhalational, and gastrointestinal. Anthrax has gained much attention for its potential use as a biological weapon. *Bacillus anthracis* is an encapsulated Gram-positive, nonmotile, aerobic, spore-forming bacterial rod with a spore size of approximately 1 x 2 μm.

CUTANEOUS ANTHRAX

This is the most common form of anthrax seen in the natural setting. Initial infection occurs when an individual comes into contact with an infected animal or an animal product, or is involved in a bioterrorism event. The incubation period is 3 to 7 days, and lesions develop on exposed skin surfaces (hands, face, neck). The lesion initially forms as a papule, progresses through a vesicular stage, and evolves into a black depressed necrotic ulcer (eschar), which is painless. Edema, redness, and/or necrosis without ulceration may occur. Regional lymphadenopathy may be appreciated. The lesions resolve slowly over a 2- to 6-week period of time. If untreated, infection may become systemic. Untreated, mortality approaches 25%; treated, this decreases to 1%. The differential diagnosis includes ulceroglandular tularemia, scrub typhus, orf, plague, and strep or staph infections of the skin.

INHALATIONAL

Occurs with direct inhalation of spores, often from animal hides or as a potential biological weapon. The incubation period is often only several days, though it can be

*Department of Emergency Medicine and Division of Infectious Diseases, St. Luke's/Roosevelt Hospital Center, New York

longer. After inhalation, spores are engulfed by macrophages and have a predilection for the mediastinal and peribronchial lymph nodes. During this time a brief prodromal viral-like illness develops: fever, malaise, and an unproductive cough. Clinically, this rapidly leads to dyspnea and hypoxia, which may lead to respiratory failure. Hemorrhagic mediastinitis, thoracic hemorrhagic lymphadenitis, and pleural effusions may develop. Hematogenous spread and meningitis can also be seen. Even when treated, mortality rates approach 95%. Pathologically, anthrax does not cause a classic bronchopneumonia appearance. On radiographic studies of the thorax, infiltrates are not typical; however, a widened mediastinum and pleural effusions can often be appreciated. Clinically, multiple patients presenting with pneumonia and no obvious infiltrate with mediastinal widening and pleural effusions should be considered to have inhalational anthrax. Pneumonic tularemia can also present in a similar fashion.

GASTROINTESTINAL

This variant is uncommon and primarily seen in Africa when an individual eats infected undercooked meat. Vomiting, hematemesis, abdominal pain, and diarrhea may develop. This may be followed by signs of fever and sepsis. Sometimes oropharyngeal ulcers and cervical lymphadenopathy can occur. Mortality rates can be quite significant and approach 50%.

DIAGNOSIS

Clinically, the diagnosis can be suggested, but laboratory confirmation is of utmost importance, particularly in the context of a bioterrorism event. Body fluids (blood and CSF) and skin lesions can be Gram stained, looking for encapsulated, broad, Gram-positive bacilli. It may also be cultured on sheep's blood agar cultures.

Most department of health laboratories would confirm the diagnosis with the growth of virulent strains on nutrient agar in the presence of 5% carbon dioxide (or other basal mediums supplemented with 0.8% sodium bicarbonate), which produces heavily encapsulated bacilli that may be visualized with India-ink staining. Additional criteria for confirmation include susceptibility to lysis by gamma phage or direct fluorescence-antibody staining of cell-wall polysaccharide antigen. Rapid screening assays for use directly on clinical specimens (including nasal swabs) and environmental samples are investigative tools; they include nucleic acid signatures and antigen detection (enzyme-linked immunosorbent assay [ELISA] for protective antigen and capsule).

Nasal-swab culture to determine whether there may have been inhalational exposure to *B. anthracis* is an investigative tool and is not known to accurately predict the risk of subsequent clinical illness. Its use should be limited to public health teams at present.

Serologic testing is useful only retrospectively and requires specimens from the acute and convalescent phases of illness for comparison.

TREATMENT

Stable Cutaneous Anthrax or When Switching to Oral Treatment

Adults

Ciprofloxacin 500 mg po BID or Doxycycline 100 mg po BID

Children

Ciprofloxacin 10-15 mg/kg po every 12 hours
or
Doxycycline
>8 yr and >45 kg, 100 mg po BID
>8 yr and <45 kg, 2.2 mg/kg po BID
<8 yr 2.2 mg/kg po BID

Pregnant Women

Same treatment as nonpregnant. Severe Cutaneous Anthrax infection should be treated with intravenous antimicrobials, follow guidelines for inhalational treatment

Inhalational

Adults

Ciprofloxacin 400 mg IV BID or Doxycycline 100 mg IV BID
Plus the addition of one or two antimicrobials: rifampin, vancomycin, penicillin, ampicillin, chloramphenicol, imipenem, clindamycin, or clarithromycin.

Children

Ciprofloxacin 10-15 mg/kg IV every 12 hours
or
Doxycycline
>8 yr and >45 kg, 100 mg IV BID
>8 yr and <45 kg, 2.2 mg/kg IV BID
<8 yr 2.2 mg/kg IV BID

Pregnant Women

Same treatment as nonpregnant. For all infected individuals treatment is 60 days, and switch to oral treatment when stable.

CHEMOPROPHYLAXIS

Although experience using chemoprophylactic agents for potential anthrax exposure is limited, it may be indicated in certain individuals. Those with clear exposure to a release should be started initially on Ciprofloxacin 500 mg po BID for sixty days. Once sensitivities are known, an alternative antibiotic such as Doxycycline or Amoxicillin may be used.

PREVENTION

A vaccine is available against anthrax and in the past was only indicated for high-risk groups: certain military forces, veterinarians, wool mill workers, livestock handlers, and laboratory workers. The vaccine consists of a noninfectious sterile culture filtrate of an attenuated strain of *B. anthracis* adsorbed to an aluminum hydroxide adjuvant. It is administered subcutaneously on days 0, 14, and 28, and then at 6, 12, and 18 months. An annual booster is necessary to continue immunity.

RESOURCES

http://www.bt.cdc.gov
http://www.who.int/topics/anthrax/en/
http://www.vetmed.lsu.edu/whocc/mp_world.htm

REFERENCES

Inglesby TV, O'Toole T, Henderson DA, Bartlett JG, Ascher MS, Eitzen E, Friedlander AM, Gerberding J, Hauer J, Hughes J, McDade J, Osterholm MT, Parker G, Perl TM, Russell PK, Tonat K; Working Group on Civilian Biodefense. 2002. Anthrax as a biological weapon: updated recommendations for management. *JAMA* **287**:2236–2252.

Update: investigation of bioterrorism-related anthrax and interim guidelines for exposure management and antimicrobial therapy, October 2001. *MMWR* **50**(42);909–919.

Swartz MN. 2001. Current concepts: recognition and management of anthrax: an update. *New Engl J Med* **345**:1621–1626.

23 SMALLPOX

Fred P. Harchelroad, Jr., MD*

OVERVIEW

Smallpox (variola) had affected social and political agendas throughout the centuries in Europe and Asia until Edward Jenner developed a vaccine in 1796. Smallpox decimated the native American population following European exploration in the 1600s. October 26, 1977 marked the date of the last naturally occurring smallpox infection. Smallpox was officially declared eradicated by the World Health Organization in 1980. A case of confirmed smallpox seen today should be considered a bioterrorism event until proven otherwise.

ETIOLOGY

Variola is a member of the Orthopoxvirus genus of which cowpox, monkey pox, orf, and molluscum contagiosum are also members. Pox viruses are the only viruses that can replicate in cell cytoplasm without the need of a nucleus.

INCIDENCE AND PREVALENCE

Since the last documented case of wild smallpox in 1977, only two deaths from smallpox have been reported. These occurred in 1978 secondary to laboratory exposure. There is no prevalence to the disease based on race, gender, or age. Approximately 30% of contacts will become infected with classic smallpox.

PATHOGENESIS

The variola virus is acquired from inhalation, after which replicates in the epithelial cells of the respiratory tract. Massive asymptomatic viremia ensues, resulting in focal infection of skin, intestines, lung, kidneys, and brain. Rapid multiplication in

*Department of Emergency Medicine, Drexel University College of Medicine, Pittsburgh

skin epithelial cells allows the rash to be noticed progressing into pustules about 14 days after inoculation. Pustule formation is a cell mediated immune response.

PRESENTATION

Incubation Period/Time of Onset

The incubation period ranges from 7 to 17 days. Asymptomatic viremia occurs 72 to 96 hours after infection.

Signs and Symptoms

A second viremia results in fever, myalgias, headache, rigors, and backache. Rigors and vomiting are present in more than 50% of patients, and delirium in 15%. Ten percent of patients have a fleeting erythetamous exanthem before the typical cutaneous manifestations. Initial lesions often begin around the oral mucosa, spreading to the face, then forearms, hands, and eventually to the trunk and lower limbs. Lesions favor the ventral surfaces, sparing the axilla, palms, and soles.

DIAGNOSIS

Laboratory

A viral swab of the pharynx may isolate the infection, but this should only be performed in a bio-safety level IV laboratory. Currently these include the CDC in Atlanta, Georgia, and the US Army Medical Research Institute of Infectious Diseases in Fort Dietrich, Maryland.

Physical

The oral mucosa is affected first, then the face, forearms, and hands, and finally the trunk and lower limbs. Lesions favor ventral surfaces and progress from macule to papule to vesicle, to umbilicated papule, and finally to crusted lesions. The exanthem of varicella is synchronous, unlike that of varicella. The rash settles centrifugally, sparing the axilla, palms, and soles.

DIFFERENTIAL DIAGNOSIS

Monkey pox
Chicken pox
Disseminated herpes zoster
Disseminated herpes simplex
Secondary syphilis
Hand, foot, mouth disease
Erythema multiforme
Bullous pemphigoid
Hemorrhagic varicella
Ehrlichiosis

TREATMENT

Immediate contact and droplet isolation and quarantine of the patient.

Immediate notification of local health authorities.

Vaccinia (smallpox) vaccine and vaccinia immune globulin (VIG) are available only through the CDC and state health agencies.

There are no FDA-approved drugs for smallpox treatment; nevertheless, in-vitro studies have demonstrated some efficacy of Cidofovir in a dose of 5 mg per kg intravenously over 1 hour.

PROGNOSIS

Thirty percent of susceptible contacts become infected. Pregnant women have a higher morbidity: 27% in vaccinated patients and 61% in unvaccinated pregnant patients with classic smallpox; compared to 6% morbidity of vaccinated, and 35% morbidity of unvaccinated patients. Four types of variola presentations exist: classic, hemorrhagic, malignant, and modified. The hemorrhagic variety has a higher mortality than classic. The malignant or flat form of variola occurs about 6% of the time and the mortality rate approaches 100%. The modified form of smallpox consists of those previously vaccinated individuals, and death is not expected.

RESOURCES

www.emedicine.com.
www.bt.cdc.gov/agent/smallpox/index.asp
www.usamridd.army.mil

REFERENCES

Henderson DA, Inglesby TV, Bartlett JG, Ascher MS, Eitzen E, Jahrling PB, Hauer J, Layton M, McDade J, Osterholm MT, O'Toole T, Parker G, Perl T, Russell PK, Tonat K. 1999. Smallpox as a biological weapon: medical and public health management. *JAMA* **281**(22):2127–2137.

24 PLAGUE

Mara Aloi, MD*

OVERVIEW

Yersinia pestis, the Gram-negative bacillus responsible for the plague, has killed nearly 200 million humans throughout history. It is endemic on all continents except Australia and Antarctica. There have been three pandemics thus far, the best known being the epidemic that afflicted Western Europe in the 14th–18th centuries when the plague became known as the Black Death and wiped out nearly a third of the affected population. Globally, approximately 2000 cases of human plague are reported to the World Health Organization annually. *Y. pestis*, a Category A agent of bioterrorism, is an attractive agent for bioterrorist activities because of its widespread availability, high fatality rate, and potential for secondary spread resulting in epidemics. It may have been the first bacteriologic agent used in warfare. Historical accounts of Tartar soldiers catapulting plague-infected corpses over the city walls of Kaffe (Crimea) date back to 1346. Plague-infected fleas were disseminated over China to cause outbreaks of the disease during World War II. The United States and Soviet biological weapons programs reportedly developed mechanisms to aerosolize *Y. pestis* in the 1950s and 1960s, and this technology may still be available today. Use is limited, however, by its fastidious nature and the fact that it is an obligate parasite. The organism is susceptible to destruction by heat, drying, and ultraviolet radiation and, therefore, has a very short lifespan of 1 hour outside a host. Plague is universally infectious to humans. Those at greatest risk of infection live in endemic areas, usually with low standards of housing and hygiene that predispose to a higher rodent and flea populations.

*Department of Emergency Medicine, Drexel University College of Medicine, Pittsburgh

PATHOGENESIS

Approximately 30 species of fleas worldwide serve as major vectors for transmission of *Y. pestis*. Wild animal reservoirs include cats, coyotes, prairie dogs, squirrels, marmots, and other small rodents. Fleas ingest organisms during a blood meal from one of these host mammals. The organism then multiplies in the flea gut and expresses a coagulase, which results in clotting of ingested blood. Gut motility is effectively blocked, and at subsequent feedings infectious blood is regurgitated into a new host. In most cases, the rodent hosts are relatively resistant, but during epizootic plague depopulation of these animals may occur. In this situation, fleas are forced to look for alternative hosts, posing a serious health concern to humans. Therefore, human outbreaks are usually preceded by epizootic outbreaks.

PRESENTATION

The clinical course of plague varies depending on the route of exposure.

Bubonic Plague

The most common form, bubonic plague is acquired through the bite of an infected flea. Organisms spread to regional lymph nodes, which become swollen and exquisitely tender. These lesions, known as buboes, develop within 1–8 days, and their location is usually proximal to the site of inoculation. They are non-fluctuant, warm, and surrounded by considerable edema without associated lymphangitis. A flu-like syndrome of fevers, myalgias, headache, and malaise precedes the development of buboes by 24 hours. Gastrointestinal symptoms such as diarrhea, nausea, and vomiting are also frequent manifestations. The disease can progress to septicemia if not treated. Between 5 and 15% of cases are complicated by secondary plague pneumonia, which can result in direct person-to-person transmission of highly virulent organisms.

Septicemic Plague

This results in *Y. pestis* bacteremia and endotoxemia with a lack of pneumonia or characteristic buboes. It may result from handling or eating contaminated animals or as a complication of bubonic plague. The incubation period is 1–4 days. The clinical course is similar to sepsis with other Gram-negative organisms, and complications include disseminated intravascular coagulopathy, meningitis, and multi-organ system failure. Plague received its nickname, "black death," because of the appearance of massive ecchymoses and acral necrosis with gangrene of distal extremities seen with septicemic plague.

Pneumonic Plague

The pneumonic variety results from inhalation of live organisms. The infectious dose needed to cause this form is estimated to be only 100–500 organisms. After an incubation period of 1–3 days, an initial flu-like illness manifesting with high fevers, chills, and malaise is seen, rapidly followed by development of respiratory symptoms, characteristically a cough productive of watery, blood-tinged sputum. Gastrointestinal symptoms such as diarrhea, vomiting, and abdominal pain are prominent and may lead to initial misdiagnosis. Buboes are rarely seen and, when present, are cervical in location. Secondary pneumonic plague results from seeding of the lungs in patients with bubonic or septicemic forms of the disease.

Person–person transmission of bubonic and septicemic plague does not occur, but pneumonic plague is highly contagious. A World Health Organization committee in 1970 estimated that 50 kg of aerosolized *Y. pestis* over an area with a population of 5 million could result in 36,000 deaths and up to 100,000 hospitalizations. An intentional dissemination of pneumonic plague should be suspected if large numbers of previously healthy people present with severe respiratory symptoms and hemoptysis and have a fulminant course with high mortality.

Other Variants

Meningeal plague is an uncommon manifestation of the disease. It usually results from inadequate treatment of the bubonic form. Pharyngeal plague presents with sore throat, fever, and cervical lymphadenitis. It may be indistinguishable from other infectious causes of pharyngitis. Cervical buboes are sometimes present.

DIAGNOSIS

Clinicians should start treatment based on clinical suspicion if the diagnosis is going to be delayed for any reason. Immediate notification of local or state health laboratory is recommended so that confirmatory testing, not widely available, can be arranged.

Rapid Screening Tests

- Peripheral blood smears and sputum exam: bipolar or "safety pin" morphology seen on Gram's, Wayson's, or Wright-Giemsa stain.
- Direct fluorescent antibody staining of the capsular antigen of *Y. pestis*. Only expressed at 37°C. False negative results possible if specimen refrigerated for more than 30 hours or incubated at cooler temperatures.
- Antigen dipstick test: detects *Y. pestis* F1 capsular antigen; less expensive and faster results than currently available techniques. May be available soon.

Confirmatory Tests

- Culture of blood, sputum, bubo aspiration, and CSF specimens on blood agar are positive by 48 hours (colonies described as "hammered metal" in appearance).
- Serology: Antibodies against *Y. pestis* F1 antigen are present by the end of the 1st week of illness. A titer of >1:10 is evidence of presumptive infection in those not previously infected or vaccinated. A >1:28 titer is required for confirmation.
- ELISA

Adjunctive Tests

- Complete blood count will show a leukocytosis with neutrophil predominance.
- Liver enzyme levels: elevated.
- Coagulation studies: evidence of coagulopathy.
- Chest x-ray: usually unilateral infiltrate progressing to patchy diffuse pattern seen with primary pneumonic plague. Bilateral process seen initially if secondary form.

Do not incise and drain buboes because of the significant risk of aerosolization of live organisms. Needle aspiration is preferred (use a 20-gauge needle on a 10-ml syringe containing 1–2 ml sterile saline to infuse the bubo).

DIFFERENTIAL DIAGNOSIS

Bubonic Plague

- Streptococcal or Staphylococcal adenitis
- Tularemia
- Cat scratch disease

Septicemic Plague

- Sepsis from other gram-negative organisms

Pneumonic Plague

- Severe community-acquired pneumonia
- Tularemia
- Hantavirus
- Inhalational anthrax

TREATMENT

In a contained casualty situation, parenteral antimicrobial therapy is recommended. In a mass casualty situation, where large numbers of patients present for treatment and threaten to overwhelm medical resources, oral therapy may be recommended as an alternative to parenteral therapy.

Adults

- Streptomycin 1 gram IM BID for 10-14 days
- Gentamicin 5 mg/kg IM or IV once daily for 10–14 days or 2 mg/kg loading dose followed by 1.7 mg/kg TID
- Doxycycline 200 mg IV daily OR 100 mg IV BID until clinically improved then 100 mg PO BID for total of 10–14 days
- Ciprofloxacin 400 mg IV BID until clinically improved; then 750 mg PO BID for total of 10–14 days
- Chloramphenicol 25 mg/kg IV QID for 10 days (for plague meningitis)

Children

- Streptomycin 15 mg/kg IM BID for 10 days (maximum 2 g daily)
- Gentamicin 2.5 mg/kg IM or IV TID for 10 days
- Doxycycline 2.2 mg/kg PO or IV BID for 10 days (use for weight <45 kg) (maximum daily dose 200 mg)

Mass Casualty Situation

- Doxycycline 100 mg PO BID for 10 days (2.2 mg/kg PO BID for children <45 kg)
- Ciprofloxacin 500 mg PO BID for 10 days(20 mg/kg PO BID for children)
- Chloramphenicol 25 mg/kg PO QID for 10 days

Chemoprophylaxis

- Doxycycline 100 mg PO BID for 7 days or duration of exposure (use pediatric treatment dose for children)
- Ciprofloxacin 500 mg PO BID for 7 days
- Tetracycline 500 mg PO QID for 7 days

PROGNOSIS

The mortality rate of untreated bubonic plague is 40–60%. While bubonic plague is fairly amenable to treatment, the mortality rate of septicemic plague is still 30–50% even with optimum antimicrobial therapy. Pneumonic plague has a high mortality rate of nearly 100% if treatment is not started within 24 hours of symptom onset.

PREVENTION

An effective plague vaccine is not currently available for widespread use. Subunit vaccines using the F1 and V antigens of *Y. pestis* are in development. In areas of epidemics broad use of insecticides should precede rodenticidal activities. If not, the death of the preferred rodent host will force infected fleas to seek alternative hosts, thereby potentially worsening a human epidemic. Infected patients should be in isolation until completion of at least 2 days of antibiotics. Medical personnel should practice barrier and droplet precautions. Post-exposure antimicrobials should be administered to the following:

- Those having unprotected direct contact, defined as contact within 6 feet, with persons with untreated pneumonic plague
- Those with known aerosol exposure (i.e. biological warfare)
- In an epidemic setting, any person developing a fever >38.5°C or new cough, or infants developing tachypnea

RESOURCES

www.cdc.gov/ncidod/dvbid/plague/index.htm

www.bt.cdc.gov/agent/plague/trainingmodule
www.who.int/inf-fs/en/fact267.html
www.idsociety.org/bt/ToC.htm
www.hopkins-biodeefense.org/pages/agents/tocplague.html

REFERENCES

Chanteau S, Rahalison L, Ralafiarosa L, Foulon J, Ratsitorahina M, Ratsifasoamanana L, Carniel E, Nato F. 2003. Development and testing of a rapid diagnostic test for bubonic and pneumonic plague. *Lancet* **361**(9353):211–216.

Darling RG, Catlett CL, Huebner KD, Jarrett DG. 2002. Threats in bioterrorism I: CDC category a agents. *Emerg Med Clin North Am* **20**(2):273–309.

Inglesby TV, Dennis DT, Henderson DA, Bartlett JG, Ascher MS, Eitzen E, Fine AD, Friedlander AM, Hauer J, Koerner JF, Layton M, McDade J, Osterholm MT, O'Toole T, Parker G, Perl TM, Russell PK, Schoch-Spana M, Tonat K. 2000. Plague as a biological weapon: medical and public health management. *JAMA* **283**(17):2281–2290.

Loiez C, Herwegh S, Wallet F, Armand S, Guinet F, Courcol RJ. 2003. Detection of *Yersinia pestis* in sputum by real-time PCR. *J Clin Microbiol* **41**(10):4873–4875.

Rollins SE, Rollins SM, Ryan ET. 2003. *Yersinia pestis* and the plague. *Am J Clin Pathol* **119**(suppl):S78–S85.

Titball RW, Williamson ED. 2003. Second- and third-generation plague vaccines. *Adv Exp Med Biol* 529:397–406.

25

TULAREMIA

Tracy H. Zivin-Tutela, MD*

OVERVIEW

Historical Significance

Hare-associated illness compatible with tularemia has been known in Japan since 1818, and perhaps the earliest written description of a patient with unmistakable tularemia was provided by Homma-Soken in 1837. *Francisella tularensis* was incorporated as a weapon in the biological warfare program of the United States during the decades of the 1950s and 1960s.

Etiology

Tularemia is caused by *Francisella tularensis* and is one of the most infectious bacteria known. Inoculation or inhalation with only 10 organisms can cause disease! It is a small, nonmotile, aerobic, Gram-negative coccobacillus. It can survive for several weeks at low temperatures in water, moist soil, hay, straw and decaying carcasses.

Incidence and Prevalence

The worldwide incidence of naturally occurring tularemia is not known. Tularemia can cause widespread disease in animals. Prior to the 1950s several thousand human cases were reported yearly; however, only about 200 cases per year are currently reported in the United States. It is likely that this disease is underrecognized and underreported. Tularemia occurs throughout North America, Europe, and Asia. In the United States, most human cases have been reported during June–September in the south-central and western states. All states have reported disease except Hawaii.

*Division of Infectious Diseases, St. Luke's/Roosevelt Hospital Center, New York

Risk Factors

Nearly all cases of tularemia occur in rural areas. *F. tularensis* can be recovered from contaminated water, soil, and vegetation. Natural reservoirs for infection include: voles, mice, water rats, squirrels, rabbits, and hares. These animals acquire infection through various bites, e.g., tick, fly, and mosquito. Humans can become infected by inhaling bacteria from laboratory accidents, bites by arthropods, handling infectious animals, or direct contact, or ingestion of food, water, or soil.

PATHOGENESIS

Pathogenesis to humans occurs through the skin, mucous membranes, gastrointestinal tract, and lungs. Human-to-human transmission does not occur. Once infected, the major affected areas are the lymph nodes, lungs, pleura, spleen, liver, and kidneys.

PRESENTATION

Incubation Period

The onset of symptoms usually occurs 3 to 5 days after bacterial exposure, but it has been reported to take as long as 14 days.

Signs and Symptoms

The signs and symptoms depend on the exposure to *F. tularensis*. If inoculation is by inhalation, symptoms include abrupt fever, headache, chills, rigors, body aches (especially lower back), joint pain, dry cough, and progressive weakness. If exposure to tularemia occurs by direct contact, bite, or ingestion, possible symptoms include conjunctivitis, skin or mouth ulcer, swollen and painful lymph nodes, pharyngitis, nausea, vomiting, or diarrhea. Pneumonia can develop, and symptoms include a dry or slightly productive cough, hemoptysis, substernal chest pain, dyspnea, tachypnea, and respiratory failure.

DIAGNOSIS

Laboratory

Growth of *F. tularensis* in culture is the definitive diagnostic test. The organism can be grown from pharyngeal washings, sputum and gastric aspirates. Direct examination using Gram stain, direct fluorescent antibody, or immunohistochemical stains can identify *F. tularensis*. A designated reference laboratory in the National Public Health Laboratory Network can use a fluorescent-labeled antibody as a rapid diagnostic procedure. These results can be available within a few hours, though this rapid diagnostic test is not widely available. Blood cultures only rarely reveal the organism.

DIFFERENTIAL DIAGNOSIS

Tularemia could be indistinguishable from Q-fever if it was attained by mild inhalation of bacteria. Plague and anthrax would cause a faster progression of illness and a higher case fatality rate than tularemia.

TREATMENT

Antibiotics for treating tularemia in a bioterrorist event are included in the national pharmaceutical stockpile maintained by the Centers for Disease Control.

Adults: Streptomycin 1 g IM twice daily or Gentamicin 5 mg/kg IM/IV daily is recommended. Alternative choices include Doxycycline 100 mg IV twice daily or Chloramphenicol 15 mg/kg IV four times daily or Ciprofloxacin 400 mg IV twice daily.

Children: Streptomycin 15 mg/kg IM twice daily (not to exceed 2 g/d) or Gentamicin 2.5 mg/kg IM/IV three times daily. Alternative choices include Doxycycline 100 mg IV twice daily if greater than 45 kg, 2.2 mg/kg IV twice daily if less than 45 kg, or Chloramphenicol 15 mg/kg IV four times daily, or Ciprofloxacin 15 mg/kg IV twice daily (not to exceed 1 g/d).

Pregnant women: Gentamicin 5 mg/kg IM/IV once daily or Streptomycin 1 g IM twice daily is recommended. Alternative choices include Doxycycline 100 mg IV twice daily or Ciprofloxacin 400 mg IV twice daily.

Treatment with Streptomycin, Gentamicin, or Ciprofloxacin should be continued for 10 days. Treatment with Doxycycline or Chloramphenicol should be continued for 14–21 days to prevent relapse. Treatment with parenteral antibiotics can be switched to oral equivalents once clinically indicated. Since drug-resistant organisms may be utilized in a bioterrorist attack, antimicrobial susceptibility testing should be conducted quickly and treatments altered accordingly.

PROGNOSIS

If tularemia is treated with appropriate antibiotics, the mortality rate is under 10%; if not treated, over 30%. According to the Centers for Disease Control and Prevention (CDC): "If 100,000 people were exposed to a 'tularemic cloud,' 82,500 cases (an 82.5% attack rate) with 6188 deaths (6.2% death rate) would be expected. The medical costs of tularemia from this bioterrorist attack would be between $456 million and $561.8 million."

PREVENTION

Post-exposure prophylaxis for a bioterrorist attack in which individuals have not become ill should include either Doxycycline or Ciprofloxacin orally for 14 days. If an attack is discovered after illness has occurred, persons exposed with unexplained fever or flu-like symptoms should begin treatment with the above antibiotics. Close contacts do not need post-exposure prophylaxis because person-to-person transmission does not occur.

In the United States, a live attenuated vaccine has been used to protect laboratory workers but it is not currently available. This vaccine is currently under review by the Food and Drug Administration.

SPECIAL CONSIDERATIONS

A small number (10 to 50) of organisms can cause disease. If *F. tularensis* is used in the form of a biological weapon, it would likely be in airborne form. Release of the organism in a populated area would result in an abrupt, large number of acute, nonspecific febrile illnesses beginning several days after exposure, with a significant proportion of cases occurring in the following weeks.

RESOURCES

Centers for Disease Control, www.bt.cdc.gov/agent/tularemia; CDC hotline: (888) 246-2675
World Health Organization, Department of Communicable Disease Surveillance and Response, www.who.int

REFERENCES

Dennis DT, Inglesby TV, Henderson DA, Bartlett JG, Ascher MS, Eitzen E, Fine AD, Friedlander AM, Hauer J, Layton M, Lillibridge SR, McDade JE, Osterholm MT, O'Toole T, Parker G, Perl TM, Russell PK, Tonat K. 2001. Tularemia as a biological weapon: medical and public health management. *JAMA* **285**:2763–2773.

Franz DR, Jahrling PB, McClain DJ, Hoover DL, Byrne WR, Pavlin JA, Christopher GW, Cieslak TJ, Friedlander AM, Eitzen EM Jr. 1997. Clinical recognition and management of patients exposed to biological warfare agents. *JAMA* **278**:339–411.

Kaufmann AF, Meltzer MI, Schmid GP. 1997. The economic impact of a bioterrorist attack: are prevention and postattack intervention programs justifiable? *Emerg Infect Dis* **3**:83–94.

26 VIRAL HEMORRHAGIC FEVERS

Amesh Adalja, MD*

A viral hemorrhagic fever is best described as an acute febrile illness characterized by malaise, prostration, generalized signs of increased vascular permeability, and abnormalities of circulatory regulation.

MICROBIOLOGY/EPIDEMIOLOGY

Viral hemorrhagic fevers consist of viruses from four families: Bunyaviridae, Arenaviridae, Flaviviridae, and Filoviridae. Each viral family has its own unique epidemiology and clinical manifestations.

Each of the VHFs share certain microbiological characteristics. They are all negative-stranded RNA-enveloped viruses. Most VHF infections are a zoonosis often depending on vector transmission. Human infection can also occur from the excretions of infected animals or humans. Natural hosts and reservoirs range from arthropod insects to rodents to primates. Except for Dengue Fever, humans are not the natural host of these viruses. The natural host has still not been elucidated for all the VHFs.

The VHFs' striking pathology and high case fatality rate make them candidates for weaponization, and indeed evidence is present indicating they have been explored for use in this capacity.

Bunyaviruses

The chief VHFs that belong to the Bunyaviridae family are: Crimean-Congo Hemorrhagic Fever (CCHF), Hantavirus, and Rift Valley Fever. CCHF is transmitted by the bite of a tick, Hantavirus through aerosolization and exposure to rodent urine,

*Departments of Emergency Medicine and Internal Medicine, Allegheny General Hospital, Pittsburgh

and the Africa-indigenous Rift Valley Fever via the mosquito or aerosolization. RVF is also known to infect livestock, and contact with slaughtered animals may be another mode of infection. CCHF and Hantaviruses have a wide geographic range: CCHF is found in Africa, Asia, and Europe, while Hantaviruses are thought to have worldwide distribution.

Arenaviruses

Arenaviruses are all associated with a rodent reservoir. The viruses of note in this family include: Lassa virus, Junin (Argentine Hemorrhagic Fever), Machupo (Bolivian Hemorrhagic Fever), Sabia (Brazilian Hemorrhagic Fever), and Guanarito (Venezuelan Hemorrhagic Fever). Transmission is via aerosolization or exposure to rodent urine.

Lassa Fever is characteristically found in West Africa, while the other members of this family congregate in their respective South American namesake countries.

Flaviviruses

The family Flaviviridae contains the mosquito-borne Yellow Fever and Dengue Fever/Hemorrhagic Fever viruses as well as the tick-borne Kyasanur Forest virus and the Omsk Hemorrhagic Fever virus. Yellow Fever is found in tropical Africa and South America; Dengue in the Americas, Asia, and Africa; Kyasanur Forest virus in India; and Omsk Hemorrhagic Fever in the former Soviet bloc.

Filoviruses

Both the Marburg virus and the Ebola virus belong to the family Filoviridae. There are no identifiable vectors or reservoir for this family of virus. Outbreaks of these viruses have been limited to Africa.

CLINICAL FEATURES

After an incubation period that can range from a minimum 2 days (RVF) to a maximum of 35 days (Hantaviruses), a nonspecific clinical picture of fever, myalgia, and prostration emerges. Subsequently, devolution to florid shock and multi-system organ failure may occur. A petechial rash can also be a leading clue to the presence of a VHF. Hepatic inflammation/dysfunction can be seen as well.

Important distinguishing features can be used to delineate the various hemorrhagic fever viruses. The vascular bed is a major target for all these viruses.

Arenaviruses

After an incubation period of 3 to 16 days, an illness with an insidious onset ensures. Fever, chills, malaise, and retroocular pain herald the initial symptoms. Lassa is known to cause a purulent pharyngitis and aphthous ulcers. Conjunctivitis and exanthem of the face, upper thorax, and neck may be seen. However, hepatosplenomegaly is not observed. After a week of illness, symptom severity intensifies, culminating in hemorrhaging from the gums, nose, stomach, intestines, urinary tract, and uterus. Death ensues as the result of renal failure or hypovolemic shock. If the fever should break, recovery may follow.

Lassa Fever does not have a pronounced hemorrhagic component (17%), and neurological impairment is rare except for sensorineural deafness (the most common cause of deafness in West Africa). On the other hand, Bolivian Hemorrhagic Fever has neurological impairment as a prominent feature (headache, tremor, encephalitis).

Laboratory abnormalities include leukopenia, thrombocytopenia, and albuminuria. However, with Lassa Fever leukocytosis and liver function test (LFT) abnormalities can be present. Case fatality rates range from 10 to 30%.

Bunyaviruses

Crimean-Congo Hemorrhagic Fever. A sudden onset of fever, chills, and myalgias heralds the onset of this disease after an incubation period of 2 to 9 days. Sore throat, conjunctivitis, photophobia, and diarrhea may also be present. The patient may exhibit a labile mood. Three to six days into the illness, the hemorrhagic manifestations may erupt. A petechial rash and hemorrhage from most orifices and organ systems can ensue as disseminated intravascular coagulation (DIC) emerges. The liver may be enlarged and tender. Resolution of the rash may be a sign of recovery. Leukopenia, thrombocytopenia, abnormal LFTs, and abnormal clotting tests will be present. The case fatality rate is between 30 and 50%.

Rift Valley Fever. Most infections with this virus are mild self-limited febrile illnesses; however, 1–2% of patients develop hemorrhagic complications or fatal encephalitis.

Hantavirus

Hantavirus infection is responsible for two distinct clinical entities: Old World Hemorrhagic Fever with Renal Syndrome (HFRS) and New World Hantavirus Pulmonary Syndrome (HPS).

Hemorrhagic Fever with Renal Syndrome. HFRS occurs upon infection with the Hantaan (or related) subtype Hantavirus. The incubation of this illness can last up to 42 days, and 80% of the cases are mild to moderate; however, 20% progress to severe illness.

The illness can be broken into five phases: febrile, hypotensive, oliguric, diuretic, and convalescent. The febrile phase lasts 5 days. Fever, backache, facial flush, and conjunctival injection are present. Petechial hemorrhages and albuminuria will appear. In the 3-day hypotensive phase the temperature can return to normal; however, nausea, vomiting, and abdominal pain will be present. Capillary leakage ensues, leading to an increased hematocrit along with severe proteinuria, leukocytosis, thrombocytopenia, and diminishing renal function. The 4-day oliguric phase is heralded by extravascular fluid resorption, resulting in hypervolemia, hypertension, metabolic acidosis, and renal failure. Pulmonary edema may also develop. Renal function may normalize in the diuretic phase, with the consequent fluid and electrolyte shifts and imbalances. The convalescent phase may last for months. Case fatality is less than 5%.

Hantavirus Pulmonary Syndrome. The Sin Nombre subtype of Hantavirus is the most common cause of this clinical syndrome. It is heralded by a nonspecific viral prodrome of symptoms, after which follows a cardiopulmonary phase of dyspnea, hypoxia, and non-cardiogenic pulmonary edema. Renal involvement is minimal.

Increased levels of LDH and abnormal liver function tests may occur, as well as thrombocytopenia and leukocytosis. Clotting abnormalities are present. Metabolic acidosis occurs in severe cases. If survival is to occur, recovery usually begins a week after onset of the cardiopulmonary phase. Case fatality is 40 to 50%.

Filoviruses

Marburg and Ebola virus infections are likely the most feared of the VHFs. The high mortality (ranging to 90%) coupled with DIC make them particularly worrisome.

After an incubation period of 3 to 9 (Marburg) or 3 to 18 (Ebola) days, an abrupt onset of headache, backache, and myalgias begins. Nausea, vomiting, and profuse watery and bloody diarrhea occur about 3 days later. A maculopapular rash erupts, and by days 4–5 diffuse hemorrhage occurs. Death occurs frequently by day 8 or 9. Leukopenia, thrombocytopenia, clotting abnormalities, proteinuria, and amylasemia will occur. EKG changes may also reflect myocardial involvement. Case fatality reaches 30% with Marburg and 90% with Ebola.

Flaviviruses

Yellow Fever. Yellow fever is named for the jaundice it causes secondary to liver dysfunction/failure. The disease has a spectrum of presentation from a "viral-like illness" to fulminant liver failure and hemorrhage leading to death. Up to 50% of infected individuals may be asymptomatic. Mild cases present with fevers, headaches, conjunctival injection, facial flushing, and a relative bradycardia. Initial infection may resolve or become biphasic with the more ominous complications: bleeding, liver failure, shock, renal failure, myocardial dysfunction, coma, seizures, and death. With severe cases mortality approaches 50%.

Dengue Hemorrhagic Fever. Dengue Hemorrhagic Fever does not occur with primary infection of Dengue Fever. At least four serotypes exist, and infection with a different serotype triggers an immunologic mechanism leading to capillary leakage, bleeding diathesis, and shock. The onset of the illness is associated with high fevers, retroorbital headaches, nausea, muscle pains, sore throat, and abdominal pain. Easy bruising, petechiae, epistaxis, and gum bleeding can also occur. Most cases are moderately severe or mild, and when the fever subsides recovery ensues. However, severe cases can be associated with shock. On laboratory findings, leukopenia, thrombocytopenia, and evidence of plasma leakage by at least a 20% increase in the hematocrit. Case fatality is between 2 and 10%.

DIAGNOSIS

"Chance favors the prepared mind." Louis Pasteur stated this famous dictum to the scientists of his day, and it applies equally well to a physician faced with a perplexing clinical dilemma. To diagnose a VHF, a high clinical suspicion is the best tool. Anyone with a severe febrile illness with signs of vascular involvement and travel to an endemic area should raise the suspicion of a VHF. A history of arthropod/animal exposures should also be sought. Military personnel or individuals in non-endemic regions manifesting with the signs of a VHF should alert the physician to the possibility of bioterrorism. Diagnosis of all VHFs relies on the use of ELISA and/or RT-PCR under the appropriate biosafety level precautions.

TREATMENT

The mainstay of treatment for VHFs is supportive care and strict infection control measures. Judicious fluid resuscitation, administration of fresh-frozen plasma (FFP) and platelets, and the use of heparin in the setting of DIC should be employed. Nonsteroidal antiinflammatories should be avoided.

Antiviral therapy has centered on the use of ribavirin. This drug has shown some benefit in the treatment of Lassa Fever, Argentinean Hemorrhagic Fever, Bolivian Hemorrhagic Fever, CCHF, RVF, and HFRS. Interferon-alpha has shown some promise with RVF and Arenavirus infections.

The only FDA-approved vaccine for a VHF is the live Yellow Fever Vaccine. Other vaccines for RVF, Argentinean Hemorrhagic Fever, Dengue Fever, and Hantavirus are in the experimental stages.

RESOURCES

http://www.bt.cdc.gov/agent/vhf/
http://www.cdc.gov/ncidod/diseases/virlfvr/virlfvr.htm
http://www.cdc.gov/ncidod/dvbid/yellowfever/index.htm

REFERENCES

Berger S, Calisher CH, Keystone JS. 2003. *Exotic Viral Diseases: A Global Guide*. London: Decker.

Goldman L, Ausiello D. 2004. *Cecil's textbook of medicine*, 22nd ed. Philadelphia: Saunders.

Jahrling PB. 1997. Viral hemorrhagic fevers. In *Textbook of Military Medicine: Medical Aspects of Chemical and Biological Warfare*. Available at http://www.nbc-med.org/SiteContent/HomePage/WhatsNew/MedAspects/co

27 BOTULISM

Rosie Monardo and Kaushal Shah, MD*

OVERVIEW

Historical Significance

Before the Gulf War, Iraq produced 20,000 liters of botulinum toxin. Warheads were created that contained the toxin as well. Many other groups have experimented with the toxin, including scientists from the former Soviet Union and members of the Aum Shinrikyo cult in Japan.

Etiology

Clostridium botulinum is a Gram-positive, spore-forming, anaerobic bacillus that produces a neurotoxin—botulinum. The toxin blocks acetylcholine release at the neuromuscular junction and the nicotinic receptors of the autonomic ganglions, resulting in neuroparalytic effects. The bacteria can be found in soil throughout the world. Each strain produces antigenically distinct toxins, types A through G. Most human cases are caused by Types A, B, and E

Transmission Categories

- Food-borne (ingestion of toxin from home-canned foods, meats and uncooked vegetables)
- Wound botulism (from soil, drug abuse and c-sections)
- Infantile illness (ingestion of spores)
- Adult intestinal colonization (newly described; occurs in presence of colitis, bowel surgery, or with change in intestinal flora)

Incidence and Prevalence

C. botulinum is present in the soil and water, particularly in Utah, California, and Pennsylvania. In 1999 there were 154 cases of botulism, 92 of which were infantile botulism.

*Department of Emergency Medicine, St. Luke's/Roosevelt Hospital Center, New York

Risk Factors

Stagnant water, undercooked food, and especially accidental ingestion of soil: particularly in Utah, California, and Pennsylvania. The classic case is an infant who has ingested unpasteurized honey.

PATHOGENESIS/LIFE CYCLE

C. botulinum is extremely toxic, with an LD_{50} of 0.001 μg/kg (100,000 times more toxic per microgram than sarin nerve gas). Spores are resilient and able to survive at 100°C, but the toxin is inactivated more easily, within a minute at 85°C. The bacteria can survive for weeks in food or stagnant water.

PRESENTATION

Incubation Period/Time of Onset

Symptoms can occur 1–5 days after exposure, but the classic presentation occurs 12 to 72 hours after exposure. Food-borne botulism usually presents over 12 to 36 hours, whereas a cutaneous infection source usually presents over several days. Death occurs 24 to 72 hours after the symptoms appear. If the disease is not fatal, the symptoms can last for months.

Signs and Symptoms

Ptosis, diplopia, dilated pupils, and extraocular muscle palsies may be present. The gag reflex may be diminished, and there is a varying degree of dry mouth followed by descending paralysis and respiratory arrest. Autonomic dysfunction, both sympathetic and parasympathetic, can be present. There is a subsequent symmetric descending paralysis of the extremities. Mental status is not affected unless paralysis leads to respiratory depression, resulting in carbon dioxide retention and altered mental status. Infants' symptoms may include poor sucking, listlessness, flaccid facial expression, constipation, regurgitation, and weakness.

DIAGNOSIS

Diagnosis is based on clinical presentation with laboratory confirmation.

Laboratory

There are no routine laboratory tests to aid in diagnosis, but the toxin may be detected by assays of serum or gastric contents. Specialized tests are done at select Level C laboratories and take several days to confirm the diagnosis.

Other

Absent light reflex may be helpful to test for botulism. Consider CSF testing (to differentiate from Guillain-Barré syndrome) and electrophysiological studies to examine nerve conduction in conjunction with evoked muscle action potentials.

DIFFERENTIAL DIAGNOSIS

Other neuromuscular disorders, specifically myasthenia gravis, Guillain-Barré (ascending paralysis), poliomyelitis, or tick paralysis (also ascending paralysis). To differentiate between myasthenia gravis and botulism, electromyography is more reliable than the edrophonium test, which may provide a false positive result.

TREATMENT

The foremost emergency treatment is ventilatory support; diaphragm paralysis is a serious complication that can lead to hypoxia and death. There are several antitoxins available that will either shorten the course of the disease or prevent progression: trivalent equine botulinum antitoxin, which contains antibodies to Types A, B and E; a monovalent human antiserum to Type A for infant botulism; and a despeciated equine heptavalent antitoxin against all seven serotypes. These antitoxins are available through the Center for Disease Control in Atlanta, GA (404-639-2206/3311). One vial should be administered IV to adults and children. Infants should not receive antitoxin. Additionally, in infants antibiotics are ineffective for eradication of the bacteria from the intestine and may cause neurological conditions to worsen due to release of toxin through bacterial cell lysis. Consider nasogastric suctioning if a profound ileus is present. In wound botulism, wound debridement should be performed.

PROGNOSIS

Most patients eventually recover after weeks to months of supportive care, but symptoms may remain for months. Damage is occasionally permanent, but recovery can occur through the formation of new synapses. *C. botulinum* has a mortality rate in 60 to 70% of untreated cases. If treated, the mortality rate is 5 to 15%.

PREVENTION

A vaccine is available for laboratory workers and those with work-related exposure (not the public). It is a pentavalent toxoid vaccine (Types A–E) that requires repeated doses to achieve immunity. Botulism is not transmitted person-to-person, so isolation is unnecessary.

SPECIAL CONSIDERATIONS

Contamination of food and aerosolization are the most likely bioterrorism dissemination routes. Since minute quantities can cause profound intoxication and death, extreme caution should be used to handle all material suspected of containing botulism toxin.

Infantile botulism is sometimes misdiagnosed as dehydration, sepsis, or Reye's syndrome and should be considered in all infant sepsis workups. Additionally, in adults aminoglycosides are contraindicated as they potentiate neuromuscular blockade.

RESOURCES

Center for Disease Control in Atlanta, GA (404-639-2206/3311)
US Army Medical Research Institute of Infectious Diseases: www.uamriid.army.mil

REFERENCES

Cox N, Hinkle R. 2002. Infant botulism. *Am Fam Physician* **65**:1388–1392.
Darling RG, Catlett CL, Huebner KD, Jarrett DG. 2002. Threats in bioterrorism I: CDC Category A agents. *Emerg Med Clin North Am* **20**(2):273–309.
Miller JM. 2001. Agents of bioterrorism: preparing for bioterrorism at the community health care level. *Infect Dis Clin North Am* **15**(4):1127–1156.

28

Q FEVER

Christopher Cammarata, MD*

OVERVIEW

Q Fever is a zoonotic disease caused by *Coxiella burnetti*, which has high infectivity. A single organism can initiate infection. It has a spore-like form that is extremely resistant to heat, pressure, dry conditions, and many antiseptic compounds, and can live on surfaces for 5 to 60 days. It requires a host cell to grow and replicate. *C. burnetti* has now been identified in at least 51 countries and on five continents.

PATHOGENESIS

A large range of mammals and arthropods have been identified as hosts. Domestic livestock including goats, cattle, and sheep are the primary reservoirs. The organism may be excreted in the milk, urine, and feces of infected animals. Also, there are high numbers of organism in the amniotic fluid and placenta of infected hosts. Humans are the only hosts that manifest an illness due to infection; however, only about half of infected humans will manifest disease. Transmission to humans most commonly occurs via inhalation. Other less common modes of transmission include ingestion of contaminated milk or food and tick bites. Human-to-human transmission is possible, but exceedingly rare.

PRESENTATION

Incubation varies from 10 to 40 days and is indirectly proportional to the size of the inoculum. The severity of disease is directly proportional to the size of the inoculum. Q fever has an acute and a chronic stage.

*Department of Emergency Medicine, Allegheny General Hospital, Pittsburgh

Acute Stage

- Onset may be abrupt or insidious.
- The most common signs and symptoms are high fever (39–40°C), chills, severe headache, general malaise, myalgias, diaphoresis, dry cough, nausea, vomiting, and diarrhea.
- Less common signs and symptoms include chest pain, arthralgias, and nonspecific skin eruptions.
- Myocarditis, pericarditis, meningitis, and optic neuritis may occur but are uncommon.
- Atypical pneumonia and granulomatous hepatitis may develop 4 to 7 days after the onset of symptoms.
- Acute Q fever has a mortality rate of 1-2%.

Chronic Stage

- May occur with or without a recognized acute phase.
- Characterized by infection that lasts more than 6 months.
- May develop as soon as 1 year or as long as 20 years after initial infection.
- Occurs in about 5% of patients with acute Q fever.
- Endocarditis, generally involving the aortic valve, is the most common manifestation of chronic Q fever.
- Chronic Q fever has a mortality rate of up to 65%.

DIAGNOSIS

Usually diagnosed via serologic testing. The most commonly used are complement fixation, indirect fluorescent antibody, and ELISA. ELISA is the most sensitive: 80–85% early in the disease, and 100% late in the disease. Other potentially helpful testing includes a CBC, platelet count, hepatic and renal function tests, and urinalysis. Possible findings include: transient thrombocytopenia, two- to threefold increase in aminotransferases, 10–15% increase in total bilirubin, normal WBC, and an elevated ESR in 33% of patients

Chest x-ray is only indicated if pulmonary symptoms are present. Abnormalities are only seen 50–60% of the time, with a lobar infiltrate being the most common finding.

DIFFERENTIAL DIAGNOSIS

There is an extremely broad differential diagnosis that is based on the clinical symptoms present.

TREATMENT

Acute Phase

Use one of the following for 15–21 days, or until afebrile for one week:

- Doxycycline 100 mg PO twice daily, or
- Ofloxacin 200 mg PO every 12 hours

Chronic Phase

Treatment ranges from 3 years to lifetime.

- Doxycycline 200 mg PO twice a day, or
- Ofloxacin 400 to 600 mg PO each day

Other drug regimens include the addition of Chloroquine or Hydroxychloroquine to the above medications.

PROGNOSIS

Only half of patients with the disease will manifest symptoms, and the majority of patients fully recover, even without treatment. Mortality for acute Q fever approaches 1–2%. The mortality rate for chronic Q fever is less than 10% when treated and up to 65% when untreated, with an overall mortality of 10–25%.

PREVENTION

An effective vaccine has been developed (*Q-Vax*) but is only commercially available in Australia. In the event of a bioterrorism attack, the standard gas mask should protect personnel from airborne *C. burnetti.*

SPECIAL CONSIDERATIONS

Because *C. burnetti* is highly infectious, rather resistant to heat and drying, and has the ability to be aerosolized, it has a potential use as a bioterrorism agent. It is a Class B agent.

RESOURCES

www.bt.cdc.gov
www.emedicine.com
www.fema.gov

REFERENCES

Dupont HT, Raoult D, Brouqui P, Janbon F, Peyramond D, Weiller PJ, Chicheportiche C, Nezri M, Poirier R. 1992. Epidemiologic features and clinical presentation of acute Q fever in hospitalized patients: 323 French cases. *Am J Med* **93**:427–434.

Fiset P, Woodward TE. 1998. Q fever. In *Bacterial infections of humans: epidemiology and control*, 3rd ed., pp. 583–595. Ed AS Evans, PS Brachman. New York: Plenum.

Fournier PE, Marrie TJ, Raoult D. 1998. Diagnosis of Q fever. *J Clin Microbiol* **36**:1823–1834.

Levy PY, Drancourt M, Etienne J, Auvergnat JC, Beytout J, Sainty JM, Goldstein F, Raoult D. 1991. Comparison of different antibiotic regimens for therapy of 32 cases of Q fever endocarditis. *Antimicrob Agents Chemother* **35**:533–537.

Marrie T.J. 1995. *Coxiella burnetii* (Q fever). In *Mandell, Douglas and Bennett's principles and practice of infectious diseases*, 4th ed, pp. 1727-1735. Ed GL Mandell, JE Bennett, R Dolin. New York: Churchill Livingstone.

Raoult D, Houpikian P, Tissot-Dupont H, Riss JM, Arditi-Djiane J, Brouqui P. 1999. Treatment of Q fever endocarditis: comparison of 2 regimens containing doxycycline and ofloxacin or hydroxychloroquine. *Arch Intern Med* **159**:167–173.

29 BRUCELLOSIS

Richard V. Hausrod, MD*

OVERVIEW

Brucellosis (undulant, Mediterranean, and Malta fever) is a systemic zoonotic disease that exists worldwide. *Brucella* species are found primarily in domestic and feral animals, including: cattle, goats, sheep, swine, dogs, caribou, foxes, antelope, camels, elk, and bison. High-risk areas are the Mediterranean Basin (Portugal, Spain, Southern France, Italy, Greece, Turkey, North Africa), South and Central America, Eastern Europe, Asia, Africa, the Caribbean, and the Middle East. In the United States, most cases are reported in Texas, California, Virginia, and Florida. Four species—*B. melitensis* (sheep, goats), *B. abortus* (cattle), *B. suis* (pigs), and *B. canis* (dogs)—are known to cause disease in humans. Humans acquire brucellosis by one of several routes: ingestion of contaminated foods (unpasteurized dairy products) or contact with infected animals or animal products (direct inoculation through cuts and abrasions, entry across mucosal surfaces, and inhalation of aerosols). Risk factors include: occupational exposure (ranchers, dairy farmers, abattoir workers, and veterinarians), consumer exposure to unpasteurized milk products and cheese, and exposure while traveling in countries where the disease is endemic. Overall incidence in the United States is low: 0.5 per 100,000, with approximately 100 cases per year. Given the ease of aerosol transmission, brucellosis became the first agent weaponized by the old US offensive biological weapons program in 1954.

PATHOGENESIS

Brucellae are small, facultative intracellular Gram-negative coccobacilli. The organism expresses smooth lipopolysaccharide (S-LPS) on its surface, an important virulence factor. After entering the skin, the bacteria are ingested by PMNs, where they survive within the phagolysosome by neutralizing toxic oxygen byproducts through production of superoxide dismutase. The bacteria then invade the lymphatic system and bloodstream, disseminating to organs such as the liver, spleen, and bone

*Department of Emergency Medicine, Allegheny General Hospital, Pittsburgh

marrow. They are ingested by resident macrophages and survive by blocking phagosome–lysosome function.

CLINICAL PRESENTATION

Infective dose is small at 10–100 organisms, with an incubation period of 3–5 days to several weeks. Patients present with a multitude of complaints, often without objective findings except fever. Physical findings, when present are usually limited to minimal lymphadenopathy and hepatosplenomegaly. The disease is defined by time from illness onset: acute (<8 weeks), subacute (<1 year), and chronic (>1 year). Onset of disease may be sudden or insidious. Signs and symptoms include: fever (may be undulant, increased in the afternoon and evening, maximum 101–104° daily), weakness, headache, sweating, chills, generalized aching, and arthralgia. Also common are: weight loss, depression, irritability, hepatosplenomegaly, hepatic dysfunction (abnormal LFTs), gastrointestinal complaints, lymphadenopathy (cervical, inguinal), orchitis, epididymitis (normal urinalysis), nephritis, prostatitis, cystitis, pulmonary (cough, dyspnea), cutaneous (rash), visual disturbances, chronic fatigue syndrome. Duration of symptoms more than 30 days before diagnosis is a major risk factor for developing focal disease. Most common sites of localization are: osteoarticular (especially sacroiliitis), genitourinary, neurobrucellosis (usually presenting as meningitis), endocarditis, and hepatic abscess.

DIAGNOSIS

Routine laboratory studies are nonspecific (anemia, leukopenia, and thrombocytopenia are common). Radiological imaging with bone scans, radiographs, computerized tomography, echocardiograms, lumbar puncture with cerebrospinal fluid analysis, and biopsy/aspiration of tissue/abscess may be helpful in isolating focal disease. The diagnosis of brucellosis is made with certainty when brucellae are recovered from blood, bone marrow, or other tissues. The rate of isolation from blood ranges from 15 to 70%. Bone marrow cultures can approach 90% accuracy. When brucellosis is suspected, the laboratory should be alerted to maintain cultures for a minimum of 4 weeks. Serologic diagnosis is the most common method for making the diagnosis. Serum agglutination titers or ELISA measure IgG and IgM antibodies against the *Brucella* species, except *B. canis.* A titer of >1:160 or a fourfold rise between acute and convalescent sera is supportive. Rising agglutinating titers or levels of IgG suggest relapse.

DIFFERENTIAL DIAGNOSIS

There is an extremely broad differential and is based on the clinical symptoms present.

- Many nonspecific systemic febrile illnesses
- Tularemia
- Psittacosis
- Rickettsial disease

- Tuberculosis
- Typhoid fever
- Influenza
- Infectious mononucleosis
- Histoplasmosis
- Coccidiomycosis
- HIV

TREATMENT

Brucellosis

Several regimens have been used to treat brucellosis. None is 100% effective since some patients will relapse after therapy. Recommended regimens for adults include:

- Doxycycline 100 mg PO BID plus Rifampin 600–900 mg PO (15 mg/kg) QD x 6 weeks
- Doxycycline 100 mg PO BID x 6 weeks plus Streptomycin 1 g IM QD for the first 14–21 days (Gentamicin can be substituted 5 mg/kg IV QD)
- Ofloxacin 400 mg PO QD plus Rifampin 600 mg PO QD x 6 weeks

Neurobrucellosis

- Use 2–3 drugs that cross the blood/brain barrier (doxycycline, rifampin, trimethoprim-sulfamethoxazole).
- Prolonged duration of therapy from 1 to 19 months.
- Corticosteroids are often recommended, but their efficacy is unproved.

Endocarditis

- Usually left sided
- Valve
  - o Previously healthy: aortic
  - o Previously diseased: mitral
- Majority of patients need surgical valve replacement followed by several weeks to months of antibiotic therapy.
- Mortality rate approaching 85%

PROGNOSIS

With appropriate treatment, complete recovery is the most common outcome. The case fatality rate in patients that go untreated is <5%.

PREVENTION

Depends on eradication or control of the disease in animals. This relies on: pasteurization of milk and dairy products for human consumption, immunization, surveillance, and testing of animals in endemic areas, and public awareness and education regarding occupational risk and appropriate dietary hygiene in travelers. No human vaccine is available.

SPECIAL CONSIDERATIONS

- Accidental animal vaccine exposure
  - The vaccines are live attenuated strains (B19, Rev-1) that can cause human disease.
  - Treat with the full therapeutic regimen.
- Relapse (5–10%)
  - Usual cause is localized sequestration of organisms or noncompliance with medications.
  - Treat with same regimen as before relapse.
- Pregnancy
  - Can result in abortion, particularly in the first trimester.
  - Brucella species may be transmitted across the placenta.
  - Treatment: Rifampin 900 mg PO QD x 6 weeks
- Pediatric
  - Presentation is similar in neonates, children, and adults.
  - Treatment: trimethoprim-sulfamethoxazole PO BID (10-12 mg/kg Trimethoprim; 50–60 mg/kg Sulfa) plus Rifampin PO QD (15-20 mg/kg) x 6 weeks

RESOURCES

CDC: http://www.cdc.gov/ncidod/dbmd/diseaseinfo/brucellosis_t.htm

REFERENCES

Abuhammour W. 2002. Brucellosis. Emedicine.com. http://www.emedicine.com/ped/topic293.htm.

Brillman R. 1998. Brucellosis. *Infect Dis Emerg Med* **8**:889–890.

Everett D. 2004. Brucellosis. *UpToDate*. 12:2. www.uptodate.com/physicians/infectious_disease_toclist.asp?usd=618287539&r=/physicians/infectious_disease_toclist.asp&server=www.uptodate.com&app=mktg.

Lisgaris M, Salata RA. 2001. Brucellosis. Emedicine.com. http://www.emedicine.com/med/topic248.htm.

Maloney G, Fraser WR. 2004. Brucellosis. Emedicine.com. http://www.emedicine.com/emerg/topic883.htm.

Rust R. 2004. Brucellosis. Emedicine.com. http://www.emedicine.com/neuro/topic42.htm.

30 ALPHAVIRUSES

Sam Shen MD, MBA*

OVERVIEW

Alphaviruses (formerly know as group A arboviruses) are a genera of arthropod-borne viruses in the Togaviridae family that give rise to a spectrum of diseases in humans ranging from asymptomatic infections to fatal encephalitis. There are 28 types of alphaviruses classified by their antigenic properties. In the context of viral bioterrorism, several alphaviruses are particularly interesting due to their susceptibility to cultivation, their ability to cause fatal or serious illness, and a lack of measures available for their control. These viruses could be weaponized through their production and stabilization in either aerosolized wet or dried forms. The specific viruses likely to be used as a bioterrorist agent are Venezuelan equine encephalitis (VEE), Western equine encephalitis (WEE), and Eastern equine encephalitis (EEE).

HISTORICAL SIGNIFICANCE

During the 1930s, the viruses that cause WEE, EEE, and VEE were isolated from affected horses and were discovered to be antigenically related. In working with these viruses, it was discovered that they are highly contagious in aerosolized form, demonstrated by the many laboratory-acquired infections that resulted. In one incident in Moscow, 20 workers were infected within 24 hours after a vial containing the virus was dropped and broken. Although many other viruses could be used as biological weapons, WEE, EEE, and VEE possess several characteristics that make it attractive for weaponization:

- Ability to be produced in large quantities inexpensively
- Ability to remain stable and infectious as aerosols
- Ability to cause serious disease
- Existence of many subtypes making vaccine development difficult

*Beth Israel Deaconess Medical Center, Harvard-Affiliated Emergency Residency, Brigham and Women's Hospital/Massachusetts General Hospital, Boston

ETIOLOGY

In nature, alphaviruses transmit their disease by vectors, mostly mosquitoes. However, it is aerosol transmission that leads to the concern of these viruses being manufactured as biological weapons since VEE, WEE, and EEE remain highly infectious in the aerosol state.

INCIDENCE AND PREVALENCE

During the past century, there have been occasional outbreaks of VEE in Latin America. The outbreaks involved tens to hundreds of thousands of equine and human cases. More recent outbreaks have occurred in Mexico. In the United States there have been periodic outbreaks of EEE in the eastern states. As the name implies, WEE occurred in the western states as early as 1930. In addition to these natural outbreaks, there have been many cases of laboratory workers being infected from mishandling of these viruses.

RISK FACTORS

Human infections are acquired in areas endemic for vectors carrying the viruses. The infection pattern is seasonal. Alphaviruses have not been reported to be transmissible between humans through normal contact. Laboratory workers that handle and work with VEE, WEE, or EEE are at high risk.

PATHOGENESIS/LIFE CYCLE

Infection is transmitted by mosquitoes. When a vertebrate host is infected, a transient viremia occurs. Dissemination of the virus occurs as infected cells are lysed, releasing the virus. A host can be infected and seroconversion can occur in the absence of clinical disease. In humans, aerosol transmission is the main concern, as this would be the modality for biological warfare.

PRESENTATION

There are two forms of the disease. The first presents with fever, headache, malaise, and symptoms of encephalitis (e.g., eastern, western, or Venezuelan equine encephalitis viruses). The other form presents as fever, rash, and arthralgia (e.g., Chikungunya, Ross River, Mayaro, and Sindbis viruses). The clinical manifestations can start as relatively mild but quickly become fulminant encephalitis, followed by coma and death in 1 to 2 weeks. Children are more likely to die from an infection than adults. In pregnant women spontaneous abortions, stillbirths, and fetal abnormalities can often occur.

INCUBATION PERIOD/TIME OF ONSET

The incubation period is 1–6 days and the time of onset is acute.

SIGNS AND SYMPTOMS

VEE, Western, Eastern

- Acute onset of malaise
- High fever (101–105°F)
- Severe headache
- Rigors
- Photophobia
- Myalgias (predominantly in legs and lumbosacral region)
- Cough
- Sore Throat
- Vomiting
- Seizures

Chikungunya, Ross River, Mayaro, Sindbis

- Fever
- Severe arthralgia (polyarticular, migratory, affecting small joints of the hands, wrists, ankles, and feet)
- Rash (flush over face and trunk followed by maculopapular rash; face, palms, and soles may be affected as well)
- Generalized myalgias

DIAGNOSIS

Diagnosis is based on clinical presentation and history of exposure to the virus or suspected bioterrorist attack. Laboratory tests can confirm diagnosis through virus isolation.

LABORATORY

Certain alphaviruses, like Venezuelan equine encephalitis, can be isolated from the blood or throat swabs during the acute phase of the illness. Blood tests can detect a specific rise in IgG or IgM antibody. Cerebrospinal fluid should also be collected from patients with neurological symptoms. CSF analysis may reveal findings consistent with encephalitis (elevated white cells/mm^3 that are predominantly mononuclear cells and elevated protein concentration). Other potential laboratory test findings include leukopenia, lymphopenia, and elevated serum glutamic oxaloacetic transaminase (SGOT).

DIFFERENTIAL DIAGNOSIS

- Influenza
- Flu-like illnesses from other potential bioterrorist agents (*Bacillus anthracis, Yersinia pestis, Coxiella burnetii*)
- Brain abscess
- Lyme disease
- Rocky Mountain spotted fever
- Meningitis/encephalitis from fungal agents
- Lupus cerebritis
- Cerebral and granulomatous arteritis

TREATMENT

Supportive care is the mainstay therapy. Attention should be paid to fluid and electrolyte balance. Analgesics should be given for headaches and myalgias. Anticonvulsants may be given to patients with encephalitis. Nonsteroidal antiinflammatory drugs should be given for arthralgias. Currently, no antiviral drugs exist for the treatment of alphaviruses, though several compounds like interferon-alpha have been reported to mitigate the disease in animal models.

PROGNOSIS

The overall case fatality rate for Venezuelan equine encephalitis is less than 1%. It may reach 20–35% in children with encephalitis.

PREVENTION

There are two main controls for the disease. The first is disease surveillance of natural hosts. This will guide in determining whether measures to reduce the population of vector mosquitoes are needed. The second control is vaccination of hosts such as humans if at high risk, and other potential animal hosts, like horses. Formalin-inactivated vaccines for some types of WEE, EEE, and VEE exist for high-risk laboratory workers.

SPECIAL CONSIDERATIONS

Patients should be put in isolation with universal as well as droplet precautions. The virus is destroyed by heat (80°C for 30 minutes) and standard disinfectants.

REFERENCES

Lam SK, Chua KB. 2004. *Alphaviruses*. Kuala Lumpur: WHO Collaborating Centre for Arbovirus Reference and Research (DF/DHF), Department of Medical Microbiology, Faculty of Medicine, University of Malaya. Available at http://www.vadscorner.com/alphaviruses.html.

Baron S, Peake RC, James DA, Susman M, Kennedy CA, Durson-Singleton MJ, Schuenke S. 1996. *Medical microbiology*, 4th ed. Galveston: The University of Texas Medical Branch.

Sidwell RW, Smee DF. 2003. Viruses of the Bunya- and Togaviridae families: potential as bioterrorism agents and means of control. *Antiviral Res* **57**:101–111.

Smith JF, Davis K, Hart MK. 1997. Viral encephalitides. In *Medical aspects of chemical and biological warfare*, pp. 561–589. Ed R Zajtchuk, RF Bellamy. Washington, DC: Office of the Surgeon General, US Department of the Army. Available at http://www.nbc-med.org/SiteContent/HomePage/WhatsNew/MedAspects/contents.html.

Weaver SC, Ferro C, Barrera R, Boshell J, Navarro JC. 2004, Venezuelan equine encephalitis. *Annu Rev Entomol* **49**:141–174.

www.tdh.state.tx.us/bioterrorism/facts/alphavirus.html.

31

RICIN

Kristin J. Kent, MD*

OVERVIEW

Ricin is on the Category B list of potential bioterrorism agents by the US Center for Disease Control and Prevention. It is of particular concern because it is available worldwide, is technically easy and inexpensive when preparing large quantities in liquid or crystal form, and the toxin is stable, as well as because ricin has received so much attention by the media.

Ricin is a potent toxin extracted from the bean of the castor plant, *Ricinis communis*. The entire castor plant contains ricin, but the greatest concentration is found in the seeds. The plant's most common use is for the production of castor oil, but it also grows uncultivated worldwide. Hexane or carbon tetrachloride is used to extract the oil from the plant, leaving a castor meal containing the toxin ricin. Then, ricin is extracted from the castor meal by a salting-out procedure. Ingestion, injection, or inhalation could produce intoxication. There is no potential for spread by human-to-human contact.

HISTORICAL SIGNIFICANCE

There have been several reports of ricin being used as a weapon both at home and abroad. A ricin-containing bomb, code-named "compound W," was developed and tested by the United States, in collaboration with Britain, before World War I. Ricin was used in injection form to assassinate Georgi Markov, a Bulgarian defector, in 1978. In 1994 and 1995, four men from a tax protest group were convicted of possessing ricin as a biological weapon. Plans linked to al Qaeda to produce ricin were found in Afghanistan in November 2001. In October 2003 a package containing ricin and a threatening note were sent to a South Carolina post office. In May and June of 2004, ground castor beans were found in jars of Gerber Banana Yogurt Dessert in California.

*Department of Emergency Medicine, St. Luke's/Roosevelt Hospital Center, New York

INCIDENCE AND PREVALENCE

Over 750 cases of ricin intoxication by ingestion have been reported. Ricin has been used as an injection in clinical trials, but reported cases of non-medicinal uses by injection are rare. In the English-speaking world there are no reports of ricin intoxication by inhalation, but there is one incidence of workers being exposed to dust from castor beans around a processing plant.

PATHOGENESIS

Ricin toxin is a globular protein consisting of an alpha chain and a beta chain connected by a disulfide bond. The beta chain allows the toxin to bind to carbohydrates on the cell surface of eukaryotic cells. This triggers internalization of the protein by endocytosis. Once the protein is in the cytoplasm, the alpha chain enzymatically cleaves an adenine residue of the 28-S ribosomal subunit of RNA, inhibiting protein synthesis by the eukaryotic cell.

PRESENTATION

Incubation Period/Time of Onset

The initial signs and symptoms of ricin intoxication occur 6 hours after ingestion. Although there are no reported cases of inhalation, it is thought that signs and symptoms would occur within 8 hours. Death could take place 36 to 72 hours after exposure, and if death has not occurred within 5 days the victim usually recovers.

Signs and Symptoms

The infective dose is thought to be 3 to 5 μg/kg. Ricin is less toxic when ingested, probably due to the poorer absorption and enzymatic degradation by digestion. In general, ricin intoxication may lead to fever, fatigue, weakness, dehydration, leukocytosis, metabolic acidosis, hematuria, and elevated liver function tests. However, the clinical signs and symptoms of ricin toxicity vary with the route of exposure.

If ingested, ricin can lead to nausea, vomiting, abdominal pain, bloody diarrhea, mydriasis, fever, thirst, sore throat, anuria, hypovolemic shock, gastric and intestinal ulcerations, lymphoid necrosis of mesenteric lymph nodes and the spleen, liver necrosis, and diffuse nephritis. In reported cases, death occurred by day 3.

In cancer patients who have received ricin as an injection in clinical trials, flu-like symptoms, fatigue, muscular pain, and, rarely, seizures occurred. In high doses (used in assassinations) there have been reports of severe local lymphoid necrosis, gastrointestinal hemorrhage, liver necrosis, diffuse nephritis, and diffuse splenitis.

One report of processing plant workers being exposed to castor bean dust led to an allergic syndrome of congestion, itchy eyes, urticaria, and chest tightness. From animal studies, it is assumed that lethal ricin inhalational exposure in humans will lead to diffuse necrotizing pneumonia, hypoxemia, acidosis, and anorexia. Cough, fever, chest tightness, and pulmonary edema may also be seen as less severe signs and symptoms.

DIAGNOSIS

The diagnosis of ricin toxin would rely heavily on recognizing the signs and symptoms from many geographically clustered patients.

Laboratory

Radioimmunoassay and enzyme-linked immunosorbent assay (ELISA) are used to detect ricin in bodily fluids. Radioimmunoassay can monitor ricin toxin to concentrations as low as 50 to 100 pg/Ml. However, identification can be difficult because ricin binds quickly and is metabolized before it is excreted.

Pathology

Necrosis of respiratory epithelium may be seen within eight hours of inhalational exposure. Lymphoid necrosis in mesenteric lymph nodes and gut-associated lymphoid tissue, Kupffer cell necrosis, and evidence of diffuse nephritis may be seen if ingested.

Radiology

Although nonspecific, pulmonary edema may be seen on chest films.

DIFFERENTIAL DIAGNOSIS

Like the signs and symptoms of ricin poisoning, the differential diagnosis differs by route of intoxication. The differential diagnosis of inhalational ricin includes staphylococcal enterotoxin B, exposure to organofluorines, oxides of nitrogen, and phosgene. The differential diagnosis of ingestion of ricin includes enteric pathogens, mushrooms, caustics, iron, arsenic, and colchicine.

TREATMENT

Treatment for ricin intoxication is supportive. One of the most important things to do when exposed is for one to leave the area, remove clothing, and wash with soap and water. In general, it is important to monitor for hypotension, hepatotoxicity, and bone marrow suppression. For pulmonary intoxication, furosemide and respiratory support, including positive end-expiratory ventilatory therapy, may be needed. If ingestion of more than one castor bean per 10 kg of body weight occurs, activated charcoal followed by magnesium citrate should be used, along with fluid resuscitation. Patients who are asymptomatic 8 hours after exposure may be discharged.

PROGNOSIS

There have been relatively few deaths from ricin intoxication and only 2 since 1930. In one review looking at 751 cases, 1.9% of patients in one study died, and only about 6% who were symptomatic. Patients usually recover if death has not occurred in 3 to 5 days. Injection of ricin in clinical trials for cancer patients has led to two deaths.

PREVENTION

Avoiding exposure to ricin is the best prevention. A protective mask is the best protection against inhalation. If exposure to skin occurs, decontaminate with soap and water. Also, hypochlorite solutions can be used to inactivate ricin. Currently, there is no vaccine for ricin.

RESOURCES

Center for Disease Control and Prevention: http://www.bt.cdc.gov/agent/ricin/facts.asp
For Spanish speakers: http://www.bt.cdc.gov/agent/ricin/espanol/facts.asp
Poison Control Center: (800) 222-1222
Agency for Toxic Substance and Disease Registry; (888) 422-8737.

REFERENCES

CDC. Ricin. http://www.bt.cdc.gov/agent/ricin/index.asp. Last accessed 1 September 2004.

Doan LG. 2004. Ricin: mechanism of toxicity, clinical manifestations, and vaccine development: a review. *J Toxicol Clin Toxicol.* **42**(2):201–208.

Franz DR, Jaax NK. 1997. Ricin toxin. In *Medical aspects of chemical and biological US warfare*, pp. 631–642. Washington: Office of the Surgeon General, Department of the Army, DC.

Greenfield RA, Brown BR, Hutchins JB, Iandolo JJ, Jackson R, Slater LN, Bronze MS. 2002. Microbiological, biological, and chemical weapons of warfare and terrorism. *Am J Med Sci* **323**(6):326–340.

Kortepeter M, Christopher G, Cieslak T, Culpepper R, Darling R, Pavlin J, Rowe J, McKee Jr K, Eitzen E, eds. 2001. *USAMRIID's medical management of biological casualties handbook.* Fort Detrick, MD: US Army Medical Research Institute of Infectious Disease.

Pollack A. 2004. FDA finds traces of poison in two jars of baby food in California; no one is harmed. *New York Times*, 29 July, p. A12.

Rosenbloom M, Leikin JB, Vogel SN, Chaudry ZA. 2002. Biological and chemical agents: a brief synopsis. *Am J Ther* **9**:5–14.

32

EPSILON TOXIN

Robert E. Antosia, MD, MPH*

INTRODUCTION

Clostridium perfringens is an anaerobic, Gram-positive, spore-forming bacteria. This ubiquitous organism is present in soil throughout the world and has been found in the stool of virtually every vertebrate organism ever tested. *Clostridium* species can produce a variety of toxins, and these are responsible for illness (Epsilon is 1 of 12 toxins). Epsilon toxin is a permease enzyme made by strains B and D of *C. perfringens*. This toxin is a CDC Category B Bioterrorism Agent since it has the potential to be aerosolized as a BT agent.

CLINICAL PRESENTATION

There are no human data for disease due to pure Epsilon toxin. If aerosolized Epsilon toxin occurs, then pulmonary edema, kidney failure, shock, and multi-organ failure may follow, based on animal studies.

DIAGNOSTIC TESTING

Growth of *C. perfringens* in culture and detection of toxin in research lab assay(s).

INFECTION CONTROL PRECAUTIONS

Universal precautions apply. Because this is a toxin-mediated syndrome, there is no potential for person-to-person spread.

*Department of Emergency Medicine, Beth Israel Deaconess Medical Center, Harvard Medical School, Boston

TREATMENT AND PROPHYLAXIS

No antitoxin or vaccine is presently available. Treatment is supportive. ICU and ventilatory support may be necessary in an aerosolized Epsilon toxin exposure or when multi-organ failure and shock are present.

REFERENCES

Moran GJ. 2002. Threats in bioterrorism, part 2: CDC category B and C agents. *Emerg Med Clin North Am* **20**:311–336.

33 STAPHYLOCOCCUS ENTEROTOXIN B

Robert E. Antosia, MD, MPH*

INTRODUCTION

Staphylococcus Enterotoxin B (SEB) is a heat-stable toxin that is a common cause of food poisoning. The toxin is secreted by the ubiquitous organism *Staphylococcus aureus* and is stable in aerosols. Although rarely fatal, it could render a high percentage of exposed individuals seriously ill within a few hours. SEB can be used as a weapon in aerosol form or by contaminating food or water supplies.

CLINICAL PRESENTATION

Symptoms begin after a brief latent period of 3 to 12 hours and will be different depending on the route of exposure. Typical symptoms include high fever, headache, myalgia, prostration, and dry cough. Vomiting and diarrhea may result from ingestion of toxin. In severe cases of inhalation, pulmonary edema, adult respiratory distress syndrome, and respiratory failure may also develop. In rare cases death may occur from dehydration.

DIAGNOSTIC TESTING

The diagnosis of SEB intoxication is primarily clinical and epidemiologic. The symptoms are generally nonspecific and overlap with many other clinical syndromes, including those of other BT agents. Because of the short incubation period, this agent is likely to lead to a sudden cluster of cases in a localized area. The toxin may be identified by ELISA of nasal swabs after aerosol exposure, or the antigen can be detected in the urine; however, neither of these tests is readily available.

*Department of Emergency Medicine, Beth Israel Deaconess Medical Center, Harvard Medical School, Boston

PROPHYLAXIS AND TREATMENT

No vaccine against intoxication from SEB currently exists; however, a vaccine is under development and is being tested. Post-exposure treatment is supportive. Some patients may require IV hydration for fluid losses, and ventilatory support may be required in severe cases. The illness can last up to 2–4 weeks.

INFECTION CONTROL PRECAUTIONS

Because this is a toxin-mediated syndrome, there is no potential for person-to-person spread and no special containment equipment is required. Responders to contaminated areas should use an N95 respirator to prevent inhalation exposure to the toxin. Healthcare workers exposed to the toxin on skin or clothing require a simple change of clothes and shower with soap and water to provide adequate decontamination. Patient care requires the use of universal precautions but does not require any special equipment. Any food or disposable equipment contaminated with SEB should be discarded.

REFERENCES

Franz DR, Jahrling PB, McClain DJ, Hoover DL, Byrne WR, Pavlin JA, Christopher GW, Cieslak TJ, Friedlander AM, Eitzen EM Jr. 1997. Clinical recognition and management of patients exposed to biological warfare agents. *JAMA* **278**:339–411.

Moran GJ. 2002. Threats in bioterrorism, part 2: CDC category B and C agents. *Emerg Med Clin North Am* **20**:311–336.

34

FOOD- AND WATER-BORNE AGENTS

Ann-Jeannette Geib, MD,* and Michele M. Burns, MD**

OVERVIEW

Advances in sanitation and food sciences have given industrialized nations a safer food and water supply; however, the complicated systems involved in their processing offer multiple opportunities for human intervention and sources for contamination. In addition, disasters causing disruption of water and food delivery infrastructures may compromise their safety for human consumption. Contamination may occur with biologic, xenobiotic, or radiologic substances and may be intentional or inadvertent. Many of the major agents discussed elsewhere in this volume could potentially be spread via contaminated food or water. This chapter focuses on pathogens not discussed in other specific chapters.

HISTORICAL SIGNIFICANCE

In 1984 a religious cult contaminated salad bars in Oregon with *Salmonella typhimurium*. The intent was to disrupt voter turnout for a local election. More than 750 persons were afflicted by diarrhea, fevers, and dehydration. Epidemiologic investigation focused on a case-control study of restaurant patrons and found 751 clinical or culture-confirmed cases. The restaurants, their banquet facilities, food products under preparation, employees, distributors and suppliers, the water supply, and restaurant equipment all were examined. A concurrent criminal investigation identified the cult's role in disseminating the pathogen. The *Salmonella* culture had been obtained from a commercial supplier and propagated in the cult's clandestine laboratory.

In January 2003 a disgruntled grocery worker tainted approximately 200 pounds of ground beef sold at a supermarket in Michigan. At least 92 patients had clinical presentations consistent with nicotine-containing pesticide intoxication. Epidemiology and lab studies confirmed that the food product had been contaminated at the level of the local grocery store, and not at a higher level in the food supply chain. Unintentional contamination with pesticides also has been reported.

*Children's Hospital, Harvard Medical School, Boston

In 1993 a malfunction at one of Milwaukee's water treatment plants caused an estimated 403,000 residents to be sickened with cryptosporidiosis. Investigators calculated that approximately 4400 were hospitalized and 69 died due to the disease during the outbreak. Economic losses due to healthcare costs and loss of productivity were estimated at greater than $96 million US.

PATHOGENESIS AND TRANSMISSION

Food-borne viral or bacterial disease typically causes a gastroenteritis-like syndrome. The onset of symptoms may be within hours if preformed toxins are present (e.g., *Staph* enterotoxin B and *Bacillus cereus*), hours to days if viral (e.g., Norwalk agent) or due to toxins formed within the alimentary tract by bacteria (e.g., enterotoxigenic *E. coli*), or days if caused by invasive bacteria (*Salmonella, Shigella, Campylobacter*, and *E. coli* spp.). Infection with *Salmonella typhi* may cause enteric fevers and generate a prolonged carrier state. Enteric bacteria and viruses also are spread silently among close contacts, food handlers, and caregivers, making their area of impact even broader.

CLINICAL PRESENTATION

Preformed bacterial toxins and viruses generally cause vomiting, crampy abdominal pain, and watery diarrhea that is self-limited. Care for these patients generally is supportive with maintenance of adequate hydration. Antiemetics offer symptomatic relief. Antiemetics with serotonin inhibition (e.g., ondansetron) may be used for persistent emesis in all age groups. Those antiemetics with dopamine antagonism (e.g., promethazine) should not be used in infants and young children due to the high incidence of side effects. Tetracycline, doxycycline, and fluoroquinolones also should not be used in children under age 18.

Some enteric bacteria invade the walls of the GI tract, causing bloody diarrhea and fevers. Systemic complications include dehydration, shock, hemorrhage, coagulopathy, sepsis, and renal failure (as in the case of HUS after *E. Coli* O157:H7 infection).

EVALUATION

Patients should be evaluated with standard laboratory evaluation, assessment of hydration status, and stool culture. Stool cultures often require special media and conditions for growth and identification. The local hospital, department of health, or reference lab should be consulted for specific transport and culture requirements. In addition, the local department of health should be contacted if a suspected food-borne incident has occurred so that epidemiologic investigations can be initiated if needed. Consider involvement of infectious disease consultants as well.

PREVENTION AND PRECAUTIONS FOR CAREGIVERS

Unless exposed to specific chemical agents, patients usually do not require decontamination prior to medical treatment. Strict hand-washing precautions should be adhered to in order to prevent spread of disease to others by rescuers, healthcare workers, or patients themselves. Security measures should be enforced surrounding watersheds, reservoirs, and water treatment plants to prevent intentional contamina-

Table 1. Common Food and Waterborne Organisms

Agent	Mechanism	Onset	Predominant sx	Treatment	Contagion
S. aureus; B. cereus	Preformed toxin	1–6 h	Vomiting; some pain & diarrhea	Supportive	Unrefrigerated food
Noroviruses (Norwalk-like viruses)	Viral	24–48 h	Vomiting; some pain & diarrhea	Supportive	Common water sources (e.g., cruise ships; hand-to-mouth; poorly cooked shellfish
Enterotoxigenic *E. coli; C. perfringens*	Toxin formed in gut	24–72 h; 8–16 h	Watery diarrhea	If severe: TMP-SMX; azithromycin; ciprofloxacin; treat x3 d	ETEC: Drink bottled water, no ice, while traveling; peel fruit & vegetables; Prophylactic antibiotics not recommended. *C. perf*: Meat, gravy, meat products
Cryptosporidium; cyclospora	Protozoan parasites	Within 7 d	Watery diarrhea (crypto worse in HIV+)	Crypto: Nitrozoxanide; paromomycin +/− azithromycin; Cyclospora: TMP/SMX x7 d	Chlorinate water; wash fruit. Crypto may last up to 20 d
Salmonella	Inflammatory	1–3 d	Mucoid diarrhea; fevers; cramps; bacteremia; osteomyelitis	Ampicillin; amoxicillin, TMP/SMX, cefotaxime, ceftriaxone if tx indicated (infants <3 mo, HIV, chronic GI disease, severe illness or bacteremia	Contact precautions for incontinent patients; or anyone w/diarrhea until 3 stool cx 48 h post-antibiotics are (−). Cook food thoroughly
Enterohemorrhagic E. coli (EHEC; Shigatoxin-producing; O157:H7)	Inflammatory toxin formed in gut	1-7 d	Bloody, mucoid diarrhea; fevers	Antibiotic tx not recommended due to risk of HUS	Contact precautions until 2 stool cx (−) Cook ground beef thoroughly; avoid unpasteurized milk & juice
Campylobacter	Inflammatory	2–5 d	Bloody/ mucoid diarrhea	Erythromycin or azithromycin; fluoroquinolones	Cook poultry thoroughly; strict hand washing; avoid contact w/sick pets
Shigella	Hemorrhagic inflammatory	2-4 d	Bloody diarrhea	Ampicillin; TMP/SMX; ceftriaxone; fluoroquinolones	Contact precautions; hand washing; clean fomites; avoid contaminated water sources
Cholera (*Vibrio cholerae*)	Secretory	1–3 d	Profuse "rice water diarrhea" +/− vomiting; no fevers	Aggressive hydration (bolus followed by maintenance) with isotonic solution (ORT or LR); monitor electrolytes; antibiotics if moderately to severely ill: doxycycline x1 dose or tetracycline x3 d, or TMP/SMX, erythro, furazolidine, or fluoroquinolone	Avoid raw fish and shellfish; water chlorination; little person-to-person spread.

Adapted from *The Red Book* (Pickering, 2003).

tion of the water supply. Likewise, agricultural, auction, distribution, and food-processing facilities should be closely supervised. Quality control and environmental testing measures help to ensure safety of food and water for consumption.

TRICHOTHECENE MYCOTOXINS

Trichothecene mycotoxins are perhaps a more obscure cause of food-borne disease of some historical importance. Produced by fungus growing at low temperatures on grain, these toxins are extremely fastidious. Trichothecene mycotoxins may affect refugee populations or those involved in disasters that interrupt the normal harvesting and processing of cereal grains. They are thought to be responsible for the illness and death of thousands in Soviet Russia during and after World War II when wheat was unable to be harvested in a timely fashion. Their resistance to degradation makes them easy to weaponize. Refugees from Cambodia and Laos after the Vietnam War have reported "Yellow Rain," possibly dropped from low-flying aircraft, causing symptoms of trichothecene mycotoxin poisoning. It also has been suggested that these toxins have been used by both the Soviets in Afghanistan and by Iraq in its battles with Iran.

Trichothecene mycotoxins produce systemic toxicity and have irritant/vesicant properties. Research has found that trichothecenes inhibit DNA synthesis, protein synthesis, ribosome function, and mitochondrial protein synthesis. In addition, they produce single-strand DNA breaks and inhibit cellular thiol enzymes. The net result is multisystem toxicity, bone marrow suppression, and immune suppression, known as a "radiomimetic" syndrome. Trichothecenes are rapidly absorbed through abraded skin, inhalation, and the GI tract. The US Army has estimated the LD_{50} at 1.2 mg/kg by the oral route.

Dermal or ocular contact will cause irritation, blistering, and eye irritation, followed by systemic toxicity. Inhalation is accompanied by eye irritation, rhinorrhea, dysphagia, dyspnea, chest pain, and hemoptysis, followed by systemic symptoms that may lead to pulmonary edema and cardiovascular collapse. Oral ingestion causes mouth and throat irritation, vomiting and diarrhea, followed by GI bleeding and systemic toxicity. Chronic ingestion (e.g., in the case of contaminated grain) will cause alimentary toxic aleukia.

Poisoning with trichothecene mycotoxins is diagnosed based on environmental findings and the patient's clinical picture. It may be differentiated from mustard gas exposure by the presence of systemic symptoms and the absence of mustard gas agents on field testing. Exposure to ricin may be ruled out by the presence of skin irritation and blistering in the patient exposed to trichothecenes. Radiation levels will not be above background in environments contaminated with trichothecenes. Currently there is no field test for trichothecenes. Samples from grain or exposed surfaces may be sent to a reference lab for confirmatory testing (e.g., gas chromatography/mass spectroscopy).

Trichothecenes and their metabolites may be detected in the serum and urine for up to 28 days after exposure. Clinical specimens should be sent to a reference lab for either antigen detection or GC/MS techniques.

If the toxin has been ingested, activated charcoal should be administered. Treatment for those with trichothecene poisoning is supportive; there is no specific antidote. Attention should be given to maintaining a patent airway, adequate respiratory effort and oxygenation, and hemodynamic status. Standard burn and wound care applies to skin wounds. Hematology/oncology consultation should be obtained for those patients exhibiting signs of coagulopathy or bone marrow suppression. Antibiotic coverage should be considered for those patients with signs of sepsis or infection.

Rescuers should wear protective chemical suits as contact with contaminated skin or clothing leads to dermal irritation. Patients should be decontaminated with soap and water. Their clothing should be removed and confiscated. Surfaces and equipment need to be decontaminated in a solution of 1% sodium hypochlorite with 0.1 M sodium hydroxide for 1 hour of contact time. There are no special precautions for health care workers once decontamination is complete.

SUMMARY

Technology has provided us with both a safer, more nutritious food supply and purified water sources. Tampering or malfunction of these processes may alter their quality with the potential for widespread outbreak of food-borne or waterborne disease. Care of these patients should focus on hydration and antibiotic therapy in certain instances. Trichothecene mycotoxicoses may be of natural or artificial origin with a clinical presentation consistent with vesicant or radiation exposure. Treatment for these cases is supportive. Decontamination of equipment status post any food or waterborne outbreak requires special attention.

RESOURCES

Virtual Naval Hospital: http://www.vnh.org/
World Health Organization: http://www.who.int/topics/food_contamination/en/

REFERENCES

Acheson DWK. 2004. Differential diagnosis of microbial food-borne disease. *Up to date.* http://patients.uptodate.com/topic.asp?file=gi_infec/11820.

Boulton M, Stanbury M, Wade D, Tilden J, Bryan D, Payne J, Eisenga B. 2003. Nicotine poisoning after ingestion of contaminated ground beef—Michigan, 2003, *MMWR* **52**(18):413–416.

Corso PS, Kramer MH, Blair KA, Addiss DG, Davis JP, Haddix AC. 2003. Cost of illness in the 1993 Waterborne Cryptosporidium outbreak, Milwaukee, Wisconsin. *Emerging Infect Dis* **9**(4):426–431.

Kortepeter M, Christopher G, Cieslak T, Culpepper R, Darling R, Pavlin J, Rowe J, McKee Jr K, Eitzen E, eds. 2001. *USAMRIID's medical management of biological casualties handbook.* Fort Detrick, MD: US Army Medical Research Institute of Infectious Disease.

MacKenzie WR, Hoxie NJ, Proctor ME, Gradus MS, Blair KA, Peterson DE, Kazmierczak JJ, Addiss DG, Fox KR, Rose JB. 1994. A massive outbreak in Milwaukee of cryptosporidium infection transmitted through the public water supply. *N Engl J Med* **331**(15):1035.

Pickering LK, ed. 2003, American Academy of Pediatrics. *Red Book: 2003 report of the committee on infectious diseases.* 26th ed. Elk Grove Village: American Academy of Pediatrics.

Provisional Committee on Quality Improvement, Subcommittee on Acute Gastroenteritis. 1996. Practice parameter: the management of acute gastroenteritis in young children. *Pediatrics* **97**(3):424–435.

Torok TJ, Tauxe RV, Wise RP, Livengood JR, Sokolow R, Mauvais S, Birkness KA, Skeels MR, Horan JM, Foster LR. 1997. A large community outbreak of salmonellosis caused by intentional contamination of restaurant salad bars. *JAMA* **278**:389-395.

Wannemacher RW, Wiener SL. 1997. Trichothecene mycotoxins. In *Medical aspects of chemical and biological warfare*, pp. 655–676. Ed FR Sidell, ET Takafuji, DR Franz. Washington, DC: Office of the Surgeon General at TMM Publications.

35 MELIOIDOSIS

Kristin J. Kent, MD*

ETIOLOGY

Melioidosis is on the Category B list of potential bioterrorism agents issued by the United States Centers for Disease Control and Prevention. It is a tropical disease caused by *Burkholderia pseudomallei*, a motile, aerobic, non-spore-forming Gram-negative bacterium found in soil and water. It is transmitted through direct contact of penetrating wounds or skin lesions with contaminated soil and water. Evidence for person-to-person transmission, inhalation of organisms, laboratory acquired infection, and vector transmission have also been documented. The clinical manifestations are widely varied, from asymptomatic to septicemia.

INCIDENCE AND PREVALENCE

Melioidosis is endemic in northern Australia and Southeast Asia. It is most common in Thailand, where the incidence is highest in rural areas and during the rainy season, and it is estimated that between two and five thousand cases of clinical melioidosis occur each year. However, the true incidence of the disease may be underestimated, as it is being more frequently recognized due to awareness and improvement in laboratory capabilities to isolate and identify the bacteria. In the United States confirmed cases are from travelers and immigrants and total 0–5 confirmed cases per year.

RISK FACTORS

Diabetes mellitus is the major risk factor for bacteremic melioidosis. Risk factors for non-bacteremic melioidosis include diabetes mellitus, occupational exposure, preexisting renal disease (most commonly renal calculi), alcoholism, and thalassemia.

*Department of Emergency Medicine, St. Luke's/Roosevelt Hospital Center, New York

Diabetic rice farmers in endemic regions have a six to nine times higher risk for developing melioidosis than non-diabetics and non-rice farmers.

PATHOGENESIS/LIFE CYCLE

B. pseudomallei is not evenly distributed within the environment in endemic areas. Optimal environmental factors include: temperatures of 37–42 °C, pH of 6.8, nitrite fertilizers, and absence of UV light. The organism is typically acquired by direct contact with soil or water, and the virulence of the strain, host immune status, and size of the inoculum play a role in whether exposure of the bacteria leads to disease.

The bacteria infect and survive inside several eukaryotic cell lines. After internalization, the bacteria escape from endocytotic vacuoles into the cytoplasm of the cell and induce actin polymerization at one pole, which forms membrane protrusions in order to spread from cell to cell. It also forms a capsule composed of hydrated glycocalyx polysaccharide, which facilitates formation of microcolonies, protecting the bacteria from antibiotics. *B. pseudomallei* is a difficult organism to kill because it is resistant to complement, lysosomal defensins, and cationic peptides, and it produces proteases, lipase, lecithinase, catalase, peroxidase, superoxide dismutase, and hemolysins.

The organism is found in the sputum, pus, urine, and feces of infected individuals, which contaminate their surroundings; however, the ability of *B. pseudomallei* to multiply once introduced into a new environment is unknown.

INCUBATION PERIOD/TIME OF ONSET

The incubation period for melioidosis can range from 2 days to many years. Infection often remains dormant in the immunocompetent individual, only to manifest itself when immunosuppression or a stressful physiological event occurs (burns/trauma).

PRESENTATION

Melioidosis has varied presentations: from no effect, asymptomatic seroconversions, and various clinically apparent infections. Acute localized infection occurs from inoculation through a break in the skin, is localized as a nodule, can produce fever and general muscle aches, and may rapidly progress to infect the bloodstream. Presentation of acute pulmonary infection may vary from mild bronchitis to severe pneumonia and is typically accompanied by a nonproductive cough or productive cough with normal sputum, high fever, headache, anorexia, and general malaise. It is not uncommon for the illness to be confused with tuberculosis. Acute bloodstream infection usually results in septic shock, is typically short in duration, abscesses are found throughout the body, and, depending on the original site of infection, can include respiratory distress, headache, fever, diarrhea, muscle tenderness, and disorientation. Chronic suppurative infection typically involves the joints, viscera, lymph nodes, skin, brain, liver, lung, bones, spleen, and parotid gland.

DIAGNOSIS/LABORATORY

Melioidosis should be suspected in any patient traveling from an endemic area who is severely ill and has a fever, especially patients with underlying predisposing conditions. The diagnosis is made by isolation of *B. pseudomallei* from blood, urine, sputum, throat, or skin cultures. Cultures should be grown on routine blood agar or MacConkey's agar and Ashdown's selective medium for respiratory tract specimens. With Wright stain, *B. pseudomallei* demonstrates a bipolar safety pin appearance.

Blood culture is the gold standard for diagnosis; however, this method of diagnosis comes with the disadvantage of being time consuming: the mean time to a result is 23.9 hours. Serological tests have the advantage of speed and can be helpful in areas where prevalence is low, but are not useful in endemic areas where the majority of the population is seropositive.

RADIOLOGY

Radiologic presentation is varied and nonspecific. With the acute form of the disease, multiple, small, irregular densities from 4 to 10 mm are the most common finding on chest radiograph. Segmental or lobar consolidation may be seen as the small nodules coalesce, and pleural effusions or empyemas may also be seen. In the subacute form of the disease, upper lobe infiltrates with cavitation are seen on chest radiograph and may be mistaken for tuberculosis. With the chronic form of melioidosis, infection is often extrapulmonary and osteomyelitis may be seen on plain films.

Abdominal ultrasound should be done on all suspected cases as abscesses are often seen in the liver and spleen. Clinically hidden sites of infection may be found with radiolabeled white-cell scanning.

DIFFERENTIAL DIAGNOSIS

The differential diagnosis of melioidosis includes tuberculosis, malaria, typhoid fever, and leptospirosis.

TREATMENT

Treatment should begin with intravenous ceftazidime, imipenem, or the newer beta-lactam/beta-lactamase inhibitors. These treatments have a significantly better survival rate and less adverse effects compared with older conventional regimens of chloramphenicol, doxycycline, and cotrimoxazole. Parenteral treatment should be given for a minimum of ten days and should continue until the patient can take oral medication and has made a clear clinical improvement. Physicians who do not have much experience with treating this disease tend to switch antibiotic treatment prematurely because of the fear of resistance, although resistance occurs in less than 3% of patients. Intravenous therapy should be followed by a 20-week course of oral therapy. Conventional drugs used include a combination of chloramphenicol, doxycycline and trimethoprim-sulphamethoxazole. With this regimen, chloramphenicol is only given for the first 8 weeks. For pregnant women and children 8 years and younger amoxicillin-clavulanate is used.

PROGNOSIS

Prognosis depends on the manifestations of the disease and proper treatment. Mortality is high in the septicemic form of the disease, with a 40 to 90% mortality rate with disseminated septicemia and a 20% mortality rate with septicemia as well as single-organ involvement. Antibiotic treatment decreases mortality, but even after treatment relapse with high mortality rates is common.

PREVENTION

Prevention of melioidosis is difficult because in endemic areas contact with contaminated soil is common. People with skin lesions and risk factors such as diabetes should avoid contact with soil and standing water in endemic areas. Avoiding contact by wearing boots during agricultural work and by using blood and body fluid precautions in healthcare settings can help prevent transmission of the disease. There is no human vaccine for melioidosis.

RESOURCES

www.cda.gov.au
www.cdc.gov/ncidod/dbmd/diseaseinfo/melioidosis_g.htm

REFERENCES

CDC. 2004. Melioidosis. www.cdc.gov/ncidod/dbmd/diseaseinfo/melioidosis_g.htm.01. Accessed August 2004.

Cieslak TJ, Talbot TB, Hartstein BH. 2002. Biological warfare and the skin, I: bacteria and toxins. *Clin Dermatol* **20**:346–354.

Dance DA. 2000. Ecology of *Burkholderia pseudomallei* and the interactions between environmental Burkholderia spp. and human-animal hosts. *Acta Trop* **74**:159–168.

Dance DA. 2000. Melioidosis as an emerging global problem. *Acta Trop* **74**:115–119.

Mukhopadhyay A, Lee KH, Tambyah PA. 2004. Bacteraemic melioidosis pneumonia: impact on outcome, clinical and radiological features. *J Infect* **48**:334–338.

Samuel M, Ti TY. 2004. Interventions for treating melioidosis (Cochrane Review). In *The Cochrane Library*, issue 3. Chichester: John Wiley & Sons.

Suputtamongkol Y, Chaowagul W, Chetchotisakd P, Lertpatanasuwun N, Intaranongpai S, Ruchutrakool T, Budhsarawong D, Mootsikapun P, Wuthiekanun V, Teerawatasook N, Lulitanond A. 1999. .Risk factors for melioidosis and bacteremic melioidosis. *Clin Infect Dis* **29**:408–413.

Tshibwabwa ET, Richenberg JL, Aziz Z. 2002. Lung radiology in the tropics. *Clin Chest Med* **23**(2):309–328.

White NJ. 2003. Melioidosis. *Lancet* **361**:1715–1722.

36 NERVE AGENTS

Frank Guyette, MD*

OVERVIEW

Chemical weapons were first used on a large scale by Germany in World War I. The atrocities witnessed on the battlefield prompted a worldwide convention prohibiting the use of chemical weapons following World War I. Despite this sanction, dozens of countries have chosen to develop and deploy nerve agents, as they are relatively inexpensive to manufacture and raw materials are readily available. Nerve agents are derivatives of the organophosphate insecticides first synthesized in the 1930s. Although initially intended to be more potent insecticides, German scientists quickly recognized the compounds as potential weapons. Weaponized organophosphates are known by common chemical names and two letter designations. The German agents are given a designation of "G" followed by a letter, which denotes their order of discovery. During the Second World War, Nazi Germany manufactured and stockpiled thousands of tons of the agents Tabun (GA) and Sarin (GB). Although the weapons were never used, the Germans continued to develop more lethal agents such as Soman (GD), which was only made in small quantities. Seizing upon this work, British and American scientists continued to refine nerve agents as weapons through the 1950s, resulting in the Viper series of nerve agents, the most common of which is VX. Although little is known about their manufacture, it is thought that the former Soviet Union had produced large quantities of even newer agents.

The first documented use of nerve agents in combat was not until the Iran–Iraq war of the 1980s, when Iraq used combinations of nerve and blister agents against Iranian troops. It is also thought that the Soviets may have used nerve agents in a limited fashion in Afghanistan, while the Serbs allegedly employed them in Bosnia.

Most recently, nerve agents have been considered a potential threat from terrorists and other extremist groups, as they are relatively inexpensive and require only rudimentary scientific expertise to produce. More importantly, many of the precursors necessary for their production can be purchased from reputable sources such as chemical and agricultural companies. In 1994 and 1995 the Aum Shinrikyo cult in Japan

*Department of Emergency Medicine, University of Pittsburgh Medical Center, Pittsburgh

exploited these circumstances, producing small quantities of liquid containing Sarin (GB). Members then released the liquid in an apartment complex and later into crowded subway terminals, killing 19 and injuring over 1300. Despite these relatively small events, the cult members were able to cause significant disruption and strike fear into hearts of millions of Japanese citizens.

PHARMACOLOGY OF CHOLINESTERASE INHIBITORS

Nerve agents exert their biological effects by inhibiting acetylcholinesterase. Acetylcholinesterase rapidly hydrolyzes the acetylcholine ester that acts at the postsynaptic neural junction to cause a nerve transmission. Inhibition of acetylcholinesterase leads to acetylcholine acting unopposed. The unopposed action of acetylcholine causes continual stimulation of skeletal muscles at the neuromuscular junction, which may result in a flaccid paralysis. Excessive acetylcholine levels in the parasympathetic nervous system causes hyperactivity of gastrointestinal motility and glandular secretion. Acetylcholinesterase is also found on erythrocytes (erythrocyte or true acetylcholinesterase) and in the serum as butyrocholinesterase (pseudocholinesterase). When a patient is exposed to nerve agents, the level of acetylcholinesterase is decreased and this can be used as an indicator of severity of exposure.

PRESENTATION

Exposure to nerve agents evokes myriad symptoms, which vary with dose and type of exposure. The agents are not gases, but liquids at room temperature, and can be inhaled as a vapor or absorbed through the skin and mucous membranes. Onset of symptoms varies from seconds, when large quantities of vapor are inhaled, to hours, when small amounts of liquid are absorbed through the skin. Absorption through the skin also varies with the ambient temperature and vascularity of the exposed surface. Following a vapor release, asymptomatic patients can be released from the emergency department immediately, while those with the potential for liquid contamination may require an observation period.

CLINICAL PRESENTATION

Low doses of nerve agent may cause nonfatal poisoning, which can present as increased production of saliva, rhinorrhea, and a feeling of pressure on the chest. The pupil becomes contracted (miosis), and accommodation is reduced so that short-range vision deteriorates. Higher doses cause the symptoms described above plus bronchoconstriction and secretion of mucus in the respiratory system with breathing difficulty. GI cramping and vomiting occur. Muscular weakness, twitching, and convulsions occur due to the effect on the neuromuscular junction by excess acetylcholine. If the dose is high, muscle paralysis occurs. Death is by suffocation due to paralysis of the muscles of respiration.

DIAGNOSIS

The diagnosis of nerve agent exposure is largely based on the history of exposure and clinical findings. It is most important that physicians obtain historical information regarding exposure to unknown substances, insecticides, or unusual odors (most nerve agents smell like fruity camphor). The history of the event also provides important information about the type of exposure. The ideal method for assessing nerve agent intoxication is to assay tissue cholinesterase levels. As this is not possible, plasma and erythrocyte cholinesterase levels can be used as surrogates. Erythrocyte cholinesterase (RBC-ChE) activity can be assessed in some hospital laboratories and is the best means for diagnosis. Inhibition of 50–90% of the enzyme activity is indicative of significant intoxication. This test is limited, however, by its availability, turnaround time, and variations in individual levels of cholinesterase.

DIFFERENTIAL DIAGNOSIS

The symptoms associated with nerve agent intoxication may be the result of other organophosphate compounds such as the carbamate insecticides. Cholinergic crisis can be the result of a variety of medication overdoses, including neostigmine, physostigmine, pyridostigmine bromide, PCP, phenothiazines, clonidine, and muscarinic mushrooms. In addition, CNS symptoms may be mimicked by stroke, seizure, or other neuromuscular disorders. Such clinical findings as rhinorrhea, lacrimation, and bronchospasm may also be present with exposure to riot-control agents.

TREATMENT

Nerve agents have a rapid effect, so that treatment must be immediate. The action of excess acetylcholine at the muscarinic receptor level can be reversed by atropine, which occupies the muscarinic sites and blocks the action of acetylcholine. However, atropine will not have any action at the nicotinic receptors such as the neuromuscular junction. Atropine will improve the effects of excessive parasympathetic stimulation (GI hyperactivity, bronchospasm, excessive glandular secretion and rhinorrhea) but will not reverse the flaccid paralysis seen with toxic doses of nerve agent. Assisted ventilation will be required for patients having such severe muscular weakness that they cannot oxygenate themselves.

Pralidoxime chloride (2-PAM) is the mostly widely available drug that can reactivate the organophosphate inhibited cholinesterases by removing the organophosphoryl moiety. Although the nerve agent initially binds reversibly to acetylcholinesterase, the binding becomes irreversible within a few minutes to several hours depending on the agent. Once "aging" has occurred, displacement of the nerve agent with drugs such as 2-PAM will not occur. Armed forces operating in potential chemical warfare environments carry Mark I autoinjectors (containing pralidoxime chloride (500 mg) and atropine (2 mg), which can be immediately used if a nerve agent is encountered).

Medical treatment depends upon the severity of the nerve agent exposure. This is gauged by the patient's symptoms as outlined below and in Table 1.

Table 1. Treatment for Nerve Agent Exposure

Severity	Vapor exposure	Liquid exposure
Mild	Observation only	2 mg atropine, 600 mg 2-PAM Cl, and observation
Moderate	2 mg atropine, 600 mg 2-PAM Cl, and observation	2–4 mg atropine, 600–1200 mg 2-PAM Cl, and observation
Severe	6 mg atropine, 1800 mg 2-PAM Cl, and 10 mg diazepam	6 mg atropine, 1800 mg 2-PAM Cl, and 10 mg diazepam

Minimal Exposure

Symptoms. With mild exposure the patient may have miosis, headache, rhinorrhea, and salivation, and complain of tightness in the chest.

Treatment. These patients may be managed by removing them from the source of exposure and that may require removal of their clothes. During the subway Sarin attack in Tokyo, patients' clothing continued to "off gas," which resulted in continued exposure of patients plus exposure to medical personnel. Most patients with mild exposure will not require treatment. If eye pain is severe, topical atropine or homatropine can be administered in the eye.

Moderate Exposure

Symptoms. These patients will exhibit all of the signs and symptoms seen with mild exposure plus increased breathing difficulty, muscular fasciculations, and severe rhinorrhea. The rhinorrhea in these patients may be so severe as to fill their gas mask if they are wearing one.

Treatment. These patients usually require atropine and pralidoxime IV or IM. The atropine and pralidoxime are dosed to clinical effect with a maximum of 1500 mg of pralidoxime being used, and the atropine dosing is administered until the patient's secretions are controlled. This will usually require 2 to 6 mg of atropine. If they were exposed to vapor, decontamination can usually be accomplished by removal of clothes. If they were exposed to liquid agent, they will require full liquid decontamination.

Severe Exposure

Symptoms. These patients will exhibit all of the signs listed above plus profound rhinorrhea, severe respiratory difficulty/arrest, flaccid paralysis, and convulsions.

Treatment. Aggressive airway management, including intubation may be warranted. Immediate antidotal therapy should be initiated using 4–6 mg atropine, 1–2 g pralidoxime, and 10 mg diazepam. Supportive ventilatory therapy may need to be maintained for a period of hours after administration of antidotal therapy. This group of patients will require full liquid decontamination.

PROGNOSIS

The prognosis of untreated nerve agent casualties varies with the severity of their exposure. However, those with severe exposures will die from respiratory arrest secondary to airway obstruction and diaphragmatic paralysis within minutes. Conversely, even patients in cardiopulmonary arrest should be treated if resources permit, because they can survive with adequate antidotal and supportive therapy. Patients with less severe exposures may survive delayed treatment but many have noted enduring neurological sequelae.

PREVENTION

The most effective prevention for nerve agent casualties occurs before the event. Few emergency responders have the proper training and equipment to deal with such a crisis. As a result, the best way of preventing casualties is to enforce bans on their manufacture and use and provide adequate intelligence and surveillance to prevent their use by rogue organizations. Other means of prevention include personal protective equipment, patient decontamination, and chemoprophylaxis. Current means of personal protection revolve around the use of protective suits and respiratory equipment. Both are necessary because of the potential hazards associated with inhalation of the vapor and skin absorption of the liquid. The minimum level of protection is level "C" PPE; surgical masks and latex exam gloves are inadequate, as demonstrated in the 1995 Tokyo Subway attack.

Chemoprophylaxis against nerve agents consists of administering reversible cholinesterase inhibitors prior to exposure to prevent binding of the irreversible inhibitors (nerve agents). This is particularly useful if the nerve agent threat is Soman (GD) or another rapidly aging agent. Chemoprophylaxis is fraught with complications, as it must be administered over a period of several hours prior to the exposure with the nerve agent and is not useful against agents with long aging times such as VX and Tabun (GA). Physostigmine and pyridostigmine bromide were both studied for their potential use as nerve agent chemoprophylaxis, but pyridostigmine is the agent of choice as it has fewer side effects. Chemoprophylaxis is of very limited utility given its side effects, its indication only for a limited number of agents, and the need to administer it prior to exposure.

SPECIAL CONSIDERATIONS

For any suspected nerve agent intoxication, an act of terrorism must be ruled out. It is imperative that precautions to prevent contamination of the facility and staff be undertaken as soon as possible. The appropriate emergency management and law enforcement officials should be alerted immediately. Once measures to protect the staff and treat the patient are undertaken, every effort should be made to facilitate public health personnel in the investigation and containment of the event. It is worth noting that the first patients are likely to present to the nearest emergency rooms within minutes, prior to any alert of the medical community. This quickly leads to the nearest facility being overwhelmed despite efforts to evenly distribute patients.

RESOURCES

CDC: www.bt.cdc.gov; Chemical, Biological, Radiological Hotline 1-888-246-2675
www.state.sd.us/doh/bioterrorism/chemical%20agents.pdf
National Response Center: Chemical, Biological, Radiological Hotline: 1-800-424-8802 to report an incident
US Army Medical Research Institute of Chemical Defense (USAMRICD): ccc.apgea.army.mil, (410)-436-2230

REFERENCES

Aas P. 2004. Future considerations for the medical management of nerve-agent intoxication. *Prehospital Disaster Med* **18**(3):208–215.

Allswede, M. 2004. *RaPiD T: WMD training for first responders*. Personal communication.

Berkenstadt H, Amitai Z, Barsuk D, Levine I, Cohen A, Vardi A. 2003. The use of advanced simulation in the training of anesthesiologists to treat chemical warfare casualties. *Anesth Analg* **96**:1739–1742.

Burns MJ, Linden CH. 2001. Chemical and biological warfare agents. In *The clinical practice of emergency medicine*, pp. 1452–1463. Ed A Harwood-Nuss, AB Wolfson, CH Linden, SM Shepherd, PH Stenklyft. Philadelphia: Lippincott, Williams and Wilkins.

Delorenzo RA. 2001. Exposed: signs, symptoms and EMS management of nerve Agent poisoning. *JEMS* **26**(6):48–56. http://www.jems.com/911/911y.html.

Keeler JR, Hurst CG, Dunn MA. 1991. Pyridostigmine used as a nerve agent pretreatment under wartime conditions. *JAMA* **266**:693–695.

Lee EC. 1993. Clinical manifestations of sarin nerve gas exposure. *JAMA* **290**:659–662.

Newmark J. 2004. Therapy for nerve agent poisoning. *Arch Neurol* **61**:649–652.

Robey III WC, Meggs WJ. 2000. Insecticides, herbicides, rodenticides. In *Emergency medicine: a comprehensive study guide*, 5th ed., pp. 1174–82. Ed JE Tintinallli, GD Kelen, JS Stapczynski. New York: McGraw-Hill.

Rotenburg JS, Newmark J. 2003. Nerve agent attacks on children: diagnosis and management. *Pediatrics* **112**:289–292.

Sidell FR. 1997. Nerve agents. In *Textbook of Military Medicine—BW and CW*, pp. 129–179. Ed FR Sidell, ET Takafuji, DR Franz. Washington, DC: US Department of the Army, Office of the Surgeon General, and Borden Institute.

37 VESICANTS

Stephen J. Traub, MD*

OVERVIEW

Historical Significance

Sulfur mustard, more commonly known as "Mustard Gas," and Lewisite are the two major vesicant gases of concern today. Sulfur mustard was used extensively during World War I, and was the chemical weapon that caused the greatest number of casualties in that conflict. Lewisite was synthesized by the United States for use in the European theater in World War I, but the war ended before it was deployed.

Physical Characteristics

Sulfur mustard (military chemical weapon designation: HD) and Lewisite (military chemical weapon designation: L) are formulated alone or in combination with other agents to be liquids over a large range of temperatures. Although they are liquids, they rapidly evaporate due to their high vapor pressure; the resultant gases are denser than air, and thus persist near the ground after release rather than dissipating into the atmosphere. This greatly increases the likelihood that they poison their intended targets.

Mechanism of Action

Vesicant agents appear to react with the DNA of epithelial cells to form chemical complexes that activate cellular repair machinery. The resultant biochemical activity and inflammatory process promotes an exudation of fluid into the subepidermal space; this fluid then forms the characteristic blisters seen with these agents.

In addition to acting as a vesicant, Lewisite may also release large amounts of arsenic when it reacts with epithelial cells, leading to systemic arsenic toxicity as well.

*Division of Toxicology, Beth Israel Deaconess Medical Center, Harvard Medical School, Boston

Presentation

Patients who have been exposed to vesicant gases may present with complaints referable to multiple symptoms, depending on which part(s) of the epithelium is involved:

Dermal toxicity. This is the hallmark of vesicant agent poisoning. Skin blisters tend to be large and painful. Patients exposed to Lewisite tend to develop blisters quickly (on the order of minutes), whereas those exposed to sulfur mustard tend to develop symptoms more slowly (over several hours). Patients exposed to massive doses of sulfur mustard, however, may develop symptoms much more quickly.

Pulmonary toxicity. Coughing, hypoxia, and airway obstruction may all be seen in vesicant gas poisoning due to the sloughing of respiratory epithelial cells.

Ocular toxicity. Ocular irritation of both the conjunctiva and cornea may occur, leading to temporary or permanent visual impairment.

DIAGNOSIS

There are no laboratory tests to assist in the diagnosis of vesicant gas poisoning. In general, a chemical weapons attack should be considered when several, several hundred, or several thousand previously healthy people, who have nothing in common but geographic proximity at a given time, present with similar symptoms. When these symptoms are dominated by dermal, pulmonary, and/or ocular complaints, special consideration should be given to vesicant gas poisoning.

Other scene clues may assist in the diagnosis of vesicant gas poisoning. The presence of a yellow gas suggests sulfur mustard. Sulfur mustard is reported to have an odor of mushroom or onions, and Lewisite an odor of geraniums; a report of either of these smells may also help make the diagnosis.

DIFFERENTIAL DIAGNOSIS

Although the classic presentation of dermal, pulmonary and ocular toxicity strongly suggests vesicant gas poisoning, several other diagnoses should be entertained when patients present with these complaints:

Irritant gases. Irritant gases such as phosgene, diphosgene, and chlorine may produce both ocular and pulmonary toxicity. These agents do not produce dermal toxicity, however.

Nerve agents. Nerve agents may produce pulmonary symptoms and airway obstruction due to increased secretions. Ocular toxicity and dermal toxicity are not expected with this poisoning, however.

Burns. Thermal injury may produce blisters that appear similar to those produced by vesicant gases. The location of the blisters differs, however; thermal burns generally occur on unprotected areas, whereas vesicant gas-induced blisters tend to occur on moist areas of the body (e.g., under the arms), even when these areas are protected by clothing.

TREATMENT

Treatment of a patient who is the victim of vesicant gas poisoning begins with removal of the patient to a safe area. Then next step consists of securing the airway, breathing, and circulation. If the patient is demonstrating apnea, or respiratory failure is imminent, or the patient cannot protect the airway, endotracheal intubation is warranted. Oxygen should be administered to all critically ill patients, especially when there is a suspected or documented hypoxia. Intravenous crystalloid should be administered to patients with hypotension or clinical evidence of hypovolemia.

Decontamination should be performed by trained personnel as soon as possible. Dilute household bleach may be used to decontaminate the skin and hair, but not the eyes. Tap water is appropriate for ocular decontamination, but may be used for skin and hair decontamination if household bleach is not available.

After aggressive skin and hair decontamination, povidone-iodine should be applied to the skin, as this agent has been shown to reduce dermal damage when applied soon after a vesicant agent poisoning.

Pulmonary toxicity is treated with standard supportive measures, including treatment for acute lung injury (ALI) or the acute respiratory distress syndrome (ARDS) should they occur.

Treatment of such patients may challenge even the most competent of physicians. Assistance in the diagnosis and management of patients poisoned by vesicant agents, as well as any other toxins, may be obtained by dialing the local Poison Control Center. In the United States, the closest Poison Control Center can be reached by dialing 1-800-222-1222 from any phone.

PROGNOSIS

The prognosis for patients with vesicant gas poisoning is variable, and depends in large part on the dose absorbed and the availability of prompt, effective medical care. Minor exposures may cause irritation but no lasting effects; severe exposures, especially in circumstances in which access to medical care is limited, may easily result in death.

PREVENTION

Prevention of vesicant gas poisoning lies first and foremost with prevention of a vesicant gas attack. Federal, state, and local government agencies, and in particular the US Department of Homeland Security, are actively working to assure that such attacks do not happen on United States soil.

Pretreatment with topical agents known as highly reactive nanoparticles may limit the toxicity of sulfur mustard. Such agents are currently experimental. Although initial results are encouraging on a scientific level, it is unlikely that pretreatment would be effective in a practical sense, as one would need to know that an attack was going to occur for pretreatment to be effective.

SPECIAL CONSIDERATIONS

Chemical weapons attacks, such as vesicant gas attacks, may generate thousands of patients in a short period of time, rapidly overwhelming even the most prepared of emergency response systems. When such an attack is suspected, the hospital disaster plan should be activated, and local, state, and federal authorities should be immediately notified. One way to be certain that these disparate groups are notified in a timely fashion is to involve the local Poison Control Center early in the event; the center can then help with issues of diagnosis and management, as well as passing information along to the relevant agencies.

SUMMARY

Vesicant agents were commonly used during World War I, and produced hundreds of thousands of casualties. Although used infrequently since that time, vesicant agents are established Weapons of Mass Destruction (WMDs), and therefore a potential tool for terrorists everywhere. Clinicians should understand the chemistry, presentation, diagnosis, differential diagnosis, and treatment in the event of vesicant gas attacks in order to be adequately prepared.

38 PULMONARY AGENTS

Ann-Jeannette Geib, MD, and Michele M. Burns, MD*

OVERVIEW AND HISTORICAL SIGNIFICANCE

Pulmonary agents were originally developed for use as chemical warfare agents in World War I. They currently are employed primarily in industrial applications either as substrates, products, or byproducts. Due to their ease of synthesis, however, their diversion to use as weapons of mass destruction (WMDs) is a very real possibility. This chapter discusses chlorine, phosgene, and nitrogen dioxide (NO_2). Generally, highly soluble gases (i.e., ammonia) produce upper respiratory tract (e.g., eyes, nose, and throat) disease since they are readily absorbed, while less-soluble gases (phosgene and nitrogen dioxide) penetrate deeper with subsequent lower respiratory tract pathology. The reader should refer to specific chapters regarding other gases.

CHLORINE (Cl_2)

Pathogenesis

This irritant gas is heavier than air and intermediately soluble in water, explaining its action as both an upper- and lower-airway irritant with delayed onset of lower-airway symptoms after exposure. Chlorine gas is readily available from several occupational sources, including building maintenance workers as well as public swimming and water purification plants. Chlorine may be formed from inadvertent mixing of an acid with household bleach (sodium hypochlorite). When inhaled, chlorine reacts with pulmonary water to form hydrochloric acid (HCl) and hypochlorous acid (HOCl) plus nascent oxygen (O^-). This combination leads to diffuse pulmonary inflammation, necrosis, acute lung injury, and oxidant injury.

Clinical Presentation

Patients characteristically present with mild eye irritation initially, followed by the onset of respiratory symptoms several hours after exposure. Due to the delayed onset

*Children's Hospital, Harvard Medical School, Boston

of pulmonary symptoms, patients may have had a prolonged period of breathing chlorine gas at moderate concentrations. Irritation of the lower airways will cause cough, dyspnea, and a sensation of chest tightness. Acute lung injury results from inflammation and noncardiogenic pulmonary edema, and is characterized by dyspnea and hypoxia; wheezing or rales may be noted on physical exam. Cough, chest pain, and frothy sputum also can be present.

Diagnostics

Chest radiographs may demonstrate bilateral alveolar infiltrates with a normal cardiac silhouette, differentiating it from congestive heart failure. Tachycardia and hypoxia can be detected with pulse oximetry. Hypoxia and metabolic acidosis may be seen on blood gas analysis.

Differential Diagnosis

Considerations in the differential diagnosis of chlorine exposure include other pulmonary irritants such as phosgene, asthma/reactive airway disease (RAD), and other causes of acute lung injury (ALI)/adult respiratory distress syndrome.

Treatment

Chlorine exposure is treated with supportive care with an emphasis on optimizing oxygen delivery. Care should be taken to ensure a patent airway, even if endotracheal intubation is required. Aerosolized bronchodilators may be required. There are insufficient data to support using parenteral steroids at this point. Treatment with aerosolized bicarbonate is controversial and has not been demonstrated to improve survival, but may provide symptomatic relief to those with mild symptoms. Skin burns are treated as thermal burns, with decontamination, wound care, and pain control. Eyes should be irrigated until a pH of 7.4 is reached and examined for signs of corneal abrasion as well as foreign particulate matter.

Prevention and Protection for Caregivers

A self-contained breathing apparatus (SCBA) may be required for rescuers at the scene.

Special Considerations

Pediatric patients are at greater risk for severe toxicity when compared to adults due to their higher minute volume per kilogram of weight as well as their short stature; these physical attributes expose them to higher concentrations of chlorine. Children more commonly develop stridor than adults due to their smaller airway size, and treatment with aerosolized racemic epinephrine should be provided if this is the case. Patients with signs of mild toxicity should be observed for up to 24 hours for the development of delayed-onset pulmonary edema. Pulmonary symptoms should resolve over the course of a month; however, a prolonged RADS-like syndrome may be present.

PHOSGENE ($COCl_2$)

Phosgene is another of the original chemical agents used in WWI, used under the designation CG. Its use currently is limited to industrial applications where organic compounds such as isocyanates are produced; it is formed from the combustion of organochlorine compounds and may be present at fire scenes, particularly in the industrial setting. It is best known for its odor of "freshly mown hay" and such an agreeable fragrance may not prompt exposed individuals to evacuate. As it is heavier than air, phosgene can cause asphyxiation if victims are found in low-lying areas. Children are more vulnerable to its toxic effects for the reasons described above.

Pathogenesis

Phosgene undergoes slow hydrolysis in the distal portions of the lungs to produce hydrochloric acid, crosslinking of cellular structures, and reactive oxygen species.

Clinical Presentation

Delayed onset (up to 24 hours) of acute lung injury is the chief manifestation of toxicity, although battlefield exposures have been reported to have onset of symptoms within 2–6 hours. As in the case of chlorine, pulmonary edema is noncardiogenic. Systemic illness and death occur because of hypoxia. Long-term effects of phosgene exposure include pulmonary scarring, emphysema, and airway reactivity.

Treatment

Treatment again consists of airway support and oxygenation. Positive pressure may be warranted. Bronchodilators should be administered if the patients exhibit any signs of respiratory distress. Patients with known exposure should be observed for a prolonged period (i.e., up to 48 hours) due to the risk of delayed-onset ALI.

Prevention and Protection for Caregivers

Rescuers should use positive pressure demand SCBA. Phosgene may cause skin burns, so chemical suits are required (Responder, Tychem 10000, or Teflon brands). If liquid phosgene is involved, then the victims' clothing should be removed and double bagged to prevent off gassing.

NITROGEN DIOXIDE (NO_2)

Nitrogen dioxide is a pulmonary irritant that is primarily associated with low-level environmental exposures but of interest to disaster medical personnel because it is created by high-temperature combustion (as in an explosion) and decay of silage (causing silo-filler's disease). At room temperature, NO_2 forms a clear to brown colored liquid. Above its boiling point (21°C), it is a reddish-brown, pungent gas. Heavier than air, nitrogen dioxide may act as a suffocant to those close to the ground and may cause more severe toxicity in children. It is likely that NO_2 will be found in mixture with other oxides of nitrogen (e.g., NO and N_2O_4) and with products of combustion (e.g., sulfur oxides, carbon monoxide, carbon dioxide, and cyanide).

Pathogenesis

Nitrogen dioxide is poorly water soluble and creates nitrous and nitric acids after contact with pulmonary water. In addition to direct corrosive effects, lung damage occurs due to the formation of reactive oxygen species and impairment of normal immune responses.

Clinical Presentation

Those exposed initially complain of mild eye and upper-airway irritation, followed by shortness of breath, cough, and chest pain. Wheezing and noncardiogenic pulmonary edema are the result. Symptoms may be delayed in onset up to 48 hours. Late effects include bronchiolitis obliterans and reactive airways disease syndrome (RADS). Exposure to admixed gases will cause methemoglobinemia, carboxyhemoglobinemia, and metabolic acidosis.

Diagnosis and Evaluation

There are no specific tests necessary for those with nitrogen dioxide exposure; however, obtaining an accurate history is paramount and the clinician should rule out other causes of shortness of breath and/or hypoxia with chest x-ray, ABG, co-oximetry, a methemoglobin level, and routine labs.

Treatment

Treatment is supportive with emphasis on stabilizing an airway and oxygenation. Bronchodilators may be used for patients with wheezing. Oxygen should be administered to any hypoxic patient. Patients should be observed for 48 hours because of the potential for delayed onset of pulmonary edema. Corticosteroids may be of benefit in reducing inflammation and preventing bronchiolitis obliterans. Skin or eye irritation is treated by having affected areas irrigated copiously with water for at least 20 minutes. Methylene blue may be required for methemoglobinemia. Hyperbaric oxygen therapy should be considered for those with carbon monoxide poisoning. After discharge, patients should be reexamined within 1 month and again at 3 months for progression to BO; pulmonary consultation may be required. Bronchiolitis obliterans is characterized by persistent cough, fever, malaise and shortness of breath after the initial insult has resolved.

Prevention and Protection for Caregivers

Rescuers should wear SCBA and chemical-protective suits. Those individuals exposed to liquid or gaseous nitrogen dioxide should be decontaminated in showers to remove any residue on skin and hair. Clothing should be double bagged and discarded in an appropriate manner, since off-gassing of any liquid NO_2 present poses a risk to healthcare personnel. Exposed or irritated eyes should be irrigated with plain water for at least 20 minutes.

SUMMARY

Exposure to irritant gases usually causes pulmonary symptoms and disease from generation of reactive species. Patients with known or suspected exposure should be observed for >24–48 hours for the development of noncardiogenic pulmonary edema.

Treatment in general is supportive with emphasis on improving bronchial airflow and optimizing oxygenation. Corticosteroids may be beneficial for prevention of bronchiolitis obliterans in those exposed to nitrogen dioxide.

RESOURCES

ATSDR Medical Management Guidelines: http://www.atsdr.cdc.gov/MHMI/mmg172.html

REFERENCES

Ainslie G. 1993. Inhalation injuries produced by smoke and nitrogen dioxide. *Respir Med* **87**:169–174.

Anonymous. 2002. Chemical Terrorism Fact Sheet. http://www.bioterrorism.slu.edu. St Louis University.

ATSDR medical management guidelines (MMGs) for nitrogen oxides. www.atsdr.cdc.gov/MHMI.

Douglas WW, Hepper NG, Colby TV. 1989. Silo-filler's disease. *Mayo Clinic Proc* **64**(3):291–304.

Mayorga M. 1994. Overview of nitrogen dioxide effects on the lung with emphasis on military relevance. *Toxicology* **89**:175–92.

Medical management guidelines for phosgene. ATSDR. http://www.atsdr.cdc.gov/MHMI/mmg176.html.

Nelson LS. 2002. Simple asphyxiants and pulmonary irritants. In *Goldfrank's toxicologic emergencies*, 7th ed., pp. 1453–1469. Ed LR Goldfrank, NE Flomenbaum, NA Lewin, MA Howland, RS Hoffman, LS Nelson. New York: McGraw-Hill.

Peterson JS, Cairns CB. 2003. Toxicity, nitrous dioxide. www.emedicine.com/emerg/topic847.htm.

Roberge RJ. 2004. Toxicity, chlorine gas. http://www.emedicine.com/EMERG/topic851.htm 2004 Jun 29.

Segal E, Lang E. 2004. Toxicity, chlorine gas. http://www.emedicine.com/emerg/topic851.htm.

Suchard JR. 2002. Chemical and biologic weapons. In *Goldfrank's toxicologic emergencies*, 7th ed., pp. 1527–1552. Ed LR Goldfrank, NE Flomenbaum, NA Lewin, MA Howland, RS Hoffman, LS Nelson. New York: McGraw-Hill.

Traub SJ, Hoffman RS, Nelson LS. 2002. Case report and literature review of chlorine gas toxicity. *Vet Human Toxicol* 44(4):235–239.

39 CYANIDES

Joshua Nagler, MD*

OVERVIEW

Historical Significance

Cyanide is often perceived as the archetypal poison, with accidental and intentional ingestions since ancient times. It is associated with the Jonestown mass-murder suicides and the Tylenol poisonings in Chicago in 1982. It was used as a military weapon in World War I and in the Nazi gas chambers during World War II. More recently cyanide-based weapons have been used during wars in the Middle East. In the last ten years, cyanide has been used by terrorists in Tokyo subways and by al Qaeda.

Sources of Exposure

Exogenous sources of cyanide include food exposures (bitter almonds, cassava, various fruit seeds/pits), medicines (Laetrile, nitroprusside), and industrial exposures (e.g., electroplating, mining, plastic manufacturing, fumigation). Smoke inhalation in building fires produces cyanide secondary to combustion of natural (e.g., wool, silk) and synthetic (e.g., polyurethane, plastic) materials. Tobacco smoke is also a source of cyanide. As military and terrorist weapons, the compounds of interest are volatile liquid hydrogen cyanide and cyanogen chloride.

Incidence and Prevalence

The incidence of cyanide toxicity is not well known. Only rarely are fatal exposures reported to the Poison Control Centers. Cyanide toxicity may be important in the approximately 10,000 deaths per year from smoke inhalation.

*Beth Israel Deaconess Medical Center, Harvard Medical School, Boston

Pathophysiology

Liquid or gaseous hydrogen cyanide and alkali salts of cyanide are rapidly absorbed through inhalation, ingestion, or absorption through the eyes and skin. Toxicity results from prevention of oxygen uptake at the cellular level. By inhibiting cytochrome oxidase, aerobic metabolism cannot occur. Organs with high-energy requirement such as the brain and the heart are most affected. Increased anaerobic metabolism leads to rapid accumulation of lactic acid and a resultant metabolic acidosis.

PRESENTATION

Time of Onset

The onset of symptoms varies based on the chemical form, the concentration or dose, and the route of exposure. Symptoms develop within seconds of inhalation of high concentrations of hydrogen cyanide, and death can occur within minutes. Cyanide salts are potent poisons and symptoms occur within minutes, and death within hours.

Signs and Symptoms

The earliest symptoms of cyanide toxicity are related to central nervous system stimulation. Headache, confusion, dizziness, and anxiety are accompanied by tachypnea, secondary to primary stimulation of the respiratory center. The earliest cardiovascular effect is tachycardia. Nausea and vomiting may occur.

Significant exposures quickly progress to stridorous breathing and CNS-based respiratory depression with hypoventilation and apnea. Bradycardia, heart block, dysrhythmias, and hypotension are late cardiovascular findings that often precede complete cardiovascular collapse. Final CNS manifestations include seizure, opisthotonos, fixed and dilated pupils, stupor, coma, and death.

DIAGNOSIS

The diagnosis of cyanide toxicity is challenging because of a lack of pathognomonic signs. The clinical toxidrome of bright red venous blood, profound metabolic acidosis, and bitter almond breath is only rarely present. Blood cyanide levels are useful in confirming toxicity; however, acute management should begin before laboratory confirmation is available.

Laboratory

Cyanide levels can be measured directly. Normal plasma cyanide levels are <0.004 μg/ml, but may be higher in smokers. Whole blood levels are higher because cyanide concentrates in red blood cells. Levels correlate with degree of symptoms.

Rapid tests have been developed, including a paper test that has been shown to detect levels over 0.5 mg/liter, and a rapid whole blood assay which may become more available in the future.

Table 1. Cyanide Level and Symptoms

Cyanide level (μg/ml)	Symptoms
<0.2	No symptoms
0.5–1.0	Flushing, tachycardia
1.0–2.5	Stupor, agitation
>2.5	Coma, potentially fatal

Surrogate tests that may suggest cyanide toxicity in an appropriate clinical context include lactate levels >10 mmol/L and a refractory anion gap acidosis. Little difference may exist between simultaneous arterial and venous pO_2 (arterialization of venous blood) secondary to decreased peripheral oxygen extraction.

Pathology

There are no specific pathologic changes that characterize cyanide toxicity. Evidence of tissue hypoxia may be seen, most notably CNS changes including necrosis and demyelination.

Radiological

There are no pathognomonic changes on radiography. Pulmonary edema may occur with significant exposures.

Other

ECG changes are nonspecific. Tachycardia and nonspecific ST-T changes reflect myocardial cellular hypoxia, and may be pronounced in those with underlying cardiovascular disease. AV block, bradycardia, and nodal or idioventricular rhythms occur with progressive cellular hypoxia.

DIFFERENTIAL DIAGNOSIS

Symptoms of cyanide toxicity are nonspecific so the differential diagnosis is broad and dependent on clinical context. With inhalation exposures, carbon monoxide and hydrogen sulfide gas impair oxygen delivery much like cyanide. The differential for anion gap acidosis is best known by the mnemonic MUDPILES (methanol, uremia, DKA, paraldehyde, INH, lactate, ethanol, salicylates).

TREATMENT

Rapid treatment of cyanide poisoning is essential for survival. Initial supportive measures should include 100% oxygen by face mask or endotracheal intubation, intravenous fluid resuscitation with addition of sodium bicarbonate for pH <7.15, and cardiac monitoring. Mouth-to-mouth resuscitation should be avoided. Hyperbaric oxy-

Table 2. Treatment Options for Cyanide Poisoning

Therapy	Mechanism	Dose	Adverse effects	Comments
Amyl nitrite perles	Methemoglobin generator; MetHgb binds cyanide as cyanomethemoglobin	Crush and inhale perle for 30 s of each minute; Replace perle every 3–4 min	Methemoglobinemia (levels of up to 5%); vasodilation; headache	Can be used in mask of spontaneously breathing or ventilatory tubing reservoir in intubated patients; use until sodium nitrite available
Sodium nitrite (3% solution)	Methemoglobin generator, MetHgb binds cyanide as cyanomethemoglobin	*Adult: 300 mg (10 ml) over 4 min; *Pediatric: 0.33 ml/kg at 2.5 ml/min (max 10 ml)	Hypotension; syncope; methemoglobinemia; headache; nausea/vomiting; use with caution with severe cardiovascular or cerebral vascular disease	For moderate to severe poisoning; goal methemoglobin level of 20%; methylene blue causes further release of cyanide, crucial to prevent excessive methemoglobinemia; use caution with smoke inhalation and associated elevated carboxyhemoglobin level
Sodium thiosulfate 25% solution)	Binds cyanide to form thiocyanate, which is renally excreted	*Adult: 12.5 g (50 ml) IV over 10 min; *Pediatric: 1.65 ml/kg (max 50 ml)	Nausea; vomiting; arthralgia; muscle cramps	Only used for known exposure; detoxification rate is slow; thiocyanate toxicity common with renal insufficiency
Hydroxycobalamin	Binds cyanide to form cyanocobalamin, which is renally excreted	*Adult: 4 g IV administered as 1-time dose; *pediatric: unknown	Volume overload	Main limitation: large volume required for treatment; not FDA approved for treatment of cyanide poisoning
Dicobalt EDTA	Chelates cyanide	Adult or pediatric: 4 mg/kg over 1 min, foll.	Hypotension; vomiting; anaphylaxis; face/neck edema;	For moderate to severe poisoning; acts more rapidly than nitrites; anaphylaxis more com-
mon		by dextrose infusion	chest pain; arrhythmias	w/o cyanide poisoning, so only use in known exposure

*May repeat half the original dose in 2 hours if persistent toxicity.

genation has been suggested but has not been proven to be effective. Gastric lavage and/or activated charcoal are indicated for ingestions within 1 hour of presentation. Hemodialysis and hemoperfusion are ineffective, except with high levels of thiocyanate, which is dialyzable. Cyanide antidote kits in the United States are composed of amyl nitrite, sodium nitrite and sodium thiosulfate. Additional agents are currently being used in parts of Europe.

PROGNOSIS

Early recognition and treatment of cyanide toxicity usually leads to a favorable outcome; however, cases are frequently not identified as cyanide toxicity until too late. There is limited data to suggest neurological morbidity—including hyperreflexia, dystonia, cognitive deficits, and parkinsonism—may occur in those surviving exposure.

PREVENTION

Removal from continued exposure is the key to preventing toxicity. Evacuation with gaseous exposures and topical decontamination for liquid exposures by removal of clothing and copious skin washing are paramount.

RESOURCES

CDC: http://www.bt.cdc.gov/agent/cyanide/index.asp.

Department of Homeland Security: http://www.nationalterroralert.com/readyguide/cyanide.htm.

REFERENCES

Ellenhorn MJ. 1997. Respiratory toxicology. In *Ellenhorn's medical toxicology: diagnosis and treatment of human poisoning*, 2nd ed., pp. 476–1484. Ed MJ Ellenhorn. Baltimore: Williams and Wilkins.

Kales SN, Christiani DC. 2004. Acute chemical emergencies. *N Engl J Med* **350**(8):800–808.

Rotenberg JS. 2003. Cyanide as a weapon of terror. *Pediatr Ann* **32**(4):236–240.

40

NUCLEAR DETONATION/ IONIZING RADIATION EXPOSURE

Robert Buckner II, MD, and Peter S. Martin, MD*

OVERVIEW

Recent terrorist threats have placed the potential use of a "dirty bomb" on center stage. "Dirty bombs" disperse radioactive particles through the use of conventional explosives. The low-level radiation contained in the particles that are used to create such a bomb make the conventional explosives the primary danger. Success in treating the victims of a "dirty bomb" attack depend upon: proper planning, identification of potential exposure, prevention of further contamination, implementation of the basic resuscitation principle, and identification of Acute Radiation Syndrome (ARS), which is unlikely in the case of such an attack. Many countries, some designated as terrorist states, have or are in the process of developing traditional nuclear weapons technology. The four types of radiation that can cause injury include alpha, beta, gamma, and neutron. Alpha particles cause no significant threat by external exposure but if taken internally can cause local injury. Beta particles are known to cause skin and eye injury with external contamination and similar damage as alpha particles when internalized. The radiation from gamma and neutron particles penetrates significantly and can cause severe whole-body exposure. High-dose exposure to radiation can lead to ARS, which causes injury to the following organ systems: hematopoietic, gastrointestinal, and central nervous system. Molecular changes within the cells that are exposed to long-term ionizing radiation can lead to the development of cancers over time.

*Department of Emergency Medicine, Allegheny General Hospital, Pittsburgh

PATHOGENESIS

Types of Radiation Injury

Irradiation. The patient is exposed to penetrating radiation from an external source that is not deposited on the body's surface. Exposure stops when the patient leaves the area of radioactive contamination. The patient is not contaminated and poses no risk to others.

External Contamination. The patient is exposed to radiation when radioactive material is deposited on the body's surface. The patient poses a risk to others and must be decontaminated.

Internal Contamination. The patient is exposed to radiation when radioactive material is incorporated into the body through ingestion, inhalation, or absorption through intact or wounded skin. The patient exposure continues until the material is expelled from the body. The patient poses a risk to others and must be externally decontaminated. Definitive treatment is specific to each radioactive material.

Prevention of Further Contamination

- Determine the source of exposure to see if irradiation or contamination has occurred. Unless the sealed container of a radioactive source is intact, assume that contamination has occurred.
- Once notified that potentially exposed patients are en route to your facility, activate your hospital emergency response plan. This often includes contacting hospital resources such as: a Radiation Safety Officer, Nuclear Medicine, Radiation Oncology, or Radiology.
- Prepare a triage site outside of the hospital near an entrance.
- Designate areas of treatment for contaminated and non-contaminated patients, separated by a buffer zone.
- If possible use separate entrances for contaminated and non-contaminated patients.
- Remove all unnecessary equipment from the contaminated treatment area and cover necessary equipment and flooring with well-secured plastic.
- Obtain baseline radiation levels of the treatment area with a radiation detection device, such as a Geiger counter.
- Although radioactive exposure from patients in the hospital is minimal, healthcare workers should utilize personal protective devices including gowns, face masks, eye protection, shoe covers, and two layers of gloves. The inner glove should be taped securely at the wrist and the outer glove should be changed between patients and frequently during the treatment of a patient to avoid recontamination.
- All staff should wear personal dosimeters.
- Patient clothing should be removed by EMS at the scene or staff prior to entering the treatment area.
- Patients should be wrapped in a clean sheet prior to all transports.
- If radioactive exposure is recognized during the treatment of a patient already in the emergency department, designate the area as the contaminated treatment area.

Presentation

ARS is caused by irradiation to all or most of the patient's body by a high dose of penetrating radiation in a short period of time (see Table 1, on acute radiation syndromes). Patients may present at any point of the syndrome. Cutaneous or local radiation syndrome presents like a thermal burn and should be treated as such. If an explosion has occurred, patients may present with blunt or penetrating trauma, thermal burns, or blindness from the flash. Significant psychological stress may be encountered, especially following a terrorist attack.

DIAGNOSIS

Obtain a history of symptoms, occupation, recent or past treatment with radiation or nuclear medicine, and if others have similar symptoms. Maintain a high index of suspicion in patients at risk who present with nausea, vomiting, and leukopenia. Contamination may be detected with a radiation detection device, such as a Geiger counter.

DIFFERENTIAL DIAGNOSIS

- Acute radiation syndrome
- Radiation Therapy-Induced Immunosuppression
- Chemotherapeutic-induced immunosuppression

TREATMENT

Initial triage and treatment is to address immediate life-threatening conditions using basic the resuscitation principle. Remember, in the case of a "dirty bomb" traumatic injuries from the blast are the most life-threatening and the radioactive contamination does not pose an immediate threat. Once the patient is medically stable, decontamination can commence.

Decontamination

- Outer clothing and shoes should have been removed prior to arrival. This can reduce contamination by 90%. Anything removed from the patient (clothing, shoes, hair, blood, urine, stool, etc.) should be double-bagged in plastic and given to the Radiation Safety Officer.
- Irrigate open wounds first with saline or water, then cover with a waterproof dressing to avoid further contamination.
- A water pick or core biopsy technique can be used for puncture wounds.
- Proceed with decontamination of the remainder of the skin, starting with the most contaminated areas. Gently wash with soap and water so as not to break or damage the skin. Skin breakage could potentially lead to internal contamination.
- Rinse eyes with saline or water.

- Wash hair with any available shampoo not containing a conditioner, as conditioners are known to bind material to the hair.
- Consider cutting hair in cases of significant contamination.
- Foreign shrapnel should be handled with forceps and treated as radioactive until proven otherwise.
- Dispose of water appropriately. If you do not have a special containment system, notify the local sewage department immediately.
- Check urine, stool, and nasal swabs (from each nostril) to determine the presence of internal contamination.
- Obtain a baseline complete blood count (CBC) with differential on presentation and every 6–8 hours for 48 hours if total-body radiation is suspected.
- Most sources recommend appropriate broad-spectrum antibiotics if signs of infection occur. These include nausea, vomiting, and diarrhea.
- Prophylactic antifungal and antiviral agents can also be considered, especially if signs of immunosuppression or pancytopenia are present.

PROGNOSIS

Depends upon the following factors: proximity to source, amount of shielding from the source, and length of exposure; in general, the earlier the onset of nausea and vomiting, the worse the prognosis (especially if <4 hours).

SPECIAL CONSIDERATIONS

- Nuclear detonation is much more devastating. Explosions such as those in Japan during the second world war included a nuclear fission reaction. This is very different from the low-level radioactive particles that would be involved in a "dirty bomb".
- "Dirty bombs" are radioactive devices in which radioactive material is dispersed without nuclear detonation but rather through the energy imparted by conventional explosives.
- Trauma from the conventional explosives and the psychological impact on the public would be the most dangerous features of a terrorist attack using a "dirty bomb".
- Nuclear reactors and radioactive material from hospital treatment areas are additional sources of radioactive material that can serve as potential terrorist targets.

RESOURCES

US Department of Energy Radiation Assistance Center Training Site (REAC/TS): http://www.orau.gov/reacts/

Centers For Disease Control and Prevention (CDC) Health Alert Network: http://www.bt.cdc.gov/

The Chemical/Biological Hotline of the National Response Center: 1-800-424-8802

Biodosimetry Assessment Tool (BAT). This is a software application that rapidly assists physicians with collection and documentation of data through the use of templates and offers diagnostic information. Can be downloaded at http://www.afrri.usuhs.mil/www/outreach/biodostools.htm.

REFERENCES

American Academy of Pediatrics Committee on Environmental Health. 2003. Radiation disasters and children policy statement. *Pediatrics* **111**(6):1455–1466. Free text available at www.pediatrics.org.

Department of Homeland Security Working Group on Radiological Dispersal Device Preparedness, Medical Preparedness and Response Sub-Group. 2003. *Medical guidelines.* http://www1.va.gov/emshg/docs/Radiological_Medical_Countermeasures_Indexed-Final.pdf.

Furlow B. 2003. Biological, chemical and radiological terrorism. *Radiol Technol* **75**(2):91–107.

Gusev IA, Guskova AK, Mettler FA. 2001. *medical management of radiation accidents*, 2nd ed. Boca Raton, FL: CRC Press.

Mettler FA, Voelz GL. 2002. Major radiation exposure: what to expect and how to respond. *New Engl J Med* **346**(20):1554–1561.

Military Medical Operations, Armed Forces Radiobiology Research Institute. 2003. *Medical management of radiological casualties*, 2nd ed. Bethesda, MD: Armed Forces Radiobiology Research Institute. http://www.afrri.usuhs.mil/www/outreach/pdf/radiologicalhandbooksp99-2.pdf.

Smith J, Spano M. 2003. *Interim guidelines for hospital response to mass casualties from a radiological incident*. Washington, DC: Department of Health and Human Services, Centers For Disease Control and Prevention. http://www.bt.cdc.gov/radiation/pdf/Mass Casualties Guidelines.pdf.

Turai I, Veress K, Gunalp B, Souchkevitch G. 2004. Medical response to radiation incidents and radionuclear threats. *Br J Med* **328**:568–572.

US Department of Defense. 2000. *Chemical and biological defense program.* Annual report to Congress. http://www.defenselink.mil/pubs/chembio02012000.pdf.

41

HAZARDOUS MATERIAL DISASTERS

Robert E. Antosia, MD, MPH*

INTRODUCTION

Disasters involving exposures to hazardous materials are relatively rare events, but they still represent one of the most common disasters in the community setting. Experts agree there are over 100,000 hazardous materials in our society. Chemicals are also effective terrorist weapons. These materials can be solids, liquids, or gases. Exposures can result in significant morbidity. Acutely, these materials can produce acute trauma such as burns, pulmonary edema, respiratory arrest, explosion injuries, and neurological injuries. Chronic effects may include progressive organ dysfunction, infertility, birth defects, and cancer.

Victims of hazardous material (HazMat) incidents often seek medical assistance and care in the emergency department. The risk of personal injury due to secondary contamination to EMTs, other pre-hospital medical personnel, and staff mandates specific policies and personal protection equipment (PPE) to prevent exposure to off-gassing chemicals and direct unprotected contact with the victim.

A hazardous material is any substance that is potentially toxic to the environment or to animals and humans. However, accurate and reliable data on the public health consequences of hazardous materials releases are difficult to obtain. Few agencies worldwide mandate reporting human exposure to hazardous materials to governmental authorities. In the United States, the Agency for Toxic Substances and Disease Registry (ATSDR) has maintained active state-based HazMat emergency event system since 1990.

ATSDR data reveal that 79% of these hazardous material releases occur at fixed sites (i.e., industrial sites, schools, farms, and manufacturing facilities) and 21% are transportation related. A single substance is released in 90% of reported events. Volatile organic compounds, acids, ammonia, pesticides, and other organic substances are most commonly involved.

*Department of Emergency Medicine, Beth Israel Deaconess Medical Center, Harvard Medical School, Boston

A patient is considered contaminated when direct physical contact with a hazardous material has occurred and the substance remains on the body or clothing. When hazardous materials are present at an emergency, incident, or disaster, patients must be decontaminated before or during medical treatment.

Many disasters are not actual chemical incidents, but involve a large number of chemically exposed patients. Examples include natural disasters, transportation accidents, and the potential of a BT attack. In these situations, victims are dispersed over a widespread area. Contamination is often discovered by EMS teams during triage. Affected patients must be removed from the source and decontaminated before they are moved to a treatment area to protect rescuers, medical personnel, and expedite patient care.

The proper personal protection equipment is essential when hazards are present, as well as appropriate reference sources including the regional poison center, or from the material safety data sheet (MSDS).

The basic principles of decontamination are summarized as follows:

- Move the patient away from further exposure
- Remove the patient's clothing and jewelry
- Wash the patient, or use dry wiping for water reactive materials.

REGULATIONS

For healthcare workers, HazMat preparedness is a matter of worker safety. Hospitals must support systems that protect ED personnel and other healthcare workers who are caring for contaminated patients. Because many contaminated patients receive initial care (i.e., decontamination) at the hospital, ED personnel, as well as the facility, are at risk of secondary contamination if victims are not treated appropriately.

OSHA regulations require workplaces to be free from recognized hazards that may cause serious physical harm or death to employers. Employers are also required to provide appropriate PPE and training to employees who may have the potential of being exposed to hazardous materials.

OSHA, the National Institute for Occupational Safety and Health (NIOSH), and the Joint Commission on Accreditation of Hospitals (JCAHO) have developed regulations and standards specific to HazMat emergencies. As a result, every ED must address certain regulatory issues specific to decontamination including the following: a written hospital emergency response plan; personal protection equipment including fitness to wear PPE; and a minimum of training to meet OSHA's First Responder Awareness Level, including an understanding of how to recognize a potential HazMat problem and respond accordingly. Specific PPE is discussed elsewhere in the text as it pertains to these standards.

In the event of a mass casualty incident (MCI) that results in HazMat contamination and poses a threat to life or health, performing emergency decontamination is necessary. Patients should be directed outside the ED near the entrance to await evaluation and decontamination. In addition, the hospital HazMat response plan should be activated. Fortunately, the vast number of exposures involve only one or two victims. However, terrorists have shown the willingness and capacity to use hazardous chemicals when attacking civilians. As such, hospitals need the assessment skills, decontamination equipment, and other appropriate resources to offer care for such patients.

REFERENCES

Hogan DE, Burstein JL, eds. 2002. *Disaster preparedness*. Philadelphia: Lippincott, Williams and Wilkins.

Smithson A. 2000. *Ataxia: the chemical and biological terrorism threat and the US response*. Report no. 35. Washington DC: The Henry L. Stimson Center.

Brennan RJ, Waceckerle JF, Sharp TW, Lillibridge SR. 1999. Chemical warfare agents: emergency medical and emergency public health issues. *Ann Emerg Med* **34**:191–204.

42

MARITIME DISASTERS

Robert E. Antosia, MD, MPH*

OVERVIEW

Disasters at sea have plagued society since ancient times. Although travel by sea is no longer as common as it was before the advent of aviation, sea disasters still occur, both with passenger and cargo vessels. According to the US Coast Guard, almost 50% of deaths and over 75% of the injuries that occur at sea are due to incidents on board that are not related to operation of the vessel (e.g., falling overboard, crush injuries, and fires). The majority of injuries and deaths are associated with ships with a high intensity of industrial activity, such as fishing vessels.

The definition of disaster takes on a relatively new meaning when applied to the maritime situation. At sea the communities are very small and resources are minimal compared to shore-side catastrophes, so not much is required to turn a shipboard emergency into a disaster.

Maritime disasters can be roughly divided into the following four groups: collisions, weather-related events, fires, and infectious diseases. Collisions between seagoing vessels are relatively uncommon. Unfortunately, a far greater number of shipwrecks are caused by rocks and reefs. Collisions occur with sudden onset and often with little or no warning. The most common cause is a combination of navigational hazards and bad weather. Receiving facilities must be prepared to handle trauma, hypothermia, and immersion injuries. Weather problems usually have a gradual onset with some warning. While bad weather is usually no surprise, its effects of capsizing and foundering usually are. The latter, foundering, is often due to a breach of the structural integrity of the ship and almost always results in loss of the vessel. In contrast, a fire may become a disaster without threatening the viability of the ship itself because of its effects on the ship's systems and inhabitants. Almost half of vessel fires start in the engine room with no warning. Fortunately, most on-board fires are easily contained, but many individuals may suffer from its effects from burns, smoke inhala-

*Department of Emergency Medicine, Beth Israel Deaconess Medical Center, Harvard Medical School, Boston

tion, and carbon monoxide (CO) poisoning. Food- and waterborne disease outbreaks are common and typically have a gradual onset with some warning. According to the Centers for Disease Control and Prevention (CDC), approximately 1 in 400 cruises has an outbreak of a diarrheal illness that is significant enough (>2%–3% of the crew or passengers) to warrant epidemiologic investigation. Overall, the Norwalk Virus is the most common cause, and facilities should be prepared to handle dehydration and electrolyte disturbance.

MARITIME DISASTER PLANNING

All ships are required to have a safety plan that includes a disaster plan in accordance with the International Maritime Organization. This includes standard procedures and drills. The medical department on cruise ships is part of this plan and is included in the drills. Lifeboat(s), stretcher team, fire and basic life support drills should be part of the safety plan. Large cruise ships also usually have their own disaster plan for which they are responsible with regard to maintenance and implementation. Such vessels also have a secondary medical space for both the storage of additional medical supplies and equipment, as well as area where medical care can be rendered if the main infirmary is overcrowded or inaccessible.

The sequence of events in a maritime disaster response is somewhat different than that in shore-side disasters. This is primarily related to location and the fact that external resources are distant. Unless the vessel happens to be in coastal waters within a few hundred miles of a Coast Guard airbase, no chance for rapid air evacuation exists and no hospital will be in close proximity. Incidents usually involve specialized response teams, and not the standard municipal police, fire, and emergency medical service (EMS) personnel. Due to environmental factors, most deaths usually result from hypothermia, shock, or drowning. Injuries may also occur from blunt or penetrating trauma, thermal burns, or from exposure to hazardous materials that may be carried as cargo, such as heavy fuel oil. Any resultant oil spill can also complicate rescue and recovery operations.

Sometimes in maritime disasters evacuation may be necessary. Radio contact with the Coast Guard is initiated, and the usual method of mass evacuation is by a military or command ship. If no outside help is available, lifeboats serve as the ambulance of last resort. According to international law, all ships must have an adequate number of lifeboats that are provisioned with food, water, and medical supplies. As a result, shore-side emergency departments and EMS systems usually have adequate time to prepare for the reception of victims from a maritime disaster.

RESOURCES

United States Coast Guard: www.uscg.mil

REFERENCES

Barnaby KC. 1968. *Some ship disasters and their causes*. New York: A.S. Barnes.

Hogan DE, Burstein JL. 2002. *Disaster medicine*, pp. 279–286. Philadelphia: Lippincott, Williams, and Wilkins.

Levinson J, Granot H. 2002. *Translation disaster response handbook*, pp. 247–252. San Diego: Academic Press, San Diego.

US Coast Guard. 1992, *Comdtist M16465.6 marine safety manual*. Washington, DC: Department of Transportation, US Coast Guard.

43

AVIATION DISASTERS

Robert E. Antosia, MD, MPH*

OVERVIEW

Crashes involving aircraft have occurred since the beginning of flight. With both the capacity and number of commercial airliners increasing, the risk of a catastrophic event involving an aircraft has multiplied. By 1997 the number of commercial air passengers had increased to 630 million, and it is expected to exceed 985 million by the year 2009. Aviation accidents have the potential for significant loss of life and for generation of a high number of casualties.

There are many causes of aviation disasters. They may result from acts of terrorism but much more frequently are related to human error (pilot or control tower), mechanical failure, or limiting factors including weather (dense fog, icing, and wind shear). Most accidents are usually the result of a combination of these factors. The majority of aviation accidents involve private aircraft (including helicopters) or smaller commercial planes. Although crashes involving large commercial aircraft represent the minority of accidents, they tend to garner more media and public attention.

Since the 1980s, aviation safety has improved dramatically, reducing the number of fatalities by 34%. The aviation community has used past experiences to improve safety aspects of modern aircraft. The US National Transportation and Safety Board (NTSB) develops regulatory and safety policies and investigates aviation incidents (an occurrence with no injury or death) and accidents (bodily harm or death). According to the NTSB, most preventable passenger deaths can be attributed to lack of familiarity with safety procedures, despite preflight instructions. In addition to aircraft crashes, other accidents include turbulence, rapid decompression, and explosions aboard the aircraft.

*Department of Emergency Medicine, Beth Israel Deaconess Medical Center, Harvard Medical School, Boston

PRE-HOSPITAL CONSIDERATIONS

From a pre-hospital perspective, the unique considerations that involve aircraft accidents must be addressed. The first consideration is access to the scene. In aviation crashes over open sea, response efforts are centered at the nearest land areas. Such crashes present unique challenges to emergency medical services (EMS), search and rescue, and primarily recovery efforts since there are unfortunately few survivors. Air crashes occurring in and around an airport will often occur within the confines of the flight line. Larger and busier airports may either suspend or continue active flight operations near the crash site. EMS units should receive prior training on responding to these situations and have established communication links with the airport control tower and fire/rescue units. A triage area should be established, and all victims should be directed to the triage area. This is important, as it improves the process of identifying and assessing all survivors. Responders need to be aware of the particular hazards associated with downed aircraft: leaking aviation fuel, potential fire hazards, toxic fumes, and scattered debris, which may be hot. Security issues and evidence preservation (terrorist events) are also concerns.

MECHANISM OF INJURY

Injuries from air crash disasters may result from: rapid deceleration, blunt trauma, penetrating trauma, burns, smoke inhalation, hazardous materials exposure, and dysbarisms due to rapid decompression and altitude changes. Rotary wing accidents due to helicopter crashes typically result in vertebral injuries and fractures. This occurs because of the intense vertical deceleration forces. Thermal injuries are infrequently seen due to the success of the crashworthy fuel systems used in helicopters. Fixed-wing aircraft fly at much greater altitudes and therefore need to have compressed cabins. Sudden changes in cabin pressure can lead to hypoxia and rapid decompression problems. The latter include clinical problems such as pneumothoraxes, hypothermia, and decompression sickness. Complications from aircraft fires are common and range from thermal injury and burns to smoke inhalation and inhalation of toxic gases including carbon monoxide and hydrogen cyanide. Additionally, the mental health impact and environmental factors associated with particular crashes, such as near-drowning, need to be considered.

PREVENTION OF INJURIES

More people are using airplanes today as a mode of transportation. For this reason, aircraft crashes require pre-hospital care providers, emergency personnel and public health agencies to make special preparations, adequate plans, and drills in order to appropriately respond to an air crash disaster. The unique hazards associated with these types of disasters should also be understood to help reduce further risk to both responders and survivors.

RESOURCES

National Transportation Safety Board, National Aviation Safety Data Analysis Center: www.nasdac.faa.gov

REFERENCES

Levinson J, Granot H, eds. 2002. *Transportation disaster response handbook*, pp. 223–245. San Diego: Academic Press.

Li G, Baker SP. 1997. Injury patterns in aviation-related fatalities. *Am J Forensic Med Pathol* **18**:265–270.

National Transportation Safety Board. 1998. *We are all safer*, 2nd ed. Washington, DC: National Transportation Safety Board. http://www.ntsb.gov/publictn/1998/SR9801.htm.

PART IV

Medical Management of Disaster-Related Injuries and Disease

IVA

Basic Emergency Medicine

44

THE ABCs AND RESUSCITATION ALGORITHMS FOR CARDIOPULMONARY ARREST

Lawrence Lo, MD, and Kaushal Shah, MD*

OVERVIEW

The healthcare provider responding to a disaster needs to be prepared to recognize and treat cardiac arrest. Several factors may play a role in deciding on resuscitative efforts in a disaster: cause of the arrest (if known), time down, size and scope of the disaster, triage protocol, and available resources. This chapter has been presented in algorithmic format for simplification

ABCs

A. Airway
   1. Open airway with chin lift or jaw thrust maneuver if c-spine compromise is suspected
   2. Remove any foreign debris

B. Breathing
   1. Assess breathing by the "look, listen, and feel" method
      — look at the chest rise
      — listen for breath sounds
      — feel breath (exhalation) from mouth/nose against your cheek
   2. Consider supplemental oxygenation via bag-valve mask ventilation or intubation

*Department of Emergency Medicine, St. Luke's/Roosevelt Hospital Center, New York

C. Circulation
 1. Check pulses (carotid/radial/femoral)
 2. Check skin color and cap refill (<2 seconds)
 3. Start CPR if no palpable pulse

D. Disability
1. Perform a quick neurologic assessment using the AVPU scale (alert, responds to verbal stimuli, responds to painful stimuli, or unresponsive)

E. Exposure
1. The patient should be completely disrobed to assess for other visible injuries (i.e., open fractures or stab wounds)

Primary Survey: the primary survey is used to quickly assess and effectively manage most immediate life-threatening issues.

PULSELESS VENTRICULAR TACHYCARDIA/FIBRILLATION

— Shock 200 J, shock 300 j, shock 360 j
— Oxygen, monitor, IV access, intubate
— Epinephrine
  - 1 mg IV
  - Alternative: vasopressin 40 Units IV x1
  - Shock 360 J
  - Continue every 3–5 minutes
  - Shock 360 J
— Amiodarone
  - 300 mg IV push (may repeat 150 mg; max 2.2 g over 24 hours)
  - Maintenance: 1.0 mg/min or 360 mg over first 6 hours, then 0.5 mg/min or 540 mg IV over 18 hours; precautions: low BP/HR
  - Shock 360 J
— Lidocaine
  - 100 mg IV (1–1.5 mg/kg) (may repeat to max of 3 mg/kg)
  - Maintenance: 1–4 mg/min
— Magnesium
  - 2 g IV (if hypomagnesemia/prolonged QT or torsades)
— Procainamide
  - Use if VF/VT breaks and recurs
  - 50 mg/min IV (max 17 mg/kg, so approx 20 min)
  - Maintenance: 1–4 mg/min
  - Precautions: low BP, double QRS, or max dose discontinue

ASYSTOLE

- CPR
- Epinephrine 1 mg IV q 3–5 min
- Atropine 1 mg IV q 3–5 min (max 0.04 mg/kg or approx 3 doses)
- Transcutaneous pacing

PULSELESS ELECTRICAL ACTIVITY (PEA)

- CPR
- Epinephrine 1 mg IV q 3–5 min
- Atropine 1 mg IV q 3–5 min (max 0.04 mg/kg or approx 3 doses)
- Correct underlying etiology

The Five "T's"
  - Tamponade
  - Tension pneumothorax
  - Thrombosis, cardiac
  - Thrombosis, pulmonary emboli
  - Tablets (overdose)

The Five "H's"
  - Hypovolemia
  - Hypoxia
  - Hydrogen ions (acidosis)
  - Hypothermia
  - Hyper/hypo K^+, Mg^{2+}, and Ca^{2+}

BRADYCARDIA

Atropine 1 mg IV
Transcutaneous Pacing
Dopamine 5–20 μg/kg/min
Epinephrine 2–10 μg/min

TACHYCARDIA

Unstable

- Shock non-sinus rhythms

Stable: Wide

- Stable VT load with amiodarone 150 mg IV over 10 minutes and magnesium 2 grams IV if polymorphic
- Supraventricular Tachycardia (SVT) with aberrancy: treat like VT (no reliable criteria to distinguish the difference!)

Stable: Narrow

- Atrial Fibrillation/Flutter: these should be thought of as the same problem
  - Less than 48 hours: cardiovert with electricity or amiodarone
  - Greater than 48 hours: rate control (beta blockers, calcium channel blocker, digoxin) and anticoagulate

- SVT: vagal maneuvers, adenosine 6 mg IV push (may repeat with 12 mg), verapamil
- Multifocal Atrial Tachycardia (MAT): rate control (calcium channel blocker preferred over beta blocker if COPD/asthma) and treat underlying disorder (usually COPD)

CLINICAL PEARLS

- Unstable may be defined as: hypotension, chest pain, dyspnea, altered mental status, and acute congestive heart failure
- Verapamil and adenosine are contraindicated for wide complex tachycardia
- Drugs that can be given through the endotracheal tube (NAVEL): naloxone, atropine, valium or vasopressin, epinephrine, lidocaine (remember to use 2–3 times the dose)
- Guidelines for Amount of Joules for Cardioversion/Defibrillation
    - o Aflutter: start 50 J
    - o VT/VF: start 200 J
    - o All other rhythms: start 100 J
- Do not cardiovert in normal sinus tachycardia! Treat underlying disorder.
- Wolf-Parkinson-White Syndrome: avoid ABCD (adenosine, beta-blockers, calcium channel blockers, digoxin) because AV nodal blockade will cause paradoxical increase in heart rate.

RESOURCE

The following website has all of the American Heart Association Algorithm: http://www.ace.cc/new%20acls%20guidelines.htm.

45

SHOCK: DIAGNOSIS AND MANAGEMENT

Kaushal Shah, MD*

OVERVIEW

Significance

The ability to diagnose and manage shock (defined as widespread inadequate tissue perfusion) is central to the practice of disaster medicine. It behooves everyone involved (EMTs, paramedics, nurses, physicians, etc.) to be able to identify the different types of shock, as it is truly a life-threatening condition. If it is not emergently reversed, systemic inflammation, organ dysfunction and death may ensue.

Etiology

Trauma and infection are the most likely etiologies of shock in the disaster setting. Trauma most commonly will cause hypovolemic shock from blood loss, but it can also result in neurogenic shock from a cervical spine injury and obstructive shock from a traumatic tension pneumothorax or cardiac tamponade. All Category A biological agents (defined by the Centers for Disease Control as those with the greatest impact on public health) can cause septic shock.

Types of Shock

- Hypovolemic: decreased intravascular blood volume, e.g., hemorrhage
- Neurogenic: vasodilatation from loss of central sympathetic tone resulting in a relative hypovolemia, e.g., cervical spine injury impinging on the spinal cord
- Obstructive: a physical obstruction to blood flow, e.g., cardiac tamponade

*Department of Emergency Medicine, St. Luke's/Roosevelt Hospital Center, New York

- Septic: severe infection causes vessel dilatation and leakage, e.g., pneumonic plague infection
- Cardiogenic: loss of forward blood flow because of inability of heart to adequately pump, e.g., massive myocardial infarction
- Anaphylactic: histamine release in response to allergen causes severe inflammation and loss of vascular tone and capacitance, e.g., peanut allergy

PRESENTATION

History

In the majority of cases, especially in disaster medicine settings, the history will identify the most likely type of shock. Severe burns and physical injuries are most likely to result in hypovolemic shock due to fluid or blood loss. Consider septic shock if there is exposure to biological agents. Neck injuries resulting in neurogenic shock are not usually subtle, but the diagnosis can be overlooked when there are multiple simultaneous injuries. Consider obstructive shock (tension pneumothorax or cardiac tamponade) with penetrating injuries.

Signs and Symptoms

The presentation of shock varies with the type and etiology. Hypotension after trauma is usually due to hemorrhage. The ensuing hypovolemic shock results in peripheral vasoconstriction to divert the reduced blood volume to the critical organs; therefore, the skin is cool and moist and the neck veins are flat. A reflex tachycardia is common. Patients usually complain of lightheadedness, especially with standing (orthostasis).

Warm skin in a trauma patient is suspicious for neurogenic shock. The body is unable to peripherally vasoconstrict due to loss of sympathetic tone.

Warm skin is expected, on the other hand, in cases of septic shock. Bacterial endotoxins cause peripheral vasodilatation and leakage. Fever (rarely hypothermia) and diaphoresis are also common. The heart initially becomes hyperdynamic to increase the circulation of a relatively reduced blood volume, resulting in tachycardia and a strong pulse. In the latter stages of septic shock, the pulse weakens and the extremities become cool.

A puncture wound to the chest should prompt inspection of the neck veins and auscultation of the heart and lungs to diagnose obstructive shock. Unilateral decreased breath sounds, low oxygen saturation, jugular venous distention, and possible tracheal deviation are signs of a tension pneumothorax; patients usually complain of shortness of breath and chest pain. In the setting of hypotension, jugular venous distention and muffled heart sounds (Beck's Triad), one should consider cardiac tamponade.

DIAGNOSIS

Empiric criteria for the diagnosis of circulatory shock requires 4 of the following: (1) ill appearing or altered mental status, (2) heart rate >100, (3) respiratory rate >22 or

$PaCO_2$ <32 mm Hg, (4) arterial base deficit <–5 mEq/L or lactate >4 mM, (5) urine output <0.5 ml/kg/hr, (6) arterial hypotension >20 minutes duration.

Once the diagnosis of shock is determined, the critical task is to identify the type of shock in order to treat appropriately.

Hypovolemic Shock

Consider in cases of suspected hemorrhage or severe burns. Tachycardia, low blood pressure, and cool, moist skin are characteristic.

Neurogenic Shock

Consider in cases of spinal cord trauma. Low blood pressure, bradycardia, and warm skin are characteristic.

Obstructive Shock

Consider in chest trauma cases. Chest pain, shortness of breath, unilateral decreased breath sounds, jugular venous distention, hypotension, tachycardia, and tracheal deviation are characteristic of tension pneumothorax. Hypotension, jugular venous distention, and muffled heart sounds (Beck's Triad) are characteristic of cardiac tamponade.

Septic Syndrome

Two or more Systemic Inflammatory Response Syndrome (SIRS) criteria (see below) in addition to hypotension or organ dysfunction (can include lactic acidosis, oliguria, or altered mental status) is considered sepsis. Hypotension despite adequate fluid resuscitation is considered septic shock. SIRS Criteria: (1) temperature >38°C or <36°C, (2) heart rate >90, (3) respiratory rate >20 or $PaCO_2$ <32 mm Hg, (4) WBC count >12,000 or <4,000 or Band neutrophilia >10%

TREATMENT

Always start with the ABCs.

Hemorrhagic Shock

1. Control hemorrhage, if possible
2. Infuse intravenous fluids (20 ml/kg) and, if available, packed red blood cells (5–10 ml/kg)

Neurogenic Shock

1. Ensure c-spine immobilization
2. Infuse intravenous fluids (20 ml/kg)
3. Treat hypotension (systolic BP < 90) and bradycardia with atropine 1 mg (may repeat to a maximum of 0.04 mg/kg)
4. Consider dopamine starting at 5-20 μg/kg/min

Obstructive Shock

1. Tension pneumothorax
   a. Needle thoracostomy of chest with 14–16 gauge needle in the second intercostal space on the mid-clavicular line provides immediate decompression
   b. Chest tube should be placed for more definitive decompression
2. Cardiac tamponade
   a. Infuse intravenous fluids (20 ml/kg) as temporizing measure
   b. Pericardiocentesis, if not stable enough for transport to the operating room
   c. Thoracotomy to open the pericardial sac and relieve the tamponade, if patient loses vital signs

Septic Shock

1. Ensure adequate ventilation and oxygenation
2. Infuse intravenous fluids (20 ml/kg initially but an adult patient may require 5–6 liters before adequate urine output is restored)
3. Antimicrobial therapy tailored to suspected source
4. If crystalloid resuscitation fails, start a vasopressor
   a. Dopamine 5–20 μg/kg/min
   b. Norepinephrine 0.1–1.0 μg/kg/min

RESOURCES

CDC website for bioterrorism: http://www.bt.cdc.gov/
US Army Medical Research Institute of Infectious Disease: http://www.usamriid.army.mil/

REFERENCES

Carcillo JA, Cunnion RE. 1997. Septic shock. *Crit Care Clin* **13**:553–574.

Karwa M, Bronzert P, Kvetan V. 2003. Bioterrorism and critical care. *Crit Care Clin* **19**:279–313.

Kline JA. 2002 Shock. In *Rosen's emergency medicine*, 5th ed., pp. 938–956. Ed JA Marx. St. Louis: Mosby.

Rivers E, Nguyen B, Havstad S, Ressler J, Muzzin A, Knoblich B, Peterson E, Tomlanovich M. 2001. Early goal-directed therapy in the treatment of severe sepsis and septic shock. *New Engl J Med* **345**(19):1368–1377.

46 INTRAVENOUS FLUID REQUIREMENTS AND BLOOD PRODUCTS

Michael Levine, MD,* and Ryan E. Braun, MD**

INTRODUCTION

Numerous bioterrorism agents can cause alterations in fluid homeostasis. Similarly, all trauma patients are at significant risk for fluid disturbances. There are numerous agents available to correct fluid disturbances. A basic understanding of physiology as well as knowledge of the various fluids available will enable the clinician to choose an appropriate fluid replacement and successfully manage these challenging patients.

FLUID COMPARTMENTS

The total body water (TBW) comprises 60% of the body's total weight in males and 50–55% in females. These values vary, however, according to age, lean body mass, and weight. The TBW is lower in young lean individuals, and is higher in older obese individuals. The TBW resides in two compartments: the intracellular fluid (ICF) and the extracellular fluid (ECF). The ICF accounts for two-thirds of the TBW (approximately 28 liters), while the ECF accounts for a third (approximately 14 L). The ECF can be further subdivided into intravascular and interstitial compartments. The intravascular and interstitial compartments account for 25% (approximately 3.5 L), and 75% (approximately 3.5 L), respectively, of the ECF.

Movement of fluid between compartments occurs via passive diffusion. Normally, the capillary membrane separating the intravascular and interstitial compartments is permeable to water, small solutes, and electrolytes. The net flow of water occurs as a result of the osmotic pressure gradient between compartments.

*Harvard-Affiliated Emergency Medicine Residency, Brigham and Women's Hospital/Massachusetts General Hospital, Boston

**Department of Anesthesiology, University Hospitals of Cleveland, Case School of Medicine. Cleveland

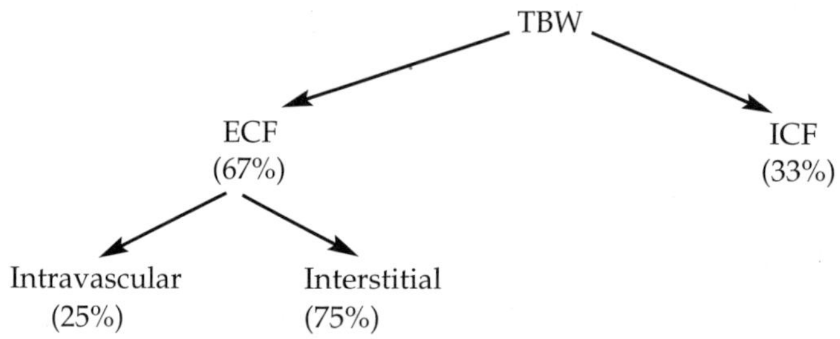

Figure 1. Total body water.

Sodium and chloride constitute more than 90% of the effective solutes in the ECF. The serum sodium concentration determines the relative amount of water and sodium in the plasma. The size of the ECF and ICF compartments are dependent on the amount of water within each compartment, while the distribution of water is dependent upon the osmolality.

FLUID REQUIREMENTS

Fluid administration should equal fluid losses. An average individual must consume enough fluid to equal the losses in urine (12–15 cc/kg/d), stool (3 cc/kg/d), and sweat (0–1.5 cc/kg/d). An additional 1 L of fluid is lost due to insensible losses from the respiratory tract (500–700 cc/d) and skin (250–350 cc/d). With rigorous energy expenditure, however, these losses can be much greater. The presence of a fever results in an additional loss of 10% fluid per °C. Thus, under normal circumstances, to maintain homeostasis, the average adult needs to consume 2–3 L of fluids per day. In addition, losses from the gastrointestinal tract due to vomiting or diarrhea, major body stressors, or hyperventilation can result in substantially larger losses.

Fluid losses can occur in several common situations. Perhaps the most obvious scenarios include hemorrhage, vomiting, or diarrhea. Other less common, but equally important, sources include nasogastric suctioning and external drainage from biliary, enteric, or pancreatic fistulas. In general, the fluid loss in these settings is isotonic with the fluid depletion initially occurring from the ECF. Fluid sequestration into the extracellular or interstitial spaces is commonly referred to as "third-spacing" and also results in isotonic loss. Common etiologies of "third spacing" include peritonitis, pancreatitis, intestinal obstructions, burns, and crush injuries. A review of hypertonic and hypotonic fluid losses is beyond the scope of this chapter.

INTRAVENOUS SOLUTIONS

If free water were infused, it would distribute proportionally throughout all fluid compartments. In clinical practice, an infusion of D5W is considered to be the most similar to free water. Ringer's lactate and 0.9% normal saline are isotonic fluids and are considered crystalloids. Crystalloids are composed of sodium, chloride, and often other small molecule solutes. Infusions of crystalloids are confined to the ECF, and dis-

Table 1. Composition of Fluids

Fluid	Na^+ (mMol/L)	Cl^- (mMol/L)	K^+ (mMol/L)	Ca^{2+} (mMol/L)	Lactate (mMol/L)	Osmolality (mOsm/L)
0.45% NaCl	77	77	0	0	0	154
0.9% NaCl	154	154	0	0	0	308
3% NaCl	513	513	0	0	0	1027
D5W	0	0	0	0	0	253
LR	130	109	4	3	28	272

NaCl = Sodium chloride (saline); LR = Lactated Ringer's.

tribute proportionately between the interstitial and intravascular compartments. Table 1 summarizes the composition of commonly used intravenous fluids.

Colloids are solutions containing high-molecular-weight substances such as proteins and polysaccharide polymers. Because of their large size, colloids stay in the intravascular space and exert an osmotic force. Common colloids in use include albumin, hydroxyethyl starch (HES, or Hetastarch), and dextran. For patients in hypovolemic shock, some authors argue that colloids should be used in addition to crystalloids. In theory, the high oncotic pressure of the colloids promotes fluid retention in the intravascular space. Despite the fact that colloids remain in the intravascular space for 3–6 hours, compared to 30 minutes with crystalloids, large trials have failed to demonstrate any clinical benefit with the use of colloids. Because colloids are much more expensive than crystalloids and the use of hespan can result in a coagulopathy, the routine use of colloids is minimal, if at all.

FLUID REPLACEMENT

Acid–base and electrolyte disturbances frequently accompany fluid loss. Without an adequate circulating volume, renal function may be altered, which impairs the kidney's ability to correct acid–base and electrolyte abnormalities. Healthy individuals can compensate for dehydration and elevated osmolality by becoming thirsty and subsequently drinking water. Seriously ill or confused patients, however, have inadequate compensatory mechanisms. If a patient has a water deficit (as evidenced by hypernatremia), and a salt deficit (as evidenced by orthostasis), 10–20 cc/kg of isotonic crystalloids should be administered. If the patient is hemodynamically unstable, these fluids should be infused as quickly as possible, and can be repeated as necessary. In hemodynamically stable individuals, the fluids should be given over an hour. Once orthostasis is corrected, if volume depletion persists, the total water deficit should be calculated. Half the total deficit should be given within the first 8 hours, with the remainder given over the subsequent 16 hours. Measuring urine output is an excellent method of ensuring adequate fluid resuscitation. The minimal acceptable urine output is 0.5 cc/kg/hr for adults and 1 cc/kg/hr for children.

In addition to correcting a fluid deficit, patients who are not able to consume oral liquids need intravenous maintenance fluids. As a general rule, maintenance fluids are based on the following formula:

1st 10 kg of body weight → 4 cc/kg/hr
2nd 10 kg of body weight → 2 cc/kg/hr
Each additional kg (beyond 20 kg) → 1 cc/kg/hr

Thus, a 60-kg individual needs (10)(4) + (10)(2) + (40)(1), or 100 cc/hr. It is important to note that this formula is a generalization and does not take into account ongoing losses. Any ongoing loss should be replaced in addition to maintenance fluids.

BLOOD

Once blood is collected from a donor, it is separated into various parts. Blood components that are available for transfusion include packed red blood cells (PRBCs), fresh frozen plasma (FFP), cryoprecipitate, platelets, and white cell preparations. (See Table 2 for a list of blood products.)

There are four main ABO groups and over 400 RBC antigens that are currently identified. Ensuring ABO compatibility is the most important step in the crossmatching procedure. Antibody screening and Rh typing are performed with a routine type and crossmatch.

The ideal transfusion involves a self-donor, where the patient donates his own blood prior to elective surgery. Patients with chest trauma may be candidates for autotransfusion. In the absence of these scenarios, however, a complete type and crossmatch should be done, if permissible. In acute hemorrhage, waiting for a full type and crossmatch may not always be feasible. In such circumstances, incomplete crossmatch, type-specific, or type O blood can be used. Type-specific blood, which can be obtained faster than a full crossmatch, involves matching the ABO and Rh group. An incomplete crossmatch involves matching the ABO and Rh groups, plus an antibody screen. Rh positive blood can safely be given to all patients except women of childbearing age.

CRITERIA FOR TRANSFUSIONS

A hemodynamically unstable patient with acute blood loss requires immediate fluid resuscitation with a 20 cc/kg bolus of crystalloids, which can be repeated as needed. If, however, a patient remains unstable after 2–3 L or 40–50 mg/kg of crystalloid, blood should also be given. As a general rule, every 1 cc of blood lost will necessitate 2–3 cc of crystalloid replacement.

For patients with acute hemorrhage, the need to transfuse blood depends on the amount of blood lost as well as the patient's comorbid conditions. Any patient with an acute blood loss of more than 15% total blood volume should be considered for blood transfusion. In general, the decision to transfuse blood should not be based solely on the hemoglobin. For example, a hemoglobin of 8 g/dl in an asymptomatic individual with no comorbid risk factors and no ongoing blood loss may not necessitate a transfusion. However, in the presence of active bleeding, cardiac or pulmonary disease, evidence of cardiac ischemia (chest pain, shortness of breath) dizziness with mild exertion, sepsis, or hemoglobinopathies, PRBCs should be transfused to achieve a hemoglobin of 10 g/dl. In general, each unit of PRBCs will raise the hemoglobin 1 g/dl, and raise the hematocrit 3%.

Table 2. Blood Products

Product	Content	General indication	Lab value change/ unit transfused
PRBCs	Red blood cells	Hypovolemia	Hgb increases 1 g/dl or Hct increases 3%
FFP	Clotting factors*	Factor deficiency, reversal of prolonged PT	PT decreases 2 s
Platelets	Platelets	Thrombocytopenia	Increases platelets by 5,000–10,000
Cryoprecipiate	Factor VIII, XIII, fibrinogen, vWF, and fibronectin	Factor VIII deficiency, hemophilia A, hypo-fibrinogenemia, bleeding in thrombolytic therapy	

*Prothrombin, fibrinogen, factors V, VII, VIII, IX, XIII, antithrombin III, and proteins C and S.

Patients who have thrombocytopenia may need platelet transfusion. As a general rule, in the absence of bleeding, platelet transfusion should occur once the platelet count is <20,000. In the presence of bleeding or coagulation disorder, or if a major procedure is anticipated, platelet transfusions should occur once the count is <50,000. On average, each unit of platelets will raise the platelet count by 5,000–10,000/mm^3. Adults, on average, require 6–10 units of platelets, while children require 1 U/10 kg body weight. Crossmatching is not necessary for platelet transfusion, but Rh-negative patients should receive Rh negative platelets.

Each unit of FFP contains prothrombin, fibrinogen, clotting factors V, VII, VIII, IX, and XIII, antithrombin III, and proteins C and S. Each milliliter of FFP contains 1 unit of activity of any clotting factor. The decision to use FFP for factor deficiency should be calculated to provide at least 30% plasma factor concentrations. Thus, usually 10–15 cc/kg of FFP is needed. For reversal of coumadin, 5–8 cc/kg of FFP is usually required, as one unit of FFP reduces the prothrombin time by 2 seconds. A crossmatch is necessary for FFP.

Cryoprecipiate contains factors VIII and XIII, von Willebrand's factor, fibrinogen, and fibronectin. Cryoprecipitate can be used to promote hemostasis in any bleeding patients, although usually FFP is preferred, as FFP contains more clotting factors. Cryoprecipiate can be given for patients with von Willebrand's disease, hypofibrinogenemia (fibrinogen <100 mg/dl), hemophilia A, and bleeding due to thrombolytic therapy.

TRANSFUSION RISKS

Transfusing blood is not without risks. While blood is screened for numerous viruses including HBV, HCV, and HIV, transmission of these viruses can still occur. Other adverse reactions to transfusions include acute hemolytic transfusion reactions, febrile transfusion reactions, allergic reactions, transfusion-related acute lung injury (TRALI), graft-versus-host disease, circulatory overload, and hemosiderosis.

MASSIVE TRANSFUSIONS

A massive transfusion is defined as replacement of more than 10 units of blood during several hours, or transfusing the entire blood volume over 24 hours. Beyond all the risks of standard transfusions, recipients of massive transfusions are also at risk to develop hypothermia, hypocalcemia, dilutional thrombocytopenia, DIC, and ventricular arrhythmias.

REFERENCES

Dronen SC, Bobek EMK. 2000. Fluid and blood resuscitation. In *Emergency medicine: a comprehensive study guide*, 5th ed., pp. 222–228. Ed JE Tintinalli, GD Kelen, JS Stapczynski. New York: McGraw-Hill.

Hoffman GL. 2002. Blood and blood components. In *Rosen's emergency medicine: concepts and clinical practice*, 5th ed., pp. 48–51. Ed JA Jarx, RS Hockberger, RM Walls. St. Louis: Mosby.

Londner J, Carr C, Kelen GD. 2000. Fluid and electrolyte problems. In *Emergency medicine: a comprehensive study guide*, 5th ed., pp. 150–169. Ed JE Tintinalli, GD Kelen, JS Stapczynski. New York: McGraw-Hill.

Miller RD, Miller ED. 2000. *Anesthesia*, 5th ed., pp. 1602–1605. Philadelphia: Churchill Livingstone.

47

DECONTAMINATION

Liudvikas Jagminas, MD, FACEP*

Decontamination is defined as the reduction or removal of chemical, biological, or nuclear agents so they are no longer hazards. Agents may be removed by physical means or be neutralized chemically (detoxification). Decontamination of the skin is the primary concern, but decontamination of other systems must also be done when necessary. To ensure appropriate and timely patient care as well as optimal response, emergency personnel must understand decontamination procedures and the proper use of personal protective equipment.

ASSESSMENT, DECONTAMINATION, AND INITIAL TREATMENT OF PATIENTS

The primary goals for emergency personnel in a hazardous materials incident include:

- Establishment of decontamination zones (see below)
- Cessation of patient exposure
- Patient stabilization
- Containment of the hazard to prevent further contamination
- Patient treatment without jeopardizing emergency personnel safety

While not all chemicals pose a hazard for secondary contamination, until the risk is known, termination of exposure is best accomplished by removing the patient from the incident area and then decontaminating the patient.

The essential requirements for any decontamination task are:

- Safe area to keep a patient while undergoing decontamination
- Method for washing contaminants off a patient
- Means of containing the rinsate
- Personal protection equipment (PPE) (see Table 1) for personnel treating the patient
- Disposable or cleanable medical equipment to treat the patient

*Department of Emergency Medicine, Memorial Hospital, Pawtucket, Rhode Island

Establishment of Decontamination Zones

Hot Zone

The Hot Zone is immediately dangerous to life or health. Accordingly, Level A personal protective equipment with self-contained breathing apparatus or supplied-air respirator is required for first responders or other personnel working inside the Hot Zone, where contact with hazardous materials is likely, including chemical gas or vapors, biological aerosols, or chemical and/or biological liquid or powder residue.

Warm Zone

The Warm Zone is an uncontaminated environment into which contaminated victims, first responders, and equipment are brought. In classic HazMat (hazardous materials) response, the Warm Zone is adjacent to and upwind from the Hot Zone. However, experience with previous disasters indicates that contaminated victims capable of fleeing the Hot Zone are likely to bypass emergency medical services and go directly to the nearest hospital, in which case the Warm Zone may occur outside the emergency department or even inside the hospital.

The protective equipment required depends on whether victims were exposed to a biological, chemical, radiological agent, or unknown agent or agents. The route of exposure may be inferred from the presence of contaminant on the clothing and skin of victims.

Vapor or aerosol exposure leaves no or minimal contaminant on victims, and material breathed into the lungs is not exhaled to contaminate others. Liquid or powder exposures may leave visible residue. In a similar manner, handling victims exposed to biological aerosols poses little risk to emergency care personnel outside the Hot Zone.

Known Biological Warfare Agent Hazards

Personnel handling victims contaminated with bioterror (BT) agents require respiratory protection. Skin protection is largely unnecessary, because these are not active through unbroken skin (with the single exception of the mycotoxins). Personnel handling victims who have been exposed to a known BT agent aerosol are not required to wear protective equipment because secondary aerosolization of residual agent from clothing, skin, or hair is insignificant. When victims are contaminated with a known liquid or powder, Level D (universal precautions) and PAPR (powered air purifying respirator) with an HEPA (high-efficiency particulate air) filter are required until decontamination is complete. Level C personal protective equipment and PAPR HEPA filter may be considered if the residue on victims is suspected of containing mycotoxins.

Known Chemical Warfare Agent Hazards

Personnel handling victims contaminated with chemical warfare agents require respiratory and skin protection. When victims are exposed to a known gas at standard temperature and pressure (such as chlorine, phosgene, oxides of nitrogen, cyanide), no personal protective equipment is required, because victims cannot breathe out hazardous gas and harm others. When victims are exposed to a known vapor from volatile liquid (such as a nerve agent or blistering vapor), PPE (personal protection equipment) is required, because responders may be exposed to low levels coming from the victims. When victims are contaminated with a known volatile liquid, Level C PPE with PAPR and chemical cartridge is required until decontamination is complete. In general, Level C PPE is used when the inhalation risk is known to be below levels expected to harm personnel and when eye, mucous membrane, and skin exposures are unlikely.

Known Radiation Hazards

When victims are exposed to external radiation but not contaminated with a radiation-emitting source, no PPE is required. If any doubt exists whether victims or their clothing are contaminated, they should be surveyed with a Geiger-Müller counter. When victims are contaminated externally with radioactive material (on their skin, hair, wounds, clothes), use Level D PPE (for example, waterproof barrier materials, such as surgical gown, mask, gloves, leg, and/or shoe coverings; universal precautions) until decontamination is complete. Double layers of gloves and frequent changes of the outer layer help reduce the spread of radioactive material.

Handle radioactive materials with tongs whenever possible. Lead aprons are cumbersome and do not protect against gamma or neutron radiation. For this reason, experts currently recommend against their use when caring for a radiation-contaminated victim. However, healthcare workers should wear radiological dosimeters while working in a contaminated environment. When victims are contaminated internally with radioactive material, wear latex gloves when handling body fluids (urine, feces, wound drainage).

Unknown Hazards (Biological, Chemical or Both)

According to current US government (OSHA) regulations, Level A PPE is required for personnel responding to an unknown hazard. Some experts maintain that Level C PPE with PAPR (with organic vapor cartridge and HEPA filter) provides adequate protection until decontamination is complete. Unfortunately, no single ensemble of PPE can protect emergency care personnel against all hazards.

Cold Zone

The Cold Zone should be completely uncontaminated. Nevertheless, victims exposed to certain biological warfare agents may develop disease that can be transmitted to others. This situation then poses a risk of secondary spread to medical personnel. The type of protective equipment required depends on the route of transmission of these infectious diseases.

Respiratory Droplet/Airborne Particles

PAPR with HEPA filter provides the greatest degree of respiratory protection against biological-associated disease spread by respiratory droplet (such as smallpox or pneumonic plague) or airborne particles (possibly smallpox) when treating victims with obvious disease. Disposable HEPA filter masks also work.

Evidence exists that smallpox may be transmitted by airborne particles under certain circumstances. Some people develop a very dense rash and severe cough when

Table 1. Personal Protection Equipment

	Description	Advantages	Disadvantages
Level A	Completely encapsulated suit and self-contained breathing apparatus (SCBA)	Highest level of protection available for both contact and inhaled threats,	Expense and training requirements restrict use to hazardous materials response teams, lack of mobility, heat and other physical stresses, limited air supply time
Level B	Encapsulating suit or junctions/seams sealed, supplied air respirator or SCBA	High level of protection adequate for unknown environment entry, supplied air ensemble with increased mobility and dexterity	Dependence on air line or limited air supply time; heat and physical stresses; expense and training significant; fit testing required
Level C	Splash suit and air-purifying respirator	Significantly increased mobility, decreased physical stress, extended operation time with high levels of protection against certain agents; no fit testing required for blood-type	Not adequate for some high concentration environments or less than atmospheric oxygen environments or high levels of splash contamination; expense and training minimal
Level D	Work clothes, including standard precautions for healthcare workers (e.g., gloves, splash protection)	Increased mobility, decreased physical stresses, extended operation time	Offers no protection against chemical or other agents; expense and training minimal

infected with smallpox. These victims are also likely to have many lesions involving the mouth and throat. During bouts of severe cough, they may shed virus into the air.

Medical personnel should wear latex gloves while handling the skin of people with smallpox, because smallpox may potentially be transmitted by contact with pox lesions that have not yet crusted over.

Blood or Body Fluid

While in contact with victims who have contracted biological-associated disease spread by blood or body fluid contact (hemorrhagic fever from Ebola, for example), Level D PPE (standard precautions) is generally protective. Higher levels of protection may be necessary, however, if such victims have coughing or extensive bleeding.

Personal Protective Equipment

Please see Table 1.

Respirators

Level C protection is the recommended minimum level of protection. Based on specific knowledge of the released agent, or if there is no information at all, then Level B protection is recommended. Powered air-purifying respirators (PAPRs) are recommended over simple air-purifying respirators. Canisters should provide HEPA filtration and protection against organic vapor and acid gases at a minimum. FR57 canisters provide NIOSH-approved protection against organic vapors, acid gases, ammonia, methylamine, chlorine dioxide, HF, and formaldehyde; they are also effective in military testing against nerve agents, mustard, riot control agents, cyanide, and acid-gas related agents.

Suits

The difference between Levels C and B has to do with the durability of the suit and the impermeability of the suit to various chemicals. If the threat is unknown, it is best to use Level B protection. An average person will take an XL suit at the smallest since flexibility of garments are minimal, and tearing is a concern if too small a suit is worn. Duct tape (or chemically resistant tape) can be used to reinforce the zipper front and crotch of the suit as additional protection. Tyvek SL offers moderate general protection against a majority of chemical agents, including nerve agents and mustard, but resistance to many organic agents is limited. This is probably a reasonable minimum level of protection for the healthcare decontamination setting. Tychem F offers improved protection against chemical and other BT agents. Tychem BR offers even a higher level of protection. For more information, visit http://personalprotection.dupont.com/protectiveapparel/products/ applications.html.

Booties

The decontamination team may need abrasion resistance, depending on the surfaces where the decontamination area is located. In general, butyl rubber booties that can be pulled over shoes will suffice. Providers should never rely on the suit-incorporated booties for adequate protection of the feet. The junctions between the suit and boot should be taped with duct tape.

Gloves

Heavy butyl over gloves and thinner nitrile inner gloves offer protection against a broad range of agents, and are inexpensive. Cuffs should be long enough to reach at least 2 inches above the sleeve cuff. Silvershield inner gloves may also be used and provide additional protection against prolonged contact with halogenated hydrocarbons. The junction between gloves and suit should be sealed with duct tape.

Radiologic

Standard suits block alpha and beta particles. Neither the suits nor radiology lead aprons are effective against gamma radiation. Inhaled radioactive dusts are generally well-controlled by a HEPA level filter. Decontamination personnel should have radiation badges or radiation pagers immediately available to their personnel as well as having G-M counters.

Prioritizing Casualties for Decontamination

Responders must prioritize victims for receiving decontamination, treatment, and medical evacuation, while providing the greatest benefit for the greatest number. Although many emergency response services prepare for such incidents, few are currently capable of treating victims inside the Hot Zone. Therefore, whenever large numbers of victims are involved, it is recommended that they be sorted into ambulatory and non-ambulatory triage categories using the START categories.

Factors That Determine Highest Priority for Ambulatory Victim Decontamination

- Casualties closest to the point of release
- Casualties reporting exposure to vapor or aerosol
- Casualties with evidence of liquid deposition on clothing or skin
- Casualties with serious medical symptoms
- Casualties with conventional injuries

Non-Ambulatory Casualties

These are victims who are unconscious, unresponsive, or unable to move unassisted. They may be more seriously injured than ambulatory victims and will remain in place while further prioritization for decontamination occurs. It is recommended that prioritization of non-ambulatory victims for decontamination should be done using medical triage systems, such as START (see Figure 1).

Gross Patient Decontamination

Primary assessment can be undertaken while simultaneously performing gross decontamination in the outer edge of the Hot Zone or in the Warm Zone. Once life-threatening matters have been addressed, rescue personnel can direct their attention to more thorough decontamination and secondary patient assessment. Appropriate personal protective equipment and clothing must be worn until the threat of secondary exposure no longer exists. If there is a risk of secondary contamination, gross decontamination should be performed simultaneously with initial patient stabiliza-

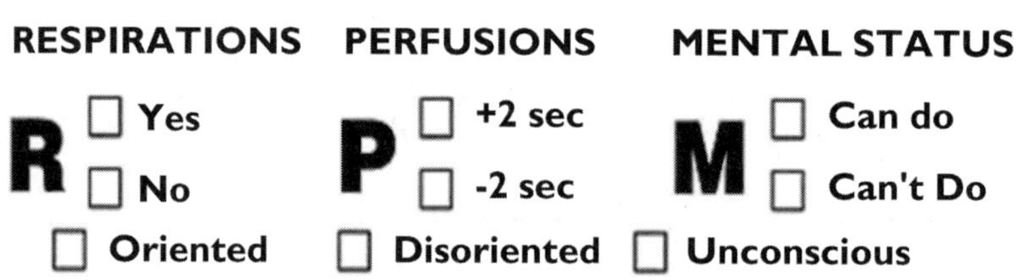

Figure 1. START categories.

tion. The sooner the patient is decontaminated, the sooner he or she can be transferred to the Cold Zone for further evaluation and treatment.

All potentially contaminated clothing, jewelry, and watches should be removed and doubled-bagged, sealed, and labeled. Any obvious contamination should be brushed or wiped off, followed by a 1-minute-long rinsing from head to toe with tepid water. If the suspected chemical is water-reactive, a longer rinsing period and a greater volume of water is required. Care should be taken to protect any open wounds from contamination by covering them with a water-repellent dressing (e.g., Chux). Throughout these procedures, every effort should be made by emergency personnel to avoid contact with any potentially hazardous substance(s).

Secondary or Definitive Decontamination

If conditions permit, a more deliberate decontamination process—known as secondary or definitive decontamination—should be initiated on each patient before transfer into the Cold Zone. This process includes washing the individual, usually with soap and water, in an organized and thorough manner. Determining the adequacy of decontamination can be very difficult, however, and is often based on a best clinical judgment rather than objective data. Detection monitors have limited value and are not generally available to most agencies. When a patient cannot be definitively decontaminated, they should be loosely wrapped in a cocoon-like fashion with a blanket or sheet prior to transfer to the Cold Zone.

The minimum equipment required for patient decontamination by emergency response personnel are listed above. These lists are not comprehensive, and are provided to guide departments in developing their own equipment lists based on community needs and requirements.

With few exceptions, intact skin is more resistant to hazardous materials than injured flesh, mucous membranes, or eyes. Therefore, secondary decontamination should begin at the head and proceed downward, with initial attention paid to contaminated eyes and open wounds. Washing should be done using warm water, soft bristle brushes or sponges, and a mild soap, such as dishwashing liquid. Decontamination of non-ambulatory patients is more difficult and labor-intensive. Invasive procedures (e.g., intubation) should not be initiated in the Contamination Reduction Zone unless absolutely necessary. All potentially contaminated patient clothing and belongings that have been removed and bagged should remain in the decontamination area.

Pediatric Decontamination Considerations

The complexity of managing a hazardous materials incident is increased when children are involved. While protective to the wearer, PPE may be frightening to a young child, resulting in less cooperation and greater psychological trauma. Whenever possible, children and parents should remain together while undergoing decontamination and medical treatment. Increased susceptibility to hypothermia is an important consideration in determining to what degree a child is decontaminated in the field as opposed to being grossly decontaminated, wrapped in a blanket for transport, and then given definitive decontamination at the hospital or other heated location.

Table 2. Antidotes and Select Pharmacologic Treatment Agents Antidote Toxicant

Atropine	Organophosphate pesticides and nerve agents
Pralidoxime chloride (2-PAM chloride)	Organophosphate pesticides and nerve agents (Atropine and 2-PAM Cl can be found combined in auto-injection kit known as Mark I)
Cyanide antidote kit	Cyanide
Methylene blue 1%	Methemoglobinemia
Calcium gluconate (Gel and IV)	Hydrofluoric acid and fluoride toxicity

Mass Population Decontamination

Certain HazMat incidents result in large numbers of patients being exposed (or potentially exposed) to a chemical agent. In this situation, it will be necessary to implement proper triage to prioritize patients entry through the decontamination process, or to quickly expand the decontamination system to clean more patients simultaneously. Large volumes of water from charged hose lines and specially mounted nozzles or deluge guns on fire engines can be used to quickly rinse large numbers of individuals. Once through the decontamination process, patients should be given towels and temporary clothing.

Patient Treatment

Some contaminated patients may require treatment with antidotes, though most cases can be handled with symptomatic care. Table 2 lists frequently used antidotes and selected other pharmacologic treatment agents.

PATIENT MANAGEMENT UNDER MASS CASUALTY CONDITIONS INVOLVING HAZARDOUS CHEMICALS

There are several important differences in disasters involving hazardous materials. A HazMat disaster may require setting up mass screening and decontamination centers. It may also be necessary to establish casualty collection points to provide stabilizing care in the field prior to transport. A major WMD/NBC incident may overwhelm any one hospital. Training in the appropriate procedures to be followed is essential for potential responders to a hazardous materials incident involving mass casualties. Triage may also be complicated for NBC exposures associated with the delayed onset of signs and symptoms of certain biological or chemical agents. If possible the patient, should be decontaminated before being transported to the emergency department to protect EMS and emergency department staff.

CRITICAL INCIDENT STRESS MANAGEMENT

Situations involving large numbers of ill or injured individuals, and which risk harm to the responder(s), are sources of critical incident stress. To minimize the occurrence of acute or long-term psychological consequences in response personnel, stress debriefing sessions should be held shortly after the incident. Acute stress reactions recognized during and after the incident should be immediately addressed by qualified peer debriefers or other mental health professionals.

REFERENCES

Burgess JL, Kirk MA, Borron SW, Cisek J. 1999. Emergency department hazardous materials protocol for contaminated patients. *Ann Emerg Med* **34**:205–212.

Cashman JR. 1995. *Hazardous materials emergencies: the professional response team*, 3rd ed. Lancaster, PA: Technomic Publishing.

Currance PL, Bronstein AC. 1994. *Emergency care for hazardous materials exposure*, 2nd ed. St. Louis: Mosby.

Haddad LM, Winchester JF. 1998. *Clinical management of poisoning and drug overdose*, 3rd ed. Philadelphia: Saunders.

Levitin HW, Siegelson HJ. 1996. Hazardous materials: disaster medical planning and response. *Emerg Med Clin North Am* **14**:327–348.

Kirk MA, Cisek J, Rose SR. 1994. Emergency department response to hazardous materials incidents. *Emerg Med Clin North Am* **12**:461–481.

Macintyre AG, Christopher GW, Eitzen E, Gum R, Weir S, DeAtley C, Tonat K, Barbera JA. 2000. Weapons of mass destruction events with contaminated casualties: effective planning for healthcare facilities. *JAMA* **4**:261–269.

US Department of Health and Human Services, Agency for Toxic Substances and Disease Registry (ATSDR). 1996. *Managing hazardous materials incidents: medical management guidelines for acute chemical exposures*, Vol. 3. Atlanta: US-DHHS.

US Department of Transportation. 1996. *1996 North American emergency response guidebook*. Washington, DC: Government Printing Office. http://hazmat.dot.gov/gydebook.htm.

US Federal Emergency Management Agency and US Fire Administration. 1999. *Hazardous materials guide for first responders*. Washington, DC: Government Printing Office.

Wetter DC, Daniell WE, Treser CD. 2001. Healthcare facility preparedness for victims of chemical or biological terrorism. *Am J Public Health* **91**:710–716.

48

ACUTE INHALATION INJURY

Dorsett D. Smith, MD, FACP, FCCP, FACOEM,*
and David J. Prezant, MD, FCCP**

OVERVIEW

Industrial societies regularly produce large amounts of potentially toxic irritant gases. Although recent events have made us all too aware that toxic gases may be used as weapons of mass destruction, accidental exposures remain the greatest threat. For example, over half a million workers are annually exposed to anhydrous ammonia. Smaller numbers are exposed to a variety of other irritant gases that are used in a multitude of industrial processes. In addition, thousands are smoke inhalation victims, exposed to toxic gases from the burning of a variety of materials. This most commonly occurs in commercial or home fires, where large amounts of carbon monoxide, hydrogen cyanide, hydrogen chloride, acrolein, sulfur dioxide, phosgene, and other irritant gases are produced. The magnitude of these exposures is quite significant. The leading cause of death from acute inhalation injury is due to carbon monoxide and hydrogen cyanide in residential exposures, and hydrogen sulfide and hydrofluoric acid in occupational exposures. Approximately 5% of workplace deaths are due to asphyxiation or poisoning. This brief review of acute inhalation injury will focus on classification, diagnosis, and treatment for asphyxiants and irritants.

ASPHYXIANT GASES

Pathology

Asphyxiant gases cause death either as simple asphyxiants, as occurs with methane gas accumulation (in a coal mine), or by causing cellular asphyxia by a chem-

*Department of Pulmonary Disease and Critical Care, University of Washington School of Medicine, Seattle

**Albert Einstein College of Medicine, Pulmonary Division, Montefiore Medical Center, Bronx, New York

ical means, as occurs with carbon monoxide. Carbon monoxide is the second most common atmospheric pollutant after carbon dioxide. It is produced by incomplete combustion from fires, faulty heating systems, volcanic eruptions, and internal combustion engines, as well as a variety of industrial processes. Carbon monoxide is an odorless, tasteless gas. Early symptoms (headache, sore throat, shortness of breath, and fatigue) can mimic the flu, especially when an entire family is affected from an exposure related to a faulty home heating system. Serious clinical effects such as tachycardia, arrhythmias, angina, and mental status changes can occur when carboxyhemoglobin concentrations exceed 20% (especially in nonsmokers) and effects are nearly always fatal when carboxyhemoglobin concentrations exceed 60%. Clinical effects may occur at lower concentrations in subjects already suffering from cardiopulmonary diseases. Carbon monoxide toxicity is related to decreased oxygen transport due to its preferential binding to hemoglobin and the resulting leftward shift of the hemoglobin oxygen dissociation curve and decreased oxygen utilization due to direct cytotoxicity by inactivating intracellular respiratory enzymes. Hydrogen cyanide is also produced by fires and manufacturing processes. Hydrogen cyanide toxicity does not affect oxygen transport but does decrease oxygen utilization due to direct cytotoxicity by inactivating intracellular respiratory enzymes.

Hydrogen sulfide (H_2S) is a gaseous asphyxiant that decreases oxygen transport by the formation of methemoglobinemia and inhibits oxygen utilization by inhibition of cellular enzymes. H_2S gas exposure is encountered in various industries, including: farming, oil and petroleum refining, rayon manufacturing, food processing, and other manufacturing processes. Exposures to very low concentrations (0.003–0.02 ppm) produce a noxious odor smelling like rotten eggs. In addition to being an asphyxiant, H_2S is also an irritant, with respiratory and eye irritation beginning around 50 ppm. Because olfactory function is lost at around 100–200 ppm, if the victim can still smell the gas the concentration is usually not high enough to cause severe injury. However, the clinical diagnosis can be aided if the healthcare provider detects the smell of rotten eggs on the victim's clothing or breath. H_2S produces intense irritation of mucous membranes and can cause pulmonary edema. Concentrations above 750–1000 ppm can cause respiratory paralysis, syncope, and sudden death. Death is due to direct central nervous system toxicity, pulmonary edema, or asphyxiation.

Diagnosis and Treatment

Although the diagnosis can be suspected by careful history, the physical examination is nearly useless as "cherry red mucous membranes" and cyanosis are only found at very high levels of carbon monoxide poisoning. High levels of carbon monoxide cause hypoxia by affecting oxygen transport and utilization. However, a carbon monoxide partial pressure of only 1 mm Hg can saturate over 50% of hemoglobin without affecting respiration and gas exchange. For this reason, measuring oxygen partial pressure is not useful in diagnosing carbon monoxide intoxication. Moreover, the spectra of oxyhemoglobin and abnormal hemoglobins such as carboxyhemoglobin are so similar that noninvasive oxygen saturation measurements are also useless in diagnosing carbon monoxide intoxication. Only direct measurements of the percent content of carboxyhemoglobin and methemoglobin (oximetry panel) can definitively make the diagnosis of carbon monoxide intoxication and H_2S intoxication, respectively. An oximetry panel should be routinely performed for patients with smoke inhalation, suspected carbon monoxide, or H_2S intoxication, and inhalation injuries of unknown type.

Carbon monoxide toxicity should be immediately treated with 100% oxygen, which reduces the half-life of carboxyhemoglobin from approximately 250 to 40 minutes. This half-life can be reduced to less than 20 minutes if treatment with hyperbaric oxygen is available. Hyperbaric oxygen therapy is recommended for patients with carbon monoxide levels exceeding 20 to 25%, or at lower levels if carbon monoxide induced cardiac or neurologic dysfunction is suspected. Hydrogen cyanide toxicity also requires confirmation with blood levels. Treatment is with a "cyanide treatment kit," containing sodium nitrite and thiosulfate solutions. H_2S toxicity if promptly diagnosed can be treated with methylene blue (1–2 mg/kg intravenously) and sodium nitrite solution, but not thiosulfate solution. Hyperbaric oxygen therapy has been suggested as an additional form of therapy for these asphyxiants.

IRRITANT GASES

Pathophysiology

The health effects of an acute exposure to an irritant gas or vapor are dependent on the physiochemical properties of that particular gas or vapor, as well as specific host factors. The extent of exposure varies considerably and is most pronounced in subjects with preexisting airway diseases. Acid and alkaline gases such as chlorine and ammonia produce extreme alterations in pH that cause tissue damage by direct contact. Other gases produce chemical reactions that cause free radical release, inflammation, and membrane damage.

The site of pulmonary injury is most dependent on the water solubility of the gas. High-solubility gases (e.g., ammonia, sulfur dioxide, formaldehyde, or methyl isocyanate) can affect all exposed mucous membranes, including: ocular (irritation, erythema, and conjunctivitis, and with heavy exposure delayed-onset of cataracts), nasal (irritation, congestion, rhinorrhea, and erythema), facial burns (skin and lip), pharyngeal (throat and tongue irritation, burns and edema), and laryngeal (burns, edema, and obstruction) injuries. Intermediate-solubility gases such as chlorine may produce upper-airway irritation, but the mucous membrane irritation is not as intense as for highly soluble gases. Because of its intermediate solubility, chlorine's effect extends more distal, producing both upper- and lower-airway injury, and pulmonary edema. Low-solubility gases, like phosgene or oxides of nitrogen, produce little in the way of upper-airway irritation, but produce intense damage to the lower airways and pulmonary edema. The low-solubility gases are more likely to produce delayed-onset symptoms and delayed-onset pulmonary edema, usually within the first 24 hours.

Several factors may influence the severity of lung injury. For the most part, pulmonary injury severity is determined by (1) gas solubility and (2) exposure duration multiplied by gas concentration. Problems in escaping the exposure due to orthopedic problems or to falling or mouth breathing due to nasal obstruction may also play important roles in determining exposure and injury severity. For example, if gas density is high (e.g., chlorine or phosgene), the gas cloud may hug the floor, thereby increasing exposure to a victim who has fallen.

Oxides of nitrogen, like nitrogen dioxide, commonly produce a triphasic illness pattern. Initial presentation may be that of cough, wheeze, dyspnea, central chest pain, fever, sweating, and weakness. Physical examination may reveal wheezes and crackles, and the patient may be hypotensive and cyanotic. The patient's x-ray may be normal or may show pulmonary edema. This phase of the illness will resolve and the patient may be relatively asymptomatic and then 2 to 8 weeks later develop symptoms of bronchiolitis obliterans. Presentation includes the late development of fevers, chills, wheeze, cough, dyspnea, and chest pain associated with wheezes and crackles on physical exam. The chest films may be normal or may show diffuse, small nodules. Chest CT scans with expiratory imaging may show air trapping, bronchial wall thickening and nodules suggestive of bronchiolitis obliterans.

Diagnosis and Treatment

The early management and treatment of acute inhalation injury from an irritant gas is summarized below and is primarily supportive, including immediately removing any contaminated clothing that might further increase the absorption of a substance through the skin.

1. Start high-flow 100% oxygen and consider arterial blood gas and co-oximetry panel.
2. Obtain history of any odors or knowledge of specific toxic agent.
3. Examine patient for eye injuries, flush eyes, and treat if inflammation is noted.
4. Examine patient for burns to face, nose, mouth, or throat.
5. If victim is hoarse, has difficulty phonating, facial burns or carbonaceous sputum, evaluate the airway with laryngoscopy or bronchoscopy and if edema is present, consider early intubation.
6. Examine chest and consider early use of bronchodilators, mucomyst, and or inhaled corticosteroids.
7. Peak flow rates and/or bedside spirometry may be helpful in diagnosing or documenting reversible bronchospasm. Full pulmonary function tests (volumes, diffusion, and/or provokability) should be reversed for a later timepoint.
8. Chest x-rays may be useful as a baseline but are generally not helpful in the acute setting unless the patient has significant hypoxemia or asymmetric breath sounds.
9. Observe patient for delayed pulmonary edema for 24 hours if the patient is hypoxemic or has been exposed to a low-solubility gas, such as phosgene.

Careful attention to the eyes is important since there may be late development of cataracts with heavy exposures. If the gas has already been identified, then knowing its solubility can help in the triage of exposed victims. For example, high-solubility gases (sulfur dioxide or ammonia) affect the upper airways and only cause lower-airway injuries when the dose effect is large. Thus, if a potential victim, exposed to ammonia, has no upper-airway signs or symptoms (watery, teary eyes, red face, rhinitis, red sore nose, erythema of the posterior pharynx or hoarseness), it is unlikely that the patient has inhaled a dose high enough to cause lower-airway injury. The patient who presents with tachypnea and stridor, particularly with some hoarseness, is at a high risk of developing progressive laryngeal edema and complete obstruction of the airway, and therefore should be considered for emergency intubation. Certainly if symptoms of upper-airway damage are present, a prompt inspection of the larynx by a laryngoscope or fiberoptic laryngoscope would be imperative, since once sufficient edema develops these patients are extremely difficult to intubate and one may have to do an emergency tracheostomy. If upper-airway edema is present, pharmacologic treatment includes nebulized racemic epinephrine and systemic corticosteroids. If edema is minimal and early intubation is not required, conservative care to maintain airflow consists of positive pressure breathing (BIPAP or CPAP) or a mixture of helium/oxygen gas that due to its lower density can improve upper-airway flow dynamics by reducing turbulence. However, in the presence of edema not immediately requiring intubation, conservative care should only be done if frequent monitoring to assess edema progression and emergent intubation is possible.

When the patient is exposed to a low-soluble gas, like phosgene, upper-airway signs and symptoms are not expected and observation is required because it may take as long as 24 hours for reactive airways dysfunction syndrome or pulmonary edema to develop. The development of reactive airways dysfunction syndrome (RADS) or asthma after exposure to irritant gases is the most common long-term complication. Early treatment with inhaled bronchodilators and inhaled corticosteroids is a well-proven treatment approach for those with symptoms and reversible bronchospasm. Reversible bronchospasm can be confirmed by documenting improvement in flow rates after treatment with either a peak flow meter or spirometry. Currently, no studies exist to determine whether early use of inhaled corticosteroids is a viable prophylactic strategy. However, the side effects of inhaled corticosteroids are minimal. Sinusitis may accompany lower-airway inflammation, and treatment with nasal corticosteroids, decongestants, nasal anticholinergic agents, and antihistamines are typical interventions.

Observation is critical if the patient complains of dyspnea or if tachypnea is noted, as these may be the earliest signs of impending pulmonary edema after acute inhalation exposure. While chest imaging is not useful in the early detection of pulmonary injury if the patient is asymptomatic, it is valuable if the patient is in respiratory distress or if pulmonary auscultation is abnormal or asymmetrical, in which case, oximetry (remember, not useful with chemical asphyxiants such as carbon monoxide and H_2S), arterial blood gases, and chest radiographs should be immediately obtained. Treatment is supportive. Abnormal gas exchange if severe should be treated with positive pressure ventilation aiming for the lowest mean airway pressure possible while still supporting gas exchange. Intubation may also be necessary if bronchial secretions are excessive and require frequent pulmonary toilet by catheter or bronchoscopic suctioning. Systemic corticosteroids are controversial for the treatment of noncardiogenic pulmonary edema and there is probably no role in the acute treatment of inhalation lung injury.

In the weeks following irritant gas exposures, the patient may continue to suffer from sinusitis, RADS, and asthma. Chronic cough syndrome may also result from irritant gas exposures. When chest radiographs and/or chest CT scans are normal, chronic cough is usually due to asthma or RADS, sinusitis, and/or gastroesophageal reflux. When chest imaging is abnormal, cough may be due to pneumonia or bronchiolitis obliterans. Prophylactic antibiotics have been suggested because sloughing of the tracheal mucosa offers a good culture media for bacteria. However, there is no evidence that prophylactic antibiotics reduce the incidence of pneumonia. Instead, antibiotics should be used only if pneumonia occurs and when possible targeted to the organisms responsible. Chest physiotherapy, high frequency percussive ventilation, bronchodilators, and frequent suctioning may be helpful in those patients with mucus plugs and thick secretions. Bronchiolitis obliterans is a serious complication that usually responds to oral steroids, but may be progressive or even fatal if not treated promptly. It is unlikely that early treatment with only antibiotics or inhaled steroids is preventive. Some might argue that, given the possibility of bronchiolitis obliterans, early treatment with oral steroids (prednisone at 40–60 mg/daily) for 8 weeks might be a reasonable prophylaxis strategy after exposure to those gases known to cause this problem, particularly in those patients with silo-filler's disease or those exposed to high doses of NO_2 or SO_2. Others believe that the occurrence of severe or life-threatening bronchiolitis obliterans after inhalation injury is too rare to warrant the routine use of oral steroids. Experimental anecdotal therapy for acute inhalation injury includes nebulized sodium bicarbonate or nebulized mucomyst (N-acetylcysteine) to break up secretion and to reduce free radical damage. The long-term consequences of irritant inhalation injury are summarized below in order of most common first:

- Complete resolution of symptoms
- Reactive airways dysfunction syndrome (RADS) or asthma
- Chronic bronchitis
- Bronchiectasis, i.e., ammonia, SO_2
- Bronchiolitis obliterans, i.e., NO_2, SO_2
- Bronchostenosis, i.e., mustard gas
- Restrictive interstitial fibrosis

SMOKE INHALATION

Pathophysiology

Inhalation injury associated with burns from fires comprises approximately a quarter of those patients admitted to a burn unit. Smoke contains toxic gases (asphyxiants and irritants) along with particulate matter that is coated with the chemicals of combustion and pyrolysis. Smoke particles cause airway damage due to direct irritation and via the toxic effects of the chemicals adsorbed to the surface of these particles. Particles greater than 10 microns in diameter cause upper-airway injury, as they typically do not penetrate into the lower airways. The subglottic or supraglottic edema following smoke inhalation (due to thermal, irritant gas, or large particles) may lead to upper-airway obstruction. Upper-airway obstruction may develop slowly over the first 12–24 hours due to initial hypovolemia and other inflammatory factors. Particles less than 3 microns in diameter cause lower-airway injury and, in fact, particles greater than 3 microns in diameter may also penetrate into the lower airways when (a) aerosolized and respired in high concentrations, (b) if the subject is a mouth breather, thereby bypassing nasal defense mechanisms, or (c) if the subject has high minute ventilation, as may be seen in firefighters. Suspicion of a smoke inhalation injury is warranted whenever there has been exposure to a fire in an enclosed space, especially if the patient displays signs of altered mental status, facial burns, stridor, carbonaceous sputum, respiratory distress, or an admission carboxyhemoglobin greater than 10%.

Diagnosis and Treatment

The most common clinical problems associated with smoke inhalation are (1) upper and/or lower-airway inflammation and (2) carbon monoxide toxicity, although hydrogen cyanide toxicity has gained recent attention. Fiberoptic bronchoscopy is very useful in evaluation of burn patients for airway injury by demonstrating carbonaceous material, airway edema, erythema, ulcerations, hemorrhage, blisters, or ischemia. During bronchoscopy, intubation should be considered, preferably over the bronchoscope, if there is evidence of upper- or lower-airway edema or if carbonaceous material has penetrated past the vocal cords. Because edema is an ongoing process in burn injuries and intubation may become increasingly difficult, it is nearly always better to intubate too soon rather than too late. Xenon-133 ventilation scanning has been used in burn patients to detect airway injury missed by fiberoptic bronchoscopy. It has a high sensitivity, but there are false positives in patients with obstructive airway disease.

All patients with a history of smoke inhalation and any of the above-noted physical signs should have direct measurement of carboxyhemoglobin and arterial blood gases, as noninvasive measures of oxygen saturation are incorrect in this setting. Chest x-rays are valuable only in those patients who have respiratory symptoms, such as tachypnea, dyspnea, and hypoxemia. Pulmonary edema is an extremely rare complication unless a specific irritant gas is a byproduct of combustion, and infiltrates usually will not be apparent without ventilation/perfusion mismatching and the consequent development of hypoxemia. In the presence of significant burn injuries, treatment with systemic corticosteroids is contraindicated, as their use has been shown to increase mortality due to sepsis. Other than the above-noted specific issues, the management and treatment of smoke inhalation and its long-term clinical consequences are no different than for other irritant gas exposures.

PULMONARY FUNCTION TESTS

Pulmonary function tests should be obtained as soon as the patient is stable. It is our practice to obtain complete pulmonary function tests (PFTs) as soon as the patient is ambulatory and no longer requiring supplemental oxygen. We obtain complete PFTs again at 3, 6, 12, and 24 months after exposure in the symptomatic patient. Spirometry frequently is normal in the presence of mild obstructive or restrictive disease from inhalation injury. Also pseudo-restriction (symmetrical reductions in forced vital capacity and forced expiratory volume at 1 s) may occur in obstructive airways disease due to air trapping. Therefore, measurement of a bronchodilator response and/or lung volumes is necessary, especially when spirometry is abnormal or at the lower limits of normal. Airflow obstruction may be due to RADS, asthma, or anatomic airway narrowing. Bronchodilator response or methacholine challenge testing can be performed to confirm obstructive airways disease and airway hyperreactivity. However, no conclusions about chronicity should occur until treatment and proven persistence are documented after at least 3 to 6 months have elapsed. Because early transient bronchial hyperreactivity may occur in the weeks following irritant gas exposures, detection of early bronchial hyperreactivity may not always predictive of long-term airway injury and irritability. However, in firefighters with heavy exposure to dust and irritant gases in the first days of the World Trade Center collapse, bronchial hyperreactivity demonstrated by methacholine challenge testing after 1 or 3 months post-exposure was predictive of persistent airway hyperreactivity and RADS. Restrictive changes in lung function progress very slowly and may not be detected until 2 or more years after the toxic exposure. The most common abnormality is an isolated reduction in residual volume. Isolated reduction in lung diffusion may occur but is usually accompanied by reduction in lung volumes. Although most patients exposed to irritant gases and/or smoke inhalation will recover completely, others may develop chronic airway hyperreactivity, obstructive lung disease (asthma, RADS, chronic bronchitis), bronchiectasis, bronchostenosis, bronchiolitis obliterans, or restrictive interstitial fibrosis.

REFERENCES

Agee RN, Long JM, Hunt JL, Petroff PA, Petroff PA, Lull RJ, Mason AD, Pruitt BA. 1976. Use of xenon-33 in early diagnosis of inhalation injury. *J Trauma* **16**:218–224.

Ainsle G. 1993. Inhalational injuries produced by smoke and nitrogen dioxide. *Respir Med* **87**:169–174.

Banauch GI, Alleyne D, Sanchez R, Olender K, Weiden M, Kelly KJ, Prezant DJ. 2003. Persistent bronchial hyperreactivity in New York City firefighters and rescue workers following collapse of World Trade Center. *Am J Respir Crit Care Med* **168**:54–62.

Douidar SM. 1997. Nebulized sodium bicarbonate in acute chlorine inhalation. *Pediatr Emerg Care* **13**:406–407.

Feldman DM, Baron S, Mueller CA, Bernard BP, Lushniak BD, Kelly KJ, Prezant DJ. 2004. Initial symptoms, respiratory function and respirator use in New York City firefighters responding to the World Trade Center (WTC) disaster. *Chest* **125**:1256–1264.

Jaffe FA. 1997. Pathogenicity of carbon monoxide. *Am J Forensic Med Pathol* **18**:406–410.

Jones GR, Proudfoot AT, Hall JI. 1973. Pulmonary effects of acute exposure to nitrous fumes. *Thorax* **28**:61–65.

Litovitz T, Oderda G, White JD, Sheridan MJ. 1993. Occupational and enviromental exposures reported to poison centers. *Am J Public Health* **83**:739–743.

Masanes MJ, Legendre C, Lioret N, Saizy R, LeBeau B. 1995. Using bronchoscopy and biopsy to diagnose early inhalation injury. *Chest* **107**:1365–1369.

Prezant DJ, Weiden M, Banauch GI, McGuinness G, Rom WN, Aldrich TK, Kelly KJ. Cough and bronchial responsiveness in firefighters at the World Trade Center site. *New Engl J Med* **347**:806–815.

Reiffenstein RJ, Hulbert WC, Roth SH. 1993. Toxicology of hydrogen sulfide. *Annu Rev Pharmacol Toxicol* **32**:109–134.

Schwartz DA, Smith DD, Lakshminarayan S. 1990. The pulmonary sequellae associated with accidental inhalation of chlorine. *Chest* **97**:820–825.

Smith DD. 1999. Acute inhalation injury. *Clin Pulm Med.*

Surunda A, Agnew J. 1989. Deaths from asphyxiation and poisoning at work in the United States, *Br J Ind Med* **46**:541–546.

49

ELECTRICAL INJURIES

Dennis Hanlon, MD*

OVERVIEW

Electrical injuries may be commonly seen in a disaster. They often occur due to damaged caused to buildings and infrastructure. Flooding also places individuals at risk, as electrical currents can readily travel through water. Individuals are at particular risk for injury during disaster recovery and cleanup. In the United States electrical injuries are the fifth leading cause of fatal occupational injury and contribute 3–6% of admissions to burn units.

DEFINITIONS

Alternating current (AC) is commonly found in households and is defined as current that changes direction on a cyclic basis. Standard household current is 60 cycles/s. Direct current (DC) travels in a constant direction and may be found in batteries, railways, and automobile electrical systems. High-voltage systems are considered those greater than a thousand volts. Ohm's law deals with the relationship between voltage and current in an ideal conductor. This relationship states that the potential difference (voltage) across an ideal conductor is proportional to the current through it. The constant of proportionality is called the resistance, R. The current flowing through the resistance is I. So Ohm's law may be stated as $I = V/R$. In the human body, resistance increases from lowest to highest as follows: nerves, vessels, muscles, skin (variable depending on moisture), tendon, fat, and bone.

INITIAL ASSESSMENT

Treat as any critically ill patient and follow general resuscitative measures: ABCs, cardiac monitor, IV fluids, and oxygen. Initial responders need to make sure that they

*Drexel University College of Medicine, Pittsburgh

do not become part of the circuit. Several types of electrical injuries may occur: true electrical injuries (victim becomes part of the circuit), arc burns (current strikes skin but does not enter the body), flame injuries (typical thermal injury), and blunt injuries (being thrown from the source).

FURTHER ASSESSMENT

Important parts of the history include: type of electrical source, duration of contact, any associated blunt trauma, factors at scene, and resuscitative measures provided. A detailed physical exam should be performed paying particular attention to the following systems:

Neurological

- Multiple presentations
  - o Acute CNS symptoms (maintain your standard differential diagnosis for these entities)
  - o Coma
- Altered mental status
- Paralysis
- Seizures
- Respiratory arrest (paralyzed respiratory center in medulla)
  - o Delayed neurological symptoms
- Mimics ascending paralysis, transverse myelitis, and incomplete cord transection
- A few days to years

Skin

- Surface burns do not predict the extent of the underlying injury.
- Entrance burns (contact or source)
  - o Small, well circumscribed, full thickness
  - o Depressed center
  - o Dry, charred appearance
  - o Most commonly on the hands
- Exit burns (ground)
  - o Exploded or blown out appearance
  - o Frequently found on the feet
- Oral commissure burns
  - o Pediatric
  - o Significant cosmetic problem
  - o Delayed labial artery hemorrhage (2 days to 2 weeks)
  - o Skin findings may be absent with current source over wide area (low-resistance/low-voltage electrical injury)
- Vascular
  - o Extensive and variable lesions
  - o Progressive necrosis
  - o High amputation rate with high-voltage injuries

Musculoskeletal

- Observe for compartment syndromes
- Fractures/dislocations (10–15%)
- Osteoschisis (longitudinal fracture from passing current)

DIAGNOSTIC STUDIES

Except for the most minor of injuries, diagnostic studies are indicated and should include: EKG, electrolytes, renal function, CPK (peak levels predict amount of muscle injury and risk of amputation), myoglobin (serum and urine), urinalysis, and radiographic studies (indicated by associated trauma).

MANAGEMENT

- ABCs (reassess)
- Cardiac monitoring
  - o Risk of arrhythmia is pathway dependent
  - o Ventricular fibrillation — AC
  - o Asystole — DC and high-voltage AC
  - o Any abnormal rhythm is possible
  - o The major cause of death is cardiac dysrhythmias.
- IV Fluids
  - o Maintain urine output at 1–1.5 ml/kg/hr
  - o Various burn formulas do not apply to electrical burns
  - o Goal is to prevent renal complications of rhabdomyolysis
- Burn care
  - o Mafenide acetate for full-thickness burns
  - o Sulfadiazine silver for extensive burns (>15% BSA)
- Extremities with burns splinted in position of function
  - o Reassess frequently
  - o Early surgical management
- Other manifestations as per standard of care for that entity.

PROGNOSIS

Only 5% in high-voltage group were able to return to their previous job.

DISPOSITION

Asymptomatic patients with a normal physical exam after low-voltage exposure may be discharged. Admission criteria include: all high-voltage injuries, intermediate-voltage injuries (>600 V), suspicion of conductive injury, dysrhythmia in pre-hospital setting or in the ED, abnormal EKG findings, documented loss of consciousness, and associated injuries that requires admission. All significant electrical injuries should be transferred to a burn center.

Table 1. High-Voltage Injuries and the Suspected Pathway of Electrical Injury

Pathway	Mortality
Hand-to-hand	60%
Hand-to-foot	20%
Foot-to-foot	5%

SPECIAL CONSIDERATIONS

- Electrical injuries are more similar to crush injuries than to typical thermal burns.
- Surface burns underestimate extent of underlying injury.
- Surface burns may be absent in the wet patient.
- Low-voltage injuries account for half of deaths due to electrical injuries.
- Massive fluid replacement is key.
- AC is more dangerous than DC.
- The current threshold of tetanic contraction is 10–15 mA.

REFERENCES

Bailey B, Gaudreault P, Thivierge RL, Turgeon JP. 1995. Cardiac monitoring of children with household electrical injuries. *Ann Emerg Med* **25**:612–617.

Fish RM. 2004. Electrical injuries. In *Emergency medicine: a comprehensive study guide*, pp. 1231–1235. Ed JE Tintinalli, GD Kelen, JS Stapczynski. New York: McGraw-Hill.

Hartman J, Cuenca P, Della-Giustina D. 2002. Electrical injuries. *J Crit Ill* **17**:94–100.

Koumbourlis AC. 2002. Electrical injuries. *Crit Care Med* **30**(12):S424–S430.

Martinez JA, Nguyen T. 2000. Electrical injuries. *South Med J* **93**(12):1165–1168.

Rabban J, Adler J, Rosen C, Blair J, Sheridan R. 1997. Electrical injury from subway third rails: serious injury associated with intermediate voltage contact. *Burns* **23**(6):515–518.

Stewart C. 2001. Electrical injuries. *Pediatr Emerg Med Rep* **6**:1–10.

Wright RK. 2001. Electrical injuries. *eMedicine* **2**:1–13; http://www.emedicine.com/emerg/topic162.htm.

50 TOXICOLOGY

Stephen J. Traub, MD*

Toxicology is the study of how toxins (street drugs, prescribed medications, occupational toxins, or chemical weapons) interact with living organisms. Fundamentally, toxicology is the discipline that concerns itself with the care of the poisoned patient.

Not only are entire textbooks written about toxicology, but they are written about specific subdivisions of toxicology: medical toxicology, environmental toxicology, regulatory toxicology, and others. A detailed discussion of the entire discipline, obviously, is beyond the scope of this introductory chapter.

Disaster medicine must concern itself with toxicology because many weapons of mass destruction and terror are toxins. A working knowledge of the principles of toxicology, therefore, is crucial for anyone who might deal with mass casualty incidents or terrorist attacks. This chapter will focus on those areas of medical toxicology that are pertinent to disaster medicine and the response to chemical or biological terrorism: identifying an incident as a toxin-mediated event, initial assessment and stabilization, post-stabilization assessment, and treatment.

IS A TOXIN INVOLVED IN THE ATTACK?

The initial key to identifying a mass toxic exposure is to have a high index of suspicion. Unless a clinician is willing to consider a poisonous gas attack as a possible etiology of unexpected pulmonary symptoms in a large number of patients, or cyanide poisoning in patients with coma and unexplained metabolic acidosis, the diagnosis will be missed.

The characteristic scenario of a mass toxic exposure is that of otherwise healthy multiple victims—several or several hundred—who develop a similar set of symptoms over a short period of time. In the case of immediately acting poisons (such as hydrogen cyanide gas), there will be little question that a toxin is involved. In cases of poisons that produce a delayed symptom complex (such as oral ricin poisoning), the diagnosis may only be made after a coordinated effort by federal, state, and local agencies.

*Beth Israel Deaconess Medical Center, Harvard Medical School, Boston

Clues on the scene may suggest a toxic exposure, and even the agent involved. The presence of an unexplained gas or mist immediately before symptoms occur suggests a toxic exposure, as does a history suggesting that symptoms are worse in those persons closest to the area from which the gas or mist emanated. Some gases have characteristic appearances and odors; a yellow gas that smells like bleach suggests chlorine gas, an odor of freshly mown hay suggests phosgene, and an odor of onions or garlic suggests a vesicant gas.

Patients' symptoms may not only help determine that a toxin is involved, but also which toxin is involved. As a general rule, toxins produce similar symptoms in all patients. Some toxins, particularly those that alter autonomic function, produce characteristic "toxidromes" (see below) that may help establish the diagnosis. In addition to the physical examination, laboratory analysis may help establish a diagnosis; cyanide, for instance, leads to a marked increase in the mixed venous oxygen saturation due to a failure to utilize oxygen on a molecular level.

INITIAL ASSESSMENT AND STABILIZATION

Assessing the patient with a potential toxic exposure follows the basic tenets of Emergency Medicine: secure the airway, breathing, and circulation. Patient decontamination may also be necessary in cases of toxin-induced disasters or chemical terrorism.

Airway

Loss of consciousness (as may be seen with cyanide), loss of muscle tone (as may be seen with botulism), or the presence of copious secretions (as may be seen with organophosphorus nerve agents) may all lead to primary airway failure. In all such patients, the airway should be secured. The preferred method of securing the airway in poisoned patients is via endotracheal intubation; as a general rule, poisons due not alter airway anatomy, although as noted above the patient may have copious secretions.

Breathing

Hypoxia may complicate any one of several toxic exposures. Vesicant gases and pulmonary agents may produce acute lung injury and hypoxia. Organophosphorus nerve agents may produce suffocating pulmonary secretions that interfere with gas exchange. Organophosphorus nerve agents or botulism may lead to diaphragmatic insufficiency and a failure of appropriate air movement into the lungs. In any case, the appropriate treatment is supplemental oxygen; a reasonable target is an oxygen saturation of greater than or equal to 95%

Circulation

Hypotension should initially be treated with intravenous crystalloid; if this fails, vasopressors should be used. Because the hypotension seen with poisoned patients is frequently the result of peripheral vascular collapse, direct acting alpha-adrenergic agonists (such as neosynephrine or norepinephrine) are usually the first-line recommendation.

Decontamination

Decontamination is a crucial intervention in the initial assessment and stabilization of a patient who is poisoned as part of a terrorist attack. In such cases, dermal decontamination is usually the focus as agents of biological and chemical terror are likely to be aerosolized. Gastrointestinal decontamination (gastric emptying and/or administration of activated charcoal), while an important intervention in the hospital-based treatment of poisoned patients, is unlikely to be helpful in the treatment of disaster-related toxic exposures, as mass exposures are unlikely to occur during the oral route. Incidents such as staphylococcal enterotoxin B poisoning, where gastrointestinal decontamination may actually be indicated, are the exception rather than the rule.

POST-STABILIZATION PATIENT ASSESSMENT

Physical Examination

A portion of the physical examination will, by necessity, be performed as part of the assessment of airway, breathing and circulation. After initial stabilization and decontamination, a more detailed examination may reveal injuries not initially suspected, such as a concussion effect from a blast that may accompany the detonation of a chemical weapon.

A more detailed physical examination may also reveal the presence of a toxic syndrome, or toxidrome, which provides a diagnosis in the absence of historical information or laboratory data. The toxidrome examination consists of assessing vital signs, mental status, pupil size, oral mucous membranes, lung sounds, bowel sounds, and the skin. Several agents that may be employed in terrorist-related disasters might be expected to produce classic toxidromes (see Table 1).

Frequent reexamination is a key component of the successful care of the poisoned patient. Patients who initially appear to be stable, such as the patient who has a mild cough and normal transcutaneous oxygen saturation after mustard gas exposure, may go on to develop acute lung injury and the acute respiratory distress syndrome several hours later. Such patients, despite their benign initial examination, may quickly deteriorate and require endotracheal intubation.

Laboratory Evaluation

The laboratory evaluation of a potentially poisoned patient is driven by the patient's symptoms and the possible agents involved. Patients who present with a mild cough after a respiratory agent attack may need no more than a chest x-ray; patients with oral ricin poisoning may need an extensive laboratory evaluation to assess for the sequelae of this disease.

One test that is unlikely to be of benefit in evaluating potential victims of toxin-related disasters is the "toxicology screen." Such screens typically test for drugs of abuse (cocaine, amphetamines, LSD, PCP, marijuana), which are unlikely to be used in terrorist attacks. Even a positive result would be unhelpful, as it would likely be an incidental finding. The "toxicology screen," therefore, really has no role in the routine management of poisoned patients in the disaster setting.

Table 1. Toxidromes that May Be Encountered in Disaster Medicine

	Nerve agents (cholinergic)	Chemical weapon BZ (anticholinergic)	Fentanyl derivatives* (opioid)
Pulse	Variable	Elevated	Normal to decreased
Blood pressure	Variable	Slightly elevated	Normal to decreased
Respiratory rate	Increase	Variable	Profoundly decreased
Temperature	Normal	Normal to elevated	Normal
Mental status	Lethargic	Confused	Lethargic
Pupils	Miotic	Dilated	Miotic
Mucous membranes	Copious secretions	Dry	Normal
Lung sounds	Rhonchorous	Normal	Normal
Bowel sounds	Hyperactive	Absent	Absent
Skin	Diaphoretic	Dry	Normal

*Fentanyl or a fentanyl derivative was used to end the Moscow Theater Siege in 2002.

TREATMENT

Contrary to popular opinion, the treatment of the poisoned patient rarely consists of finding the correct antidote. Most of the life-saving treatment of a poisoned patient consists of securing the airway, breathing, and circulation; performing adequate decontamination; and providing ongoing supportive treatment.

Occasionally, however, patients are poisoned with an agent that may be reversed with the appropriate antidote. A partial list of these poisons, with their antidotes, is provided in Table 2.

SUMMARY

Toxicology is discipline that concerns itself with patients who have been poisoned. In the field of disaster medicine, the important principles of toxicology include identifying an incident as a toxin-mediated event, initial assessment and stabilization, post-stabilization assessment, and treatment.

Table 2. Poisons that May Cause Mass Casualties and Their Antidotes

"Nerve" agents	Pralidoxime (2-PAM), atropine
Chemical weapon BZ	Physostigmine
Fentanyl derivatives	Naloxone, naltrexone
Cyanide	Amyl nitrite, sodium nitrite, sodium thiosulfate

PART IVB

Infectious Diseases of Disaster

51 MEASLES

Scott Cohen, MD*

OVERVIEW

Measles is caused by an RNA virus of the genus *Morbillivirus* in the family Paramyxoviridae. It remains a major killer of children under 5 years in the developing world, where mortality rates may approach 5–40%. Humans are the only natural hosts of the disease. Transmission is via direct contact with respiratory droplets, and airborne spread is less common. Unfortunately, 5% of vaccine recipients will not form an antibody response. Risk factors for acquiring the disease include: overcrowding, disaster or refugee camp situations, malnutrition, immunocompromised children, and unvaccinated children under 18 months of age.

PRESENTATION

The incubation period is 7 to 14 days from exposure to first signs/symptoms of disease.

Patients are contagious 1 to 2 days prior to onset of illness and until around 4 days after the rash appears.

Signs and Symptoms

The prodromal phase of the illness begins with fever and coryza (rhinorrhea) over the first 24 hours; then cough and severe conjunctivitis develop 1–2 days later. Also seen 24–48 hours after respiratory symptoms develop are Koplik spots. These are bright red spots with a gray/white center seen on the buccal mucosa (inside of the mouth). These Koplik spots, seen with any of the other symptoms, assure the diagnosis of measles. 24 to 48 hours after Koplik spots develop, a maculopapular rash develops.

*Global Pediatric Alliance, Oakland, California

Complications and Physical Findings

- Otitis Media
- Pneumonia (measles pneumonia and superimposed bacterial pneumonia) with respiratory distress
- Croup
- Diarrhea and dehydration
- Encephalitis
- Cervical adenitis
- Splenomegaly
- Corneal ulcers; keratomalacia; blindness (worsened by Vitamin A deficiency)
- Hemorrhagic measles
- Encephalitis in children older than 2 years of age (10–20% fatality; neurologic sequelae common in survivors)
- Subacute Sclerosing Panencephalitis (SSPE): very rare late complication patients 5–15 years old; slow progressive degenerative disease
- Death
- Complications are especially severe in children younger than 5 years, with no history of being immunized, who are immunocompromised (cancer, HIV), and/or malnourished.

DIAGNOSIS

Measles IgM antibody levels in serum are seen in the acute phase. Measles IgM is detectable for 1 month after onset of rash. Measles virus can be isolated from urine, blood, and nasopharyngeal secretions. In regions where no laboratory facilities are available, the clinical diagnosis, especially if Koplik spots present, is adequate and should warrant treatment.

DIFFERENTIAL DIAGNOSIS

Viral illnesses such as Roseola

TREATMENT

- Vitamin A 200,000 IU PO immediately (preserves eyesight and lowers disease severity)
- Active immunization (MMR) best if given within 3 days of exposure. MMR not to be given to children younger than 6 months of age (see "Prevention" below)
- Ophthalmic antibiotic drops or ointment
- Systemic Antibiotics for respiratory disease
- Hydration (IV or PO)
- Nutrition
- Passive immunization (immune globulin) if given less than 6 days after exposure and available.

- Criteria for immune globulin
  - o Children younger than 12 months of age and pregnant women should receive immune globulin IM (0.25 ml/kg; maximum: 15 ml) as soon as possible after exposure
  - o Immunocompromised children of any age should receive immune globulin as soon as possible after exposure (0.5 ml/kg IM; maximum: 15 ml)
  - o Infants younger than 6 months of age should receive immune globulin soon after exposure, but not the vaccine
  - o Children older than 12 months of age should receive vaccine alone within 72 hr of exposure, and not immune globulin
  - o Pregnant women and immunocompromised persons should receive immune globulin but not vaccine

PROGNOSIS

General mortality rate of 5%, which may increase to 40% during epidemics.

PREVENTION

MMR Vaccine is routinely recommended for all children worldwide by 12 to 15 months of age. It should be given as young as 6 months if there is an outbreak and exposure, but the immune response is felt to be suboptimal when given under 1 year. A second MMR vaccine is recommended routinely at 4–6 years of age but may be given at any time provided that an interval of at least 4 weeks has elapsed since the first vaccine dose. If a child receives an MMR vaccine under 1 year of age, two more doses, separated by at least 1 month, should be given after the first birthday. Contraindications to the MMR vaccine include: pregnancy, children under 6 months of age, immunodeficiency, HIV infection, cancer, and untreated active TB.

REFERENCES

Committee on Infectious Diseases, American Academy of Pediatrics. 2003. *Red book; report of the committee on infectious diseases*, 26th ed. Elk Grove Village, IL: American Academy of Pediatrics.

Eddleston M, Pierini S. 1999. *Oxford handbook of tropical medicine*. New York: Oxford UP.

Behrman RE, Kliegman RM, Jenson HB, eds. 2000. *Nelson's textbook of pediatrics*, 16th ed. Philadelphia: Saunders.

52 APPROACH TO DIARRHEA AND DYSENTERY

Tracy H. Zivin-Tutela, MD*

OVERVIEW

Historical Significance

Hippocrates said, "the influence of water upon health is very great. Such as are marshy, standing, or stagnant, must in summer be hot, thick and stinking, because there is no outflow ... In the summer there are epidemics of dysentery, diarrhea, and long quartan fever."

Outbreaks of diarrhea have historically occurred whenever there were crowded living conditions, and particularly whenever the normal patterns of trade, food supply, and social structure or governmental authority were disrupted.

Etiology

The clinical definition of diarrhea is three or more episodes of loose stool or any loose stool with blood during a 24-hour period. Chronic diarrhea is when symptoms last more than 2–4 weeks.

Incidence and Prevalence

An estimated 744 million to 1 billion episodes and nearly 5 million deaths from diarrhea occur per year worldwide.

Risk Factors

Natural and manmade disasters that produce overcrowding, a scarcity of safe drinking water, improper elimination of human waste, and the contamination of food during or after its preparation are risk factors for the spread of infectious diarrhea

*Division of Infectious Diseases, St. Luke's/Roosevelt Hospital Center, New York

PATHOGENESIS

Acute diarrhea is acquired thorough the fecal–oral route. Infectious diarrhea can be classified as noninflammatory or inflammatory. Noninflammatory diarrhea results from disturbance of absorption of fluid and electrolytes and does not involve invasion of the intestinal mucosa. The most common pathogens of noninflammatory diarrhea include viruses and protozoans. Inflammatory diarrhea results from invasion of intestinal mucosa, inducing an inflammatory response that results in colonic malabsorption and the presence of fecal leukocytes and blood. The most common pathogens include bacteria.

PRESENTATION

Incubation

Incubation varies with each implicated pathogen. Rapid onset of symptoms usually within 6 hours of ingestion suggests a preformed toxin. This includes *Staphylococcus* and *Bacillus cereus*. Onset of symptoms, more than 8 hours, suggests *Clostridium perfringens*.

Signs and Symptoms

Noninflammatory diarrhea is described as watery and voluminous. There is absence of fever and abdominal pain. Inflammatory diarrhea is described as a small volume of loose stool that may contain blood or pus. Fever as well as abdominal pain is typical.

CLINICAL PEARLS

Cholera (*Vibrio cholerae*)

It has a short incubation: usually less than 1 to 5 days. It is a dose-dependent enterotoxin-mediated infection with copious, watery, painless diarrhea also know as "rice water stools." Vomiting may occur. If not treated promptly it may quickly lead to severe dehydration and death. Monitoring of intake and outtake of fluids and electrolyte balance is important to prevent death. The treatment should involve aggressive oral rehydration; if this is not possible, then intravenous hydration.

Shigella (*Shigella dysenteriae*)

Shigella is made up of four serogroups; type one is the most virulent and the cause of epidemic dysentery. Classic symptoms include bloody diarrhea, abdominal cramps, fever, and rectal pain. Complications include seizures, renal failure, and hemolytic uremic syndrome. Fatality ranges from 5 to 15%.

Salmonella (*Salmonella species*)

The species of *Salmonella* include typhi, paratyphi, typhimurium, and choleraesuis. The incubation period ranges from 8 to 48 hours after ingestion and usually lasts

3–5 days. The symptoms include watery diarrhea, which may lead to blood dysentery, fever, crampy abdominal pain, and vomiting.

DIAGNOSIS

Laboratory

Microscopic examination is the traditional tool of investigation. Stool culture has been the mainstay in obtaining the causative agent of diarrhea. If stool is preserved for more than 24 hours, fecal leukocyte examination is unreliable. Examination of stool for ova and parasites in acute diarrhea is not cost-effective. Most parasitic infections cause a persistent or chronic clinical course.

Other

Dehydration is the main cause of morbidity and mortality in the patient with diarrhea.

Postural changes in blood pressure (decrease of 10 mm Hg) and pulse rate (increase of 10 beats/min) indicate volume depletion. Measurement of urine output, body temperature, and observation for abdominal distention and rebound tenderness are necessary for appropriate treatment. Rectal examination for occult blood is a cheap and inexpensive way to diagnose inflammatory diarrhea.

DIFFERENTIAL DIAGNOSIS

The differential diagnosis of diarrhea includes colonic neoplasm, inflammatory bowel disease, malabsorption syndromes including tropical sprue, bacterial overgrowth or celiac sprue, HIV, and lactose intolerance.

TREATMENT

Most acute diarrheal illness is self-limited, and no therapy is necessary. The goal of therapy is to restore fluid loss and prevent dehydration. In large-volume diarrhea (noninflammatory) carbonated drinks and juices should be avoided; instead, glucose-containing electrolyte repletion is recommended.

In the case of inflammatory diarrhea, antibiotics may be warranted. If suspected or culture proven *E. coli*, *Shigella*, *Salmonella*, or *Campylobacter*, the use of ciprofloxacin 500 mg orally twice daily for 3–7 days is recommended. If *E. coli* O157:H7 is suspected, no antibiotic is advised, as studies suggest it may be harmful. If *Vibrio cholerae* is suspected or culture proven, doxycycline 300 mg orally in a single dose or a fluoroquinolone in a single dose is recommended. In cases of giardiasis, treatment with metronidazole 250–750 mg orally every 8 hours is recommended for a duration of 7–10 days. If *Entamoeba histolytica* is the cause of diarrhea, then treatment with metronidazole is warranted. A common occurrence after the illness includes lactose intolerance; patients should be advised to temporarily avoid dairy products.

PROGNOSIS

The primary cause of mortality in infectious diarrhea is dehydration. Approximately 5 million deaths worldwide occur each year, and are attributable to dehydration. Through thoughtful strategies aimed at prevention and access to health care including cost-effective evaluation and treatment, there is a chance at preventing death.

PREVENTION

Prevention is achieved by protecting the water and sewage systems, avoiding overcrowding, advocating hand hygiene, and boiling contaminated water.

The traditional vaccine against cholera (based on whole, killed cells) is characterized by low levels of efficacy. It is not recommended for the control of epidemics. The new vaccines might be considered, but with these there is a rapid loss of protection, giving a false sense of security

RESOURCES

Pan American Health Organization: www.paho.org
World Health Organization: www.who.int
Centers for Disease Control: www.cdc.gov

REFERENCES

Ilnyckyj A. 2001. Clinical evaluation and management of acute infectious diarrhea in adults. *Gastroenterol Clin North Am* **30**(3):599–609.

Lim ML, Wallace MR. 2004. Infectious diarrhea in history. *Infect Dis Clin North Am* **18**(2):261–274.

53 MALARIA

John D. Cahill, MD*

OVERVIEW

Malaria has a global distribution throughout the tropics. At least 300–500 million new cases of malaria occur annually, resulting in 5 million deaths. These statistics are probably not an accurate reflection of the impact malaria has, since many of the afflicted countries do not have the proper public health surveillance systems to report and record this disease. It is important to understand the concept of stable versus unstable malaria. Stable malaria occurs in regions where the population is constantly being exposed. Therefore, much of the population will develop partial immunity by 5 years of age. In these regions mortality rates are not as high, except in the pediatric and pregnant women population. Unstable malaria occurs in regions where the disease is seasonal or sporadic; here the population is afforded no partial immunity. In these regions, malaria contributes much more significantly to morbidity and mortality. Obviously, travelers and individuals who have been away from a stable malarious for several years have no immunity. Several traits are felt to afford partial protection against malaria: sickle cell trait, SS individuals as well (usually early death), G6PD deficiency, the thalassemias, hemoglobin C, and a negative Duffy blood type (*P. vivax*: West Africa).

PATHOGENESIS

Malaria is transmitted from the bite of the female anopheles mosquito, which usually feeds from late afternoon through dawn. Other means of transmission include: blood transfusions, shared needles, airport malaria (where one is infected with a mosquito who has traveled on a plane), and (rarely) congenitally. There are four different species involved: *Plasmodium falciparum* (causes complicated malaria), *P. vivax*, *P. ovale*, and *P. malariae*. A detailed life cycle is beyond the scope of this handbook; however,

*Department of Emergency Medicine and Division of Infectious Diseases, St. Luke's/Roosevelt Hospital Center, New York

several key features will be highlighted. During a blood meal the mosquito injects the sporozoite, which makes its way to the cells of the liver, where it can replicate into a schizont or remain dormant as a hypnozoite (seen in *P. vivax* and *ovale* infection). Infected liver cells release the schizont into the bloodstream, where it attacks erythrocytes. Inside the newly infected erythrocyte an immature trophozoite develops and one of two pathways can occur. The trophozoite can mature, producing further schizonts, which eventually causes rupture of the cell and allows for other erythrocytes to become infected or the trophozoite can develop into a gametocyte that is released into the bloodstream and taken up by the mosquito during a blood meal. The gametocyte is essential for continuation of the life cycle of the parasite in the mosquito.

PRESENTATION

Depending on the species of malaria, the incubation period can be quite varied. With *P. falciparum* the incubation period is around a week; however, it sometimes can be several weeks to months. With *P. vivax* and *ovale* secondary infection with activation of the hypnozoite can occur many years later.

Although all four species clinically cause malaria, it is *P. falciparum* that causes complicated malaria and contributes significantly to the morbidity and mortality seen. Malaria always presents with cyclical fevers; other symptoms may include: fatigue, malaise, arthralgias, headache, upper respiratory complaints, nausea, vomiting, and diarrhea. On physical examination, manifestations of anemia may be noted (pale conjunctiva and tongue, increased respiratory rate, tachycardia, a new heart murmur), mild hepatomegaly, jaundice in severe cases, and splenomegaly (particularly with prolonged or repeated infections). Complications of severe malaria include: cerebral malaria (seizures, coma), anemia, congestive heart failure (secondary to anemia), pulmonary edema, jaundice, acute renal failure, metabolic acidosis, disseminated intravascular coagulation, and hypoglycemia (particularly in children).

DIAGNOSIS

There should be a high index of suspicion for malaria in all individuals presenting with a fever from the tropics. A thick and thin blood film should be obtained. The thick film is useful to screen for evidence of malaria, and if negative a thin film is not necessary. If the thick film is positive, a thin film should be performed to identify the species and the percentage of infected red blood cells. It is important to remember that a negative blood film does not exclude the diagnosis of malaria. Rapid diagnostic dipsticks have been developed for *P. falciparum*, based upon plasmodial histidine rich protein and parasite-specific LDH. Other means to diagnosis include: fluorescence microscopy (quantitative buffy coat), DNA probes, PCR, and antibody detection (useless in acute infection). On a complete blood count, anemia and thrombocytopenia may be appreciated.

DIFFERENTIAL DIAGNOSIS

Typhoid fever
Upper respiratory infection
Viral hepatitis
Dengue fever
Acute HIV
Schistosomiasis
Brucellosis
Trypanosomiasis
Visceral leishmaniasis
Rickettsial infections
Relapsing fever

TREATMENT

Several principles determine treatment for malaria. One needs to define a case as either being complicated or uncomplicated. Complicated cases would be those with evidence of significant systemic involvement (cerebral malaria, acute renal failure, pulmonary edema, metabolic acidosis, DIC), severe anemia, significant other comorbid problems, and those unable to tolerate oral medication. As soon as a patient shows signs of improvement and is able to tolerate oral medication, they should be switched over from intravenous therapy. If an individual has been infected from a chloroquine-sensitive region (Central America, Haiti, Dominican Republic, and pockets of the Middle East), chloroquine should still be mainstay treatment. Ideally, patients receiving intravenous quinine/quinidine should be place on a cardiac monitor. Rapid administration of either agent may cause hypoglycemia. Supportive treatment is also important: blood transfusions, hydration, nutrition, treating other underlying infections, correcting hypoglycemia, and dialysis. Some of the more common treatment regimens are listed below, availability of agents will vary depending upon country.

Uncomplicated Chloroquine Sensitive

Chloroquine 500 mg PO BID x 2-3 days

Uncomplicated Chloroquine Resistant

Quinine 650 mg PO TID and Doxycycline 100 mg PO BID both for 7 days
Atovaquone/Proguanil 1 g/400 mg PO QD x 3 days
Mefloquine 750 mg PO then 500 mg PO 12 hr later
Halofantrine 500 mg PO x 3 doses

Complicated Malaria

Intravenous quinine 20 mg/kg in dextrose loading dose given over 4 hours, then 10 mg/kg TID given over 2 hours, switch to oral quinine when able to tolerate, for a total treatment length of seven days
Intramuscular quinine (same dose as above)

Quinidine is used as first line treatment in the United States, instead of quinine. Intravenously it is administered as a loading dose of 10 mg/kg salt over 1–2 hours and then as a continuous infusion of 20 μg/kg/min salt. Alternatively, a loading dose of 24 mg/kg salt over 4 hours followed by 12 mg/kg over 4 hours every 8 hours. Switch to oral quinine when able to tolerate, for a total treatment length of 7 days.

Artesunate 3.2 mg/kg IM on day 1, then 1.6 mg/kg IM QD. Switch to an oral agent when able to tolerate.

Artesunate 2.4 mg/kg IV on day 1, then 1.2 mg/kg IV QD. Switch to an oral agent when able to tolerate.

Eradication of the Hypnozoite form of P. vivax and ovale

Check glucose phosphate dehydrogenase status prior to treatment

Primaquine (15 mg base) PO QD x 14 days

PROGNOSIS

Early diagnosis and prompt treatment favor a good prognosis. Unfortunately, many times the diagnosis of malaria is not entertained or treatment is delayed, contributing significantly to the mortality seen. It should be remembered that once the onset of symptoms of *P. falciparum* develop death may occur within 12 hours.

PREVENTION

Four measures can significantly decrease the chance of acquiring malaria. Mosquito nets are imperative when sleeping in the tropics, unless excellent screening is in place. The use of an insect repellant containing between 25 and 50% DEET on exposed skin surfaces. Treating one's clothes and mosquito net with permethrin. Lastly, using an appropriate antimalarial for chemoprophylaxis. A detailed discussion on chemoprophylaxis is beyond the scope of this handbook; however, it is important to remember that failure of a properly prescribed antimalarial for chemoprophylaxis is rare, whereas noncompliance is very common. Options include:

Chloroquine (in sensitive regions) 500-mg tab, 1 week prior to travel, once a week while in a malarious endemic region, and once a week for 4 weeks afterwards.

Mefloquine (suitable everywhere, except along the Thailand/Cambodia border) 250 mg tab, 1 week prior to travel, once a week while in a malarious endemic region and once a week for 4 weeks afterwards.

Atovaquone/proguanil 250/100 mg tab, 1 day prior to traveling, once a day while in a malarious endemic region and once a day for 7 days afterwards.

Doxycycline 100 mg tab, 1 day prior to traveling, once a day while in a malarious endemic region and once a day for 4 weeks afterwards.

RESOURCES

http://www.cdc.gov/malaria/references.htm
http://www.who.int/topics/malaria/en/

54 MENINGITIS AND ENCEPHALITIS

Catherine James, MD*

INTRODUCTION

Meningitis is an inflammation of the membranes of the brain or spinal cord that may be caused by bacteria, viruses, mycoplasma, spirochetes, fungi, or parasites. Pathogens gain access to the CSF either by hematogenous spread or by direct extension from a purulent parameningeal focus.

BACTERIAL MENINGITIS

Epidemiology

The epidemiology of bacterial meningitis changed dramatically between 1985 and 1995. The total number of cases decreased by 55%, to about 5800 cases per year, and the median age increased to 25 years. This is due to routine childhood vaccination with a conjugate vaccine to *H. influenza* type B. Mortality varies by causative pathogen and is highest for meningitis due to *S. pneumoniae*. Likely bacterial pathogens depend on the patient's age and underlying health status:

- Age less than 3 months: group B strep, Gram-negative enteric bacilli, *L. monocytogenes*
- Age 3 months to 18 years: *N. meningitides, S. pneumoniae, H. influenzae*
- Age 18 to 50 years: *S. pneumoniae, N. meningitidis*
- Age greater than 50 years: *S. pneumoniae, L. monocytogenes*, Gram-negative bacilli
- Immunocompromised: *L. monocytogenes* or Gram-negative bacilli
- Head trauma, neurosurgery, or with CSF shunt: Staphylococci, Gram-negative bacilli, *S. pneumoniae*

*Harvard Medical School, Boston

Diagnosis

Clinical presentation varies by the patient's age. Older children and adults present with fever, headache, photophobia, and nuchal rigidity. Kernig and Brudzinski signs may be present. Patients may also have lethargy, malaise, vomiting, altered mental status, and seizures. Skin findings include petechiae and purpura. Shock and cardiovascular collapse may be present. Neonates and infants present with fever, irritability, altered sleep patterns, vomiting, and poor feeding. A bulging anterior fontanel may be present on exam. Elderly patients may present with only altered mental status.

Lumbar puncture is the mainstay of diagnosis and should be performed as promptly as possible in patients with suspected CNS infection unless there is concern for increased intracranial pressure (see below). Cerebrospinal fluid should be sent for cell count with differential, protein, glucose, Gram stain, and bacterial culture. Other tests such as India ink stain, VDRL, Lyme titer, stain for acid-fast bacteria, PCR for herpes, cryptococcal antigen, or cultures for anaerobic bacteria, viruses, mycoplasma, and fungi should be performed as indicated. Cell counts in acute bacterial meningitis are usually markedly elevated (greater than 500 cells/mm^3), with a predominance of neutrophils. Gram stain may show bacteria. Protein is elevated and glucose is decreased. Bacterial antigen detection may be useful for patients who received antibiotics prior to LP.

Computerized tomography (CT) scanning should be performed before lumbar puncture in patients with focal neurologic deficits, papilledema, seizures, evidence of head trauma, or altered mental status, which preclude careful neurologic examination to avoid the risk of cerebral herniation. When head CT is indicated, it should be performed after blood cultures have been drawn and empiric antibiotic therapy started.

Management

Antibiotics should be instituted as soon as possible. Empiric choice of antibiotics is directed toward the most likely pathogens based on the patient's age and underlying health status:

- Age less than 3 months: ampicillin plus gentamicin or cefotaxime
- Age 3 months to 18 years: cefotaxime or ceftriaxone
- Age 18 to 50 years: cefotaxime or ceftriaxone
- Age greater then 50 years: ampicillin plus cefotaxime or ceftriaxone
- Immunocompromised: ampicillin plus ceftazidime
- Post–head trauma or neurosurgical procedure or with CSF shunt: vancomycin plus ceftazidime
- Vancomycin should be added if *S. pneumoniae* cannot be excluded

If there are identifiable bacteria on the Gram stain, therapy should be directed toward the presumptive pathogen.

- Gram-positive cocci: vancomycin plus cefotaxime or ceftriaxone
- Gram-negative cocci: penicillin G
- Gram-positive bacilli: ampicillin plus gentamicin
- Gram-negative bacilli: gentamicin plus cefotaxime or ceftriaxone

Steroids are often used to decrease meningeal inflammation and to modulate the inflammatory response caused by release of bacterial products from bacteria killed by antibiotics. Therefore, if steroid therapy is to be instituted, it should be started with or before the first dose of antibiotics. Steroids have been shown to reduce neurologic sequelae, especially hearing loss, in children aged greater than 2 months with meningitis caused by *H. influenzae*, but the decreased incidence of this infection due to the conjugate vaccine has made this pathogen uncommon, and the benefits for infections for other pathogens are not as clear. Treatment with steroids has been found to be associated with a significant reduction in mortality and in neurologic sequelae of acute bacterial meningitis in adults. Recommended dose is 0.15 mg/kg IV (10 mg in adults) given with or slightly before the first dose of antibiotics and continued every 6 hours for 2 to 4 days in patients older than 2 months of age, except in patients in septic shock, immunosuppressed patients, or patients with post-neurosurgical meningitis.

Supportive care includes the following:

- Hypotension or shock should be treated with vigorous fluid resuscitation and pressors.
- Coagulopathy should be treated if present.
- Increased intracranial pressure (ICP) may develop in patients with meningitis as a result of cerebral edema, and may lead to life-threatening cerebral herniation. Hyperventilation may be employed to decrease the $PaCO_2$, resulting in cerebral vasoconstriction. Hyperosmolar agents, such as mannitol may be used to decrease cerebral edema. Other measures, such as elevating the head of the bed to 30 degrees, antipyretics, controlling seizures, and giving lidocaine prior to endotracheal intubation are also helpful.
- SIADH may result in water retention and hyponatremia, contributing to cerebral edema. It is treated with fluid restriction and hypertonic sodium.
- Seizures: correction of hyponatremia or hypoglycemia, and anticonvulsants should be used for seizure control.

Prevention

In addition to universal precautions, droplet precautions should be used until meningococcal disease is ruled out. Household contacts of patients with meningococcal meningitis should receive rifampin (600 mg for adults, 10 mg/kg for children older than 1 year, and 5 mg/kg for children less than 1 year of age) orally every 12 hours for 4 doses, ciprofloxacin 500 mg orally for 1 dose, azithromycin 500 mg orally for one dose, or ceftriaxone 250 mg IM (125 mg for children) for one dose. Healthcare workers do not need prophylaxis unless they have had direct mucosal contact with the patient's secretions. Meningococcal vaccine is recommended for travelers to epidemic areas, military recruits, college freshman, and in established epidemics. A pneumococcal conjugate vaccine is now part of the routine childhood immunizations, though the impact this will have on pneumococcal meningitis is not yet known. The polyvalent pneumococcal vaccine should be considered for elderly or immunocompromised patients.

Epidemics

Epidemics of meningitis have been documented in areas of overcrowding due to disasters, such as refugee camps, since *N. meningitides* has airborne transmission. Mass immunization may help prevent disease. The CDC reports periodic epidemics in Sub-Saharan Africa, and an epidemic occurred in Saudi Arabia during the Hajj in 2000.

Anthrax is listed by the CDC as a potential biological weapon and can cause meningitis after inhalation. The widely publicized cases of inhalational anthrax in the United States in 2001 that were disseminated through the mail are an example of how this could be used.

ASEPTIC MENINGITIS

Aseptic meningitis is an inflammation of the meninges that occurs in the absence of growth on routine culture media. The signs and symptoms are similar to those of bacterial meningitis, but are usually not as severe. The neurologic exam is usually normal. The prognosis for viral meningitis is very good.

Causes

Causes include viruses, unusual bacteria (such as TB), fungi, spirochetes, and parasites. Enteroviruses are the most common cause of aseptic meningitis, especially in the summer months. Tuberculous and fungal meningitis are more common in immunosuppressed patients.

Diagnosis

Diagnosis is similar to that of bacterial meningitis, though other CSF studies such as India ink stain, VDRL, Lyme titer, stain for acid-fast bacteria, PCR for herpes, cryptococcal antigen, or cultures for anaerobic bacteria, viruses, mycoplasma, and fungi may be required. A PPD should be placed on all patients with meningitis from areas where TB is endemic, or if history or symptoms suggest TB infection. Lyme disease may be suggested by history or characteristic rash, and should be considered in endemic areas.

Management

Management is supportive for viral infections, though antibiotics should be started until bacterial culture results are obtained if the diagnosis is not clear. Treatment for tuberculosis, fungi, parasites, or Lyme disease should be instituted if appropriate. Some experienced clinicians may choose not to hospitalize clinically stable patients with a clear diagnosis of aseptic meningitis, but hospitalization is necessary for more ill patients or those in whom the diagnosis is not certain.

ENCEPHALITIS

Encephalitis is an inflammation of the brain parenchyma. It can be caused by infectious (usually viral) agents or due to immunologic mechanisms, as in post-infectious encephalitis. Approximately 20,000 cases occur per year in the United States, most of them mild. Viruses enter the host through the skin or through the respiratory, gastrointestinal or urogenital tracts. The virus then enters the CNS either by hematogenous spread, by retrograde transmission along neuronal axons, or by direct invasion following infection of the nasal mucosa. Viral replication in neural cells leads to cell dysfunction and death, with resulting cerebral edema and increased ICP.

Causes

Herpes simplex virus (HSV) is the most common cause of viral encephalitis in the United States (about 10% of cases). Disease in neonates is often caused by HSV type 2 acquired from perinatal transmission, but HSV type 1 is the most common cause in all other patients. The mortality rate is greater than 70% if left untreated, but is approximately 30% with treatment. Survivors commonly have significant neurologic sequelae.

Other viruses include arboviruses (such as St. Louis encephalitis, eastern or western equine encephalitis, West Nile encephalitis, LaCrosse encephalitis), rabies, mumps, measles, and varicella. The arthropod-borne encephalitides are transmitted by mosquitoes from a host, such as wild birds, to horses or humans. Outbreaks occur periodically in the United States in the summer and fall.

Post-infectious encephalomyelitis may follow infection with various viruses, most commonly varicella and influenza in the United States, but measles is the most common cause worldwide. It often follows a vague viral syndrome, usually of the respiratory tract, and occurs days to weeks after the preceding illness. It is thought to be an autoimmune phenomenon that is initiated by the viral pathogen. Demyelination is a prominent pathological finding of this disease.

Diagnosis

Clinical manifestations include headache, fever, altered level of consciousness, disturbances in behavior and speech, and generalized seizures. Focal neurologic findings generally indicate HSV infection and include ataxia, cranial nerve defects, hemiparesis, or focal seizures. Skin lesions such as the characteristic exanthem of varicella or vesicles that suggest HSV type 1 or 2 may be present. History may reveal the bite of a potentially rabid animal, and knowledge of disease outbreaks in the community (such as mosquito-borne viruses) may help to guide diagnosis. Differential diagnosis includes metabolic diseases, toxic disorders, mass lesions, and acute demyelinating disorders.

Laboratory Evaluation

Cerebrospinal fluid must be obtained to exclude bacterial meningitis. CSF should be sent for cell count, protein, glucose, Gram stain, bacterial and viral cultures, and HSV PCR. In viral encephalitis, CSF cell count usually shows fewer than 500 cells/mm^3, with a mononuclear prominence, though the cells may be predominantly polymorphonuclear early in the course of illness. CSF protein is normal to moderately elevated and glucose is usually normal. Detection of herpes virus by polymerase chain reaction (PCR) of CSF leads to a rapid diagnosis of HSV infection. Viral isolation from other body sites, such as the nasopharynx, skin lesions, urine, and feces may aid in diagnosis. Blood samples for CBC with differential, platelet count, electrolytes, BUN, creatinine, glucose, blood culture, and viral titers should be obtained. Detection of viral antibodies does not aid in acute diagnosis or management, but may be useful later to clarify the cause of the infection.

CT or MRI may show focal parenchymal involvement or temporal lobe edema in HSV encephalitis. EEG shows characteristic periodic spike wave temporal lobe activity and slow wave complexes in HSV encephalitis. It is usually normal in other encephalitides.

Management

Management of non-herpes viral encephalitis is supportive, though herpes simplex virus and varicella-zoster encephalitis are treated with acyclovir, 30–60 mg/kg/day divided q 8 h, in addition to supportive measures. Acyclovir should be administered until the virus is identified, especially if there is evidence of focality on physical or neurodiagnostic evaluation. Antibiotics should also be given until a bacterial etiology is excluded. Medical management of rabies is prevention of infection by the administration of rabies vaccine and rabies immune globulin after an exposure to a potentially rabid animal. Once infection occurs, it is uniformly fatal. Arboviral infections can be prevented by using insect repellents and protective clothing to avoid mosquito bites. Treatment of infection is supportive.

Epidemics

Epidemics of arthropod-borne encephalitis can occur during natural disasters if heavy rainfall and flooding lead to increased numbers of mosquitoes, or if insect control measures are disrupted. There have been recent epidemics of West Nile virus in the United States. In addition, the CDC lists Venezuelan, eastern, and western encephalitis as potential biological weapons. An unexplained large number of cases should raise suspicion for a potential act of bioterrorism.

RESOURCES

www.cdc.gov for information on epidemiology, disease outbreaks.
www.aapredbook.org for pediatric infectious disease information and treatment

REFERENCES

Fleisher GR. 2000. Central nervous system infections. In *Textbook of pediatric emergency medicine*, 4th ed., pp. 730–736. Ed GR Fleisher, S Ludwig. Philadelphia: Lippincott Williams and Wilkins.

Gorelick MH. 2000. Encephalitis. In *Textbook of pediatric emergency medicine*, 4th ed., pp. 708–710. Ed GR Fleisher, S Ludwig. Philadelphia: Lippincott Williams and Wilkins.

Greenough PG. 2002. Infectious diseases and disasters. In *disaster medicine*, pp. 23–33. Ed DE Hogan, J Burstein J. Philadelphia: Lippincott Williams and Wilkins.

Hasbun R, Abrahams J, Jekel J, Quagliarello VJ. 2001. Computed tomography of the head before lumbar puncture in adults with suspected meningitis. *N Engl J Med* **345**:1727–1733.

Lavoie FW, Saucier JR. 2002. Central nervous system infections. In *Rosen's emergency medicine: concepts and clinical practice*, 5th ed., pp 1527–1541. Ed JA Marx. St. Louis: Mosby.

Quagliarello VJ, Scheld WM. 1997. Treatment of bacterial meningitis. *N Engl J Med* **336**:708–716.

Schuchat A, Robinson K, Wenger JD, Harrison LH, Farley M, Reingold AL, Lefkowitz L, Perkins BA. 1997. Bacterial meningitis in the United States in 1995. *N Engl J Med* **337**:970–976.

Van de Beek D, de Gans J, McIntyre P, Prasad K. 2004. Steroids in adults with acute bacterial meningitis: a systematic review. *Lancet Infect Dis* **4**:139–143.

Whitley RJ. 1990. Viral encephalitis. *N Engl J Med* **323**:242–250.

55

TUBERCULOSIS

John D. Cahill, MD*

OVERVIEW

Although tuberculosis (TB) is not a top priority in initial disaster response, healthcare providers need to be familiar with the disease. Many disasters occur in regions of the world where the disease is endemic and contributes significantly to morbidity and mortality. TB has been called by many names throughout the centuries and notoriously is known as the disease of consumption (progressive wasting away of the body). In the last twenty years, the disease has gained significant attention with the problem of multi-drug-resistant TB and co infection with HIV.

EPIDEMIOLOGY

Tuberculosis has a global distribution and is highly prevalent throughout the tropics. The World Health Organization estimates that an individual in the world is newly infected with TB every second and that, overall, one-third of the world's population is currently infected. Factors that increase the transmission or incidence of TB include: the global trend of urbanization, overcrowding (prisons, low-income housing, and institutions), immigrants relocating from endemic regions, HIV, noncompliance with treatment, and multi-drug-resistant strains of TB.

PATHOPHYSIOLOGY

TB is caused by the bacteria *Mycobacterium tuberculosis* and occasionally from *Mycobacterium bovis* and *Mycobacterium africanum*. The infective agent is the tubercle bacilli, which can remain dormant in the body for many years. Infection typically occurs when the bacilli are dispersed into the air when an individual with active pul-

*Department of Emergency Medicine and Division of Infectious Diseases, St. Luke's/Roosevelt Hospital Center, New York

monary TB coughs. The droplet nuclei remain suspended in the air for a prolonged period of time and can survive in a dark environment. The bacilli are small enough that they escape being trapped by the protective respiratory mechanisms and end up in the terminal alveoli. Five minutes of direct sunlight kills the bacilli. Therefore, infection usually occurs in a closed environment.

During primary infection the bacilli multiply within the lung and form a Ghon focus. The primary complex is the Ghon focus along with the hilar lymphadenopathy that occurs. In the normal immunocompetent individual, the body mounts a significant hypersensitivity/cellular reaction against the primary complex to kill the bacilli and contain the infection. This usually occurs within 4 to 6 weeks of infection. However, a few dormant bacilli may persist, with the only evidence being a positive tuberculin skin test. In some individuals the primary complex is not contained and they may develop tuberculous pneumonia that may be complicated by pleural effusions and collapse of the lung tissue. Cervical lymphadenopathy, meningitis, pericarditis, hypersensitivity reactions (e.g., erythema nodosum) and miliary spread may also occur in uncontained primary infection.

Post-primary TB occurs when there is reactivation and/or reinfection with bacilli. Reactivation may be triggered by a weakening of the immune system (age, HIV, other co-infections, malnutrition, as well as other causes). The immune reaction this time is localized and can be quite destructive. In the lungs extensive damage and cavitation may occur in the upper lobes. Pleural effusion, empyema, and pneumothorax are well-described complications. Extrapulmonary TB can potentially occur in any part of the body and hence the name the "great imitator."

CLINICAL

Pulmonary

The patient presenting with pulmonary TB often gives a history of fever, night sweats, weight loss, productive cough for more than 2 to 3 weeks, dyspnea, and sometimes hemoptysis. Patients who are HIV positive may have a nonclassic presentation.

Central Nervous System

TB meningitis is most commonly seen in infants and young children. It often presents in a more chronic nature than bacterial meningitis. There is the gradual onset of headache and meningeal signs with eventual decreased mental status. Secondary to the significant inflammatory reaction that occurs at the base of the brain, cranial nerve involvement is not uncommon, particularly of the optic and auditory nerves. Obstructive hydrocephalus may develop, leading to an increase in intracranial pressure. Spinal meningeal involvement may lead to paralysis. In infants the initial presentation may be failure to thrive. Diagnosis is made by lumbar puncture, where a high opening pressure may be noted, with white cells being predominantly lymphocytes (however, polymorphs may be noted in early infection), an elevated protein, and a low glucose. A fibrin web may develop if the CSF is allowed to stand. The CSF should be examined for evidence of AFB and cultured if possible. A lumbar puncture should never be performed in the patient with evidence of raised intracranial pressure, seizures, or focal neurological findings. Although a subject of much controversy, steroids appear to be of benefit in TB meningitis.

Tuberculomas may also develop and present with symptoms consistent with an intracranial lesion. Diagnosis is made with CT scan or MRI of the brain.

Lymph Node (Scrofula)

Tuberculous lymphadenitis occurs most commonly in the cervical region, but may present anywhere in the body. Initially the nodes are firm and tender and then become fluctuant and matted together. Sinus tracts may develop as the lymph node undergoes necrosis. Diagnosis is made by biopsy of the lymph node. In the clinical setting of TB; however, this may not be necessary.

Pericardium

In the tropics, TB is the most common cause for a pericardial effusion. Patients present with chest pain, shortness of breath, and dizziness. On physical exam, hypotension, elevated JVP, evidence of right-sided heart failure, a pericardial rub, and distant heart sounds may be appreciated. Cardiac tamponade can develop if untreated. Besides clinical findings, the diagnosis can be made by: an enlarged globular heart on chest x-ray, low voltage on ECG, and by echocardiogram. Pericardiocentesis should be performed only under experienced hands.

Spine (Pott's Disease)

Very common in the tropics and if unrecognized/untreated can result in devastating paralysis. The lower thoracic and lumbar regions of the spine are most commonly affected; however, it can occur anywhere. Patients present with chronic pain of the vertebral region involved, limitation of movement, and sometimes with an acute neurological finding. Tenderness to the affected spine and a gibbus deformity may be noted on physical exam. Diagnosis is made by plain films and biopsy/culture. Besides chemotherapy, surgical stabilization may be required.

Gastrointestinal

Intestinal involvement can occur from ingestion with *Mycobacterium bovis*. Peritoneal involvement occurs from post-primary spread. Patients may have nonspecific abdominal complaints: weight loss, anorexia, abdominal pain, nausea, vomiting, and diarrhea. Intestinal obstruction may develop secondary to stricture formation. Ascites is common as the disease progresses. Diagnosis can occasionally be made by paracentesis, but peritoneal biopsy is preferred.

Genitourinary

Involvement of the kidneys can lead to dysuria, nocturia, hematuria, flank pain, and less commonly acute renal failure secondary to tuberculous interstitial nephritis. On examination of the urine, a sterile pyuria is found. It is uncommon to find AFB in the urine. Cultivation of the bacilli confirms the diagnosis. In males chronic epidymitis or orchitis may develop. Female genital tract involvement presents with pelvic pain, possible vaginal bleeding, and infertility. It may be mistaken for pelvic inflammatory disease. In both sexes the diagnosis is made by biopsy and culture.

Miliary

Can potentially go anywhere in the body affecting any or multiple organ systems.

HIV Co-Infection

Infection with both rapidly accelerates the disease process of both HIV and TB. It is important to remember that atypical presentations of TB may occur and miliary disease is more common. A high index of suspicion for co-infection needs to be held for all patients with TB.

DIAGNOSIS

Microscopy

For individuals with suspicion for pulmonary TB, three sets of sputum samples should be obtained over a several-day period. Chest physiotherapy can be performed to improve sputum production. A Ziehl-Neelsen stain can be used to look for evidence of the red-staining acid-fast bacilli. A sputum is considered positive when 10,000 bacilli per ml of sputum are noted. In an advanced facility a fluorochrome stain may also be used. Aside from sputum, other clinical specimens may be examined: bronchoalveolar lavage, gastric lavage (may be an alternative in children who cannot produce sputum), pleural effusions, peritoneal fluid, CSF, lymph node biopsies, and bone marrow aspirate.

The classic histological findings in a tissue biopsy are a region of centralized caseous necrosis that may be surrounded by histiocytes, Langhans giant cells, and lymphocytes.

Culture

If facilities are available the gold standard for diagnosis is to culture the bacilli. The usual culture medium is Lowenstein Jensen; however, liquid culture and automated systems can be used if available. *Mycobacterium tuberculosis* is very slow growing, and it may take up to 8 weeks to develop a positive culture.

Molecular

Several molecular techniques using nucleic acid amplification have been developed. These tests are highly sensitive and specific, and several commercial kits are available.

Radiographic

Radiographic studies can be helpful in making the diagnosis of TB. Chest x-rays in post-primary TB may show apical/upper unilateral or bilateral infiltrates, cavitations, and calcifications. Pleural effusions can also be seen. Some patients (particularly HIV and immunocompromised) will have minimal changes or nonspecific findings on chest x-ray. Where CT scan of the chest is available, this may further help in the evaluation of questionable findings on a chest x-ray.

Tuberculin Skin Test

This test relies on a hypersensivity reaction that occurs 24–72 hours after intradermal placement. The test does not necessarily indicate active infection, just that the individual has been exposed to the bacilli. The test may be negative in infected individuals who have the following conditions: malnutrition, severe infection, military TB, HIV, cancer, or other immunosuppressive conditions.

A test is considered negative in a normal immunocompetent individual if the induration measures less than 10 mm. In a child who has received the BCG vaccine, up to 15 mm is considered negative.

TREATMENT

The cornerstone of successful TB treatment is compliance, and this is best achieved by DOT (directly observed therapy/treatment). To ensure successful treatment, a population needs to be stationary for 6 to 9 months. This can be a challenge in refugee camps and during the acute phase of an emergency. Therefore, treatment for TB should not be started unless one can adhere to DOT or ensure compliance and full completion of chemotherapy. Another principle of treatment is to use several agents for synergism and to decrease drug resistance. Treatment for TB is prolonged compared to many other infectious diseases. The common agents used for treatment will be briefly discussed. Several of these agents are available in a combination pill.

Streptomycin was the first agent used to treat TB. It is bactericidal and belongs to the aminoglycoside family and is given intramuscularly. Adverse reactions include ototoxicity and nephrotoxicity.

Isoniazid is bactericidal and adverse reactions include peripheral neuropathy and hepatitis. Pyridoxine is given to avoid the neurotoxic adverse reactions.

Rifampin is bactericidal and adverse reactions include turning body fluids a pinkish color, hepatitis, and gastrointestinal upset.

Pyrazinamide is bactericidal and adverse reactions include joint pains and hepatitis.

Ethambutol is bacteriostatic and may cause optic neuritis.

Thiacetazone is bacteriostatic and may cause a life-threatening Steven Johnson-like reaction in HIV positive individuals.

Regimens

Can vary depending upon availability of agents and drug resistance patterns. An initial phase is typically four agents for 2 months: isoniazid, rifampin, pyrazinamide, and ethambutol. Within 2 weeks of treatment most infectious patients become noninfectious. The continuation phase is usually from 4 to 6 months depending on the site and new vs. recurrent case. A typical regimen during this period may include isoniazid and rifampin.

Supportive treatment for TB is also of great importance. Proper nutrition and weight gain take high priority. Other co-infections should be addressed and treated whenever possible.

PREVENTION

Whenever possible, respiratory and isolation precautions should be taken when treating actively infected individuals. Ideally, these patients should be kept in a separate ward until they have received at least 2 weeks of treatment. As mentioned earlier, direct sunlight kills the bacilli.

The BCG vaccine is a live attenuated vaccine derived from *M. bovis*, which is given intradermally. It should be part of the childhood vaccine series in countries with a high prevalence of TB. Children benefit the most from this vaccine when it can decrease the incidence of disseminated and severe TB. It affords little protection to adults.

RESOURCES

The online version of *TB/HIV: a clinical manual* may be found at: http://whqlibdoc.who.int/publications/2004/9241546344.pdf

REFERENCES

Koch R. 1882. Die atiologic der tuberkulose. *Berliner Klin Wochensch* **15**:221–30.

World Health Organization. 2004. *TB/HIV: a clinical manual*, 2nd ed. Geneva: WHO. http://whqlibdoc.who.int/publications/2004/9241546344.pdf.

World Health Organization. 2004. *Tuberculosis*. Fact Sheet No. 104. Revised March 2004. Geneva: WHO.

56 HUMAN IMMUNODEFICIENCY VIRUS, TYPE 1, AND AIDS

George F. McKinley, MD*

OVERVIEW

In 1981 a previously unrecognized syndrome of oral candidiasis, severe ulcerative genital herpes, and repeated episodes of *Pneumocystis carinii* pneumonia was first described in North America and Western Europe. At the same time, a syndrome of chronic diarrhea and wasting, called "slim disease," was being reported from Sub-Saharan Africa. The original patients in North America and Western Europe were predominantly homosexual men, but cases had also been recognized in intravenous drug users and in hemophiliacs and others who had received transfused blood or blood products. In Africa women and infants appeared as likely as men to be affected, but the elderly and prepubescent children were spared. These observations strongly supported modes of sexual and blood-borne transmission of a newly prevalent but still unknown infectious agent.

By 1984, the etiologic agent of the acquired immune deficiency syndrome had been identified as a human T-lymphotropic retrovirus, the human immunodeficiency virus (HIV). In almost all cases, the cause of AIDS is HIV type-1, or HIV-1. HIV-2, another human retrovirus, first identified in Portugal and France, with origins traced to West Africa, appears to be a much less aggressive pathogen, though it has been occasionally associated with AIDS.

EPIDEMIOLOGY

The incidence and prevalence of HIV/AIDS vary widely by continent, with the highest number (and concentration) of cases found in Sub-Saharan Africa. Of note, in recent years there have been encouraging signs that a few hard-hit African countries (e.g., Uganda with a seroprevalence as high as 20%) have begun to lower the rate of

*Department of Clinical Medicine, Columbia University, College of Physicians and Surgeons, New York

new infections with education and increased availability and use of barrier contraception (condoms). HIV/AIDS has a well-established though relatively low and stable (<1%) prevalence in the Americas, Western Europe, and Australia/New Zealand, where an astonishing degree of progress has been made with respect to diagnosis, management, and treatment of the underlying viral infection. In Eastern Europe and many parts of Asia, reliable data are difficult to obtain. Given the increasing prevalence of intravenous drug use in some countries, the likely wide dissemination of HIV infection through sharing of needles and secondarily through sexual partners will set the stage for many new AIDS cases the coming decades.

PATHOGENESIS

HIV-1 is an enveloped virus, approximately 100 nm in diameter, with a cone-shaped nucleocapsid containing a diploid, positive-, single-stranded RNA and multiple proteins. The virion contains a virus-encoded reverse transcriptase, which, once the virus has gained access to the host cell, synthesizes a DNA copy of the RNA genome. This DNA copy can then integrate into the host cell genome as a 9.7-kilobase segment and begin the process of viral replication. Crucially, this target cell is the primary regulatory agent of specific cellular immunity, the CD4 T-lymphocyte. The steady destruction of this CD4 T-lymphocyte population by repeated cycles of viral replication creates the immunodeficient state that manifests clinically as AIDS.

Once the etiologic agent of AIDS was identified, the cornerstone of sound public health policy and appropriate medical intervention was the validation of reliable and specific diagnostic testing. This was the HIV-1 ELISA screening test followed by western blot confirmation. This technology, first licensed in 1984, coupled with a policy of "donor-at-risk" self-exclusion, has helped to eliminate HIV from the world's supply of blood and blood products.

CLINICAL

Since the process from infection to clinical disease can take as long as 14 years (average: about 7 years), knowing an infected person's CD4 T-lymphocyte count is invaluable in determining what treatments or interventions may be necessary or beneficial. If the patient's CD4 T-lymphocyte count is less than 150 cells/mm^3, prophylactic therapy to prevent *Pneumocystis carinii* pneumonia is indicated, and multiple drugs are available for this purpose, including trimethaprim-sulfamethoxasole, dapsone, clindamycin, and atovaquone. When the CD4+ count declines below 50 cells/mm^3, preventive therapy with a macrolide (azithromycin or clarithromycin) or rifabutin is also indicated to forestall the onset of disseminated *Mycobacterium avian*-complex (MAC), often heralded by fevers, night-sweats, weight loss, and weakness; and accompanied by anemia and sometimes pancytopenia and abnormal liver function tests. Fungal infections (such as thrush and cryptococcal meningitis) or viral infections (such as cytomegalovirus [CMV] retinitis or ulcerative genital herpes) are treated when diagnosed and then prevented with secondary prophylaxis, but primary prophylaxis, even at low CD4 T-lymphocyte counts (i.e., <50 cells/mm^3), has not been deemed a cost-effective intervention.

Primary HIV infection is most often asymptomatic. Occasionally, an "acute retroviral syndrome" has been identified involving fever, morbilliform rash, acute mononucleosis-like symptoms (sore throat, lymphadenopathy) or sometimes aseptic meningitis. This acute illness occurs 1 to 6 weeks after infection, and seroconversion to positive HIV ELISA may take another 2 to 6 weeks after the acute syndrome. After exposure to HIV infection by the sexual or parenteral route, seroconversion takes place within 3 months, and a negative test at 3 months can be accepted as evidence that HIV infection has not occurred.

When an individual has been identified as HIV seropositive (whether asymptomatic or with clinical disease), medical management of the infection/illness involves a staging determination of the absolute CD4 T-lymphocyte count and the plasma HIV "viral load" (expressed as genome copies per microliter) by the branched-chain DNA (bDNA) or polymerase chain reaction (PCR) technology. These two laboratory values, considered in the context of the patient's clinical state and willingness to initiate anti-infective (including antiretroviral) therapy, help to determine which prophylactic medicines are indicated as well as the appropriate time to begin antiretroviral therapy. Initiation of antiretroviral therapy should be strongly considered when the patient's absolute CD4 T-lymphocyte count is between 200 and 350 cells/microliter and/or the viral load is greater than 60,000 genome copies/microliter on repeated determinations. Patients who do not meet these criteria, and do not have significant clinical disease, may be safely followed without antiretroviral therapy, having laboratory parameters determined serially at three to six month intervals.

AIDS must be considered in any of the following clinical presentations: oral candidiasis (thrush) with or without dysphagia and weight loss; large, painful genital or perianal ulcers (herpes simplex); dyspnea, dry cough, and fevers, often of gradual onset, associated with clear or diffuse interstitial pattern on chest x-ray, arterial blood hypoxia, and exertional arterial oxygen desaturation (*Pneumocystis carinii* pneumonia). Cryptococcal meningitis can be a very indolent disease with subtle symptoms of mild headache or photophobia and can present with fever and progress to profound obtundation. Asymptomatic cases of disseminated cryptococcosis have occasionally been diagnosed on the basis of a persistently positive serum cryptococcal antigen tests. Chronic unrelenting diarrhea with weight loss and wasting has long been identified as a classic presentation of AIDS, and the list of possible etiologies is extensive, with cryptosporidiosis, microsporidiosis, cytomegalovirus colitis as but a few prominent examples. The deadly synergy between AIDS and tuberculosis has been observed in Sub-Saharan Africa and the inner cities of North America, where HIV-infected persons with active tuberculosis harbor greater numbers of tubercle bacilli while others are rendered more susceptible to tuberculosis when exposed.

Clinically, the presence of diffuse lymphadenopathy in an individual with appropriate risk factors is considered a marker of recent or immunologically "controlled" infection, and rapid involution of lymphadenopathy (in the absence of highly active antiretroviral therapy) can be a harbinger of clinical AIDS. Elegant virologic and immunologic studies have subsequently provided a sound scientific explanation for what was once an ominous clinical finding. HIV-mediated destruction of CD4 T-lymphocytes in germinal centers has been shown to occur as the lymph nodes melt away.

Visual changes of any kind should prompt an immediate and detailed retinal examination by an ophthalmologist skilled in the diagnosis of AIDS-related conditions, chiefly CMV retinitis. The value of screening retinal examinations in asymptomatic patients with CD4 T-lymphocyte counts <50 is supported by many clinicians.

Fortunately, the success of antiretroviral therapy (ART) has virtually eliminated the incidence of CMV retinitis in areas where ART is widely available.

TREATMENT

As mentioned above, screening for opportunistic infections and offering chemoprophylaxis when appropriate is important. Individuals should be screened for other common co-infections (hepatitis B and C, syphilis, and tuberculosis). Proper nutrition is of utmost importance and in poorer countries may be the only available approach.

Antiretroviral therapy is a complex topic the details of which are beyond the scope of this summary account. However, the well-established and probably long-lasting (>10 years so far in some cases) benefits of ART make it imperative that the clinician who diagnoses, or strongly suspects, HIV/AIDS, initiate a care plan or refer the patient to a setting where such a plan can be devised.

Patient counseling, particularly with regard to risk reduction and contact notification, is a valuable component of clinician-supervised HIV-testing and can limit the spread of infection through identification of asymptomatic infected persons and modifying risk-related behaviors in both infected and uninfected persons.

The US government, through its Department of Health and Human Services, has established guidelines for the use of antiretroviral therapy. Multidrug regimens are required, usually at least three drugs, used in combinations supported by reliable clinical trials data. The efficacy of different recommended triple-drug regimens is really quite comparable, and in the overwhelming majority of cases success is determined by the patient's ability to tolerate and scrupulously comply with the prescribed regimen. Careful patient education is essential prior to initiation of ART, as is close follow-up in the early stages to mitigate the impact of misunderstandings or side-effects on ultimate treatment success. When treatment fails due to the emergence of resistance to antiretroviral drugs, genotype and/or phenotype testing of the patient's virus will sometimes assist the clinician in devising an alternative regimen.

RESOURCE

http://aidsinfo.nih.gov/guidelines/

57 SEXUALLY TRANSMITTED DISEASES

Anna Cheh, MD*

OVERVIEW

The most common and also curable "conventional" sexually transmitted diseases (STDs) within a disaster setting include chlamydia, gonorrhea, syphilis, chancroid, and trichomoniasis. HIV/AIDS has been addressed elsewhere in this text; however, HIV and other STDs are closely linked. Concurrent STD infection substantially increases one's risk of contracting HIV.

INCIDENCE AND PREVALENCE

Sexually transmitted diseases are among the most common yet underdiagnosed causes of morbidity throughout the world. An estimated 340 million curable sexually transmitted infections occur worldwide each year. In developing countries STDs rank among the top five reasons for seeking health care among adults. In fact, STDs and their complications are the second leading cause of morbidity and mortality among reproductive age women.

RISK FACTORS

STD epidemiology is not significantly impacted by acute terrorist attacks. However, STD infections thrive in disaster situations that lead to prolonged population dislocations and social disruption, such as within refugee camps. Social instability, poverty, and disintegration of stable relationships all contribute to increased STD risk by weakening sociocultural constraints that ordinarily govern sexual behavior. The break in social norms compounded by easy access to and perforation of commercial sex activity also increases STD risk. Women and children are at special risk of being victims of sexual coercion to obtain their most basic needs. Sexual violence is a

*Beth Israel Deaconess Medical Center, Harvard Medical School, Boston

well-documented aspect of civil conflicts. This is of particular importance, as approximately 75% of refugees worldwide are women and children.

PRESENTATION AND TREATMENT

The spectrum of sexually transmitted diseases, as well as their presentations and long-term complications, is notably broad. While simple diagnostic tests exist to confirm a specific infection, limited resources and disjointed medical care make this technique less feasible during a massive disaster. In general, however, early symptoms are largely genitourologic in nature. These common traits have led the World Health Organization (WHO) to advocate for the Syndromic Approach (SA) in treating STDs within refugee settings. SA has several potential benefits over traditional diagnostic modalities:

- SA focuses on the most common and curable STDs. WHO estimates that approximately 6 of every 10 STD patients harbor two or more co-infections. Syndromic approach allows the most common infections to be grouped together and targeted with the most effective drugs, ultimately saving cost and reducing morbidity.
- SA allows identification of infected individuals during their first visit. Within a setting of high population mobility, it is imperative that patients be identified and treated at the first opportunity.
- SA is appropriate for settings with limited diagnostic resources. This facilitates implementation in areas where medical services might otherwise be limited.
- SA is user-friendly. Personnel can be rapidly trained in its utilization, allowing recruitment from local populations. This is crucial for rapid mobilization of care.

Using this method, the United Nations Populations Fund (UNFPA) estimates the pharmaceutical cost of effectively treating STDs in a population of 200,000 to be approximately $10,000.

DIFFERENTIAL DIAGNOSIS

Familiarity with other infectious etiology for similar symptoms would be beneficial if treatment based on SA fails.

PROGNOSIS

Sexually transmitted diseases have excellent prognosis if detected and treated early.

PREVENTION

Treatment of STD extends beyond diagnosis and medical treatment. The key to reducing STD infections among dislocated populations is prevention and early iden-

Table 1. WHO Syndromic Approach to the Treatment of Sexually Transmitted Diseases

	Syndrome	Suspected infection	Treatment
Men	Urethral discharge	Gonorrhea Chlamydia	Ciprofloxacin 500 mg x1 Doxycycline 100 mg BID x7 days
Women	Lower abdominal pain	Gonorrhea Chlamydia	
	Vaginal discharge	Cervicitis: Gonorrhea/chlamydia	Ciprofloxacin 500 mg x1 Doxycycline 100 mg BID x7 days
		Vaginitis: Trichomoniasis/candidiasis	Metronidazole 2 g Nystatin 2p/day x 14 days
Men/women	Genital ulcers	Syphilis, chancroid, and genital herpes (if vesicles present)	Benzathine benzyl PCN 2.4 MU x1 Erythromycin 500 mg TID x7 days

tification. During a disaster/refugee crisis, it is imperative to treat sexually transmitted diseases as a public health issue. Local authorities must become involved in the formulation and execution of STD management protocols. Integration of STD services should be considered as standard components of refugee/disaster health care services. The WHO describes an effective prevention strategy as encompassing "Information, Education and Communication" (IEC). Effective communication involves understanding not just the medical but also the complex social dynamics involved in displacement:

- *Assessment of risk*: The prevalence of STDs in the host and home country should be obtained. It is wrong to assume the vector of transmission will be unidirectional.
- *Treating the invisible patient*: Partners of STD patients should be encouraged to access care and empirically treated.
- *Education*: Areas of high risk (e.g., bars), prostitution, and alcohol use should be identified and targeted for prevention and information campaigns. Patients should be educated about safe sexual habits. Access to discounted and/or free condoms should be widely publicized to both the host and refugee community.
- *Understanding local customs*, beliefs, and attitudes concerning sexuality and STDs is pivotal. Identification and further training of people within the refugee population in STD prevention and education are also necessary. Non-clinicians can be invaluable in working directly with the community to gather data and to disseminate information in a manner patients find comfortable and trustworthy. Also be aware that a refugee population is often not homogeneous. Disasters often throw together groups who have had minimal interactions in the past, altering disease epidemiology.

SPECIAL CONSIDERATIONS

One way to directly impact STD prevalence among displaced populations is to alter their landscape of powerlessness and chaos. Creating income opportunities for women and organized social events for adolescents contribute toward lessening the impact of displacement.

RESOURCES

Reproductive Health Response in Conflict Consortium: http://www.rhrc.org
United Nations Population Fund: www.unfpa.org
World Health Organization, West Pacific Region: www.wpro.who.int/
UNAIDS Best Practice Collection, Refugees and AIDS: www.unaids.org/html/pub/publications/irc-pub04/refug-pov_en_pdf.pdf

58 SCHISTOSOMIASIS

Mara Aloi, MD*

OVERVIEW

Schistosomiasis, a parasitic disease also known as snail fever or bilharziasis, afflicts nearly 200 million people worldwide and results in more than 200,000 deaths annually. Its clinical importance is underestimated because acute disease is seen in a minority of people and symptoms may only result after years of chronic infection. There are references to schistosomiasis dating back to 1500 BCE. Hieroglyphics from ancient Egypt portray men with scrotal edema, thought to be a complication of the disease. Calcified *Schistosoma* eggs have been found in Egyptian mummy tissue. However, it was not until 1851 that the etiologic agent was identified by Theodore Bilharz, who lent his name to the disease. Over the next century, the complex life cycle was elucidated and specific antiparasitic therapy was developed to combat the disease. Transmission is limited by the need for appropriate snail populations, which can only be found in certain climates. The disease is endemic in over 77 countries. *Schistosoma japonicum* is found primarily in China, Indonesia, and the Philippines. *Schistosoma mansoni* is endemic on the Arabian peninsula and in Africa, South America, and some Caribbean islands. *Schistosoma haematobium* is limited to Africa and southwest Asia. Several species are found in the large bodies of fresh water in the United States but cause only a self-limited dermatitis, their definitive hosts being ducks. An increase in prevalence of schistosomiasis has been seen recently and is thought to be due to an increased exposure to contaminated water by human populations living in endemic areas. Adolescents have the highest prevalence and highest intensity of infection due to increased exposure combined with immature immunity.

PATHOGENESIS/LIFE CYCLE

Schistosoma are trematodes. Humans are the definitive host for *S. japonicum*, *S. mansoni*, *S. haematobium*, *S. mekongi*, and *S. intercalatum*, but several other species can

*Department of Emergency Medicine, Drexel University College of Medicine, Pittsburgh

cause human disease. Twenty other species can penetrate human skin, but disease is limited to a dermatitis. Each species differs in global distribution, snail host, and preferred organ within human hosts.

Cercariae are the infective form and are found in fresh water where there is an abundance of snails. They are released by infected snails at a set time of day depending on the schistosome species. These larval forms penetrate intact skin and invade the local microcirculation, eventually migrating to the heart, lungs and, finally, to the liver. This migration takes approximately 5–10 days. Maturation into sexual forms takes place in the liver, where the worms mate. Four to six weeks after initial skin penetration, the worms migrate to the small venules of the intestine or the bladder, depending on species preference, and there they lay eggs. Worms of *S. japonicum* species seek out the mesenteric venules of the small intestine. *S. mansoni* prefers the veins that drain the colon. *S. haematobium* resides in the venous plexus that drains the urinary bladder. Some eggs flow back to the liver, while the rest lodge in the wall of the organ they are near. They eventually penetrate into the lumen where some die, calcify, and form granulomas. The rest are excreted into the stool or urine. If the excreta encounter fresh water the eggs hatch into miracidia, which are able to infect freshwater snails, the intermediate host. Direct human–human transmission is not possible.

Adult worms can survive 3–5 years within humans and do not multiply. Thus, intensity of infection depends solely on cercariae exposure. Immunocompromised hosts do not develop an overwhelming infection. The worms cause little direct damage to the host, taking small blood meals with little appreciable result. They are covered by a tegument that shields them from immune attack.

PRESENTATION

Penetration of skin by cercariae is usually asymptomatic, but some may report a tingling or itching at the site of entry. Occasionally patients can develop a self-limited pruritic, papular rash. Most of the pathology and symptoms result from egg deposition, which elicits a granulomatous response.

Larval Pneumonitis

Self-limited; results from migration of schistosomula through pulmonary vasculature; manifested by mild cough, fever, eosinophilia, bibasilar infiltrates on chest x-ray.

Acute Schistosomiasis (Katayama Fever)

Four to eight weeks after contact a serum sickness-like illness develops with fevers, malaise, arthralgias, myalgias, diarrhea, cough, and eosinophilia. May cause hepatic tenderness with normal liver transaminases. Usually resolves and enters chronic stage, but fatality rates can be as high as 25%, especially with *S. japonicum* infection.

Cercarial Dermatitis (Swimmer's Itch)

Intense papular dermatitis resulting from death of cercariae of schistosome species unable to complete life cycle within humans; parasites die as schistosomula within the dermis. Treatment usually not needed.

Chronic Schistosomiasis: most prevalent form of disease; results from granuloma formation and scarring.

Urinary schistosomiasis (*S. haematobium*): urethritis, hematuria, ureteral scarring with obstructive uropathy, recurrent urinary tract infections, recurrent gram-negative bacteremia

Intestinal Schistosomiasis (*S. japonicum, S mekongi, S. mansoni, S. intercalatum*)

- Either presents with bloody diarrhea, tenesmus, and abdominal tenderness or asymptomatic with occult blood positive stools
- Rare: obstruction (from large mass of eggs) or intussusception (granulomas can serve as lead point)

Hepatosplenic schistosomiasis (same species as above)

- Symptoms secondary to portal hypertension from presinusoidal hepatic fibrosis (Symmer's pipestem fibrosis)
- Cirrhosis does not develop and hepatocyte function is intact
- No stigmata of hepatic insufficiency such as gynecomastia, testicular atrophy, or telangiectasias
- Usually manifested by esophageal variceal hemorrhage, hypersplenism

Schistosomal nephropathy

- End-stage renal disease from infection with *S mansoni* or *S. japonicum* resulting from circulating immune complexes.

Neuroschistosomiasis

- Results from eggs within the vertebral venous plexus which embolize to brain and spinal cord
- Cauda equina syndrome
- Transverse myelitis
- Fatal schistosomal cerebritis
- Recurrent bacteremia: enteric bacteria enter circulation via inflamed colonic mucosa

DIAGNOSIS

Suspect schistosomiasis in a traveler returning from an endemic area with a history of freshwater exposure or in those living in endemic areas having the appropriate symptoms:

- Visualization of parasite eggs: via microscopy of urine or Kato-Katz smear of stool (not part of standard O&P test; must order separately). Very specific diagnostic tool but lacks sensitivity. Egg morphology aids in species identification.
- Urine specimens taken between 10:00 AM and 2:00 PM may yield higher concentration of eggs.

- Complete blood count: degree of eosinophilia roughly parallels intensity of infection; may also see mild anemia.
- Urinalysis: mild albuminuria, microscopic hematuria.
- Rectal or bladder mucosal biopsy: very sensitive method; limited by expense and invasiveness.
- Serology: Antibodies against schistosomes remain positive despite resolution of infection; most useful for tourists coming from endemic areas as positive result confirms exposure. Tests can be obtained from the CDC (1-770-480-7775). Antibodies to keyhole limpet antigen present in those with acute schistosomiasis; tests for these are more widely available but less sensitive.
- Antigen detection: circulating anodic antigen (CAA) and circulating cathodic antigen (CCA) are released by adult worms; very sensitive and specific. Levels can be followed to indicate success of therapy.
- Ultrasonography: to assess sequelae of chronic schistosomiasis.

TREATMENT

- Praziquantel: 20 mg/kg orally every 4 hours for total of 3 doses
- Oxaminiquine: 15 mg/kg twice a day orally for 2 days; not for treatment of *S. haematobium* or *S. japonicum*
- Metrifonate: 7.5–10 mg/kg every 2 weeks for 3 doses (max dose 600 mg) for treatment of urinary schistosomiasis
- Add corticosteroids for the treatment of severe acute systemic disease and neuroschistosomiasis

PROGNOSIS

The prognosis of schistosomal infection is very good assuming adequate chemotherapy and prevention of reinfection. Long-term hepatosplenic schistosomiasis may cause irreversible fibrosis and portal hypertension. Bladder cancer is a potential complication of untreated chronic *S. haematobium* infection.

PREVENTION

Since snails are necessary for the life cycle of schistosomes, eradication of snail populations would be helpful but has been relatively unsuccessful thus far. Most effort is being focused on proper sewage treatment since eggs are carried in excretory waste. Unfortunately, these measures are expensive. Also, some schistosome species can infect nonhuman hosts so transmission can occur despite adequate sewage treatment. During situations of famine or war, sewage management becomes an even more formidable problem, and increased rates of transmission can be expected. Vaccines are not currently available.

RESOURCES

www.cdc.gov/ncidod/dpd/parasites/schistosomiasis/
www.who.int/tdr/diseases/schisto/diseaseinfo.htm

REFERENCES

Bica I, Hamer DH, Stadecker MJ. 2000. Hepatic schistosomiasis. *Infect Dis Clin North Am* **14**(3):583–604.

Elliott DE. 1996. Schistosomiasis: Pathophysiology, diagnosis, and treatment. *Gastroenterol Clin North Am* **25**(3):599–625.

Strickland GT, Ramirez BL. 2000. Schistosomiasis. In *Hunter's tropical medicine and emerging infectious diseases*, pp. 804–832. Ed GT Strickland GT. Philadelphia: W.B. Saunders.

59

TETANUS

Marina Del Rios, MD*

OVERVIEW

Tetanus is an acute, often fatal disease, characterized by generalized increased rigidity and convulsive spasms of skeletal muscles. *Clostridium tetani*, the tetanus bacillus, is a spore-forming, anaerobic, Gram-positive bacillus. This organism is a wound contaminant that causes neither tissue destruction nor an inflammatory response.

The introduction of the first generation of tetanus vaccines in 1927 has led to the prevention of hundreds of thousands of deaths due to the disease. In the United States, where the percentage of the population vaccinated is greater than 90%, the incidence of tetanus has decreased from 3.9 cases per million in 1947 to 0.16 cases per million in 2000. However, the annual incidence of tetanus is estimated at 700,000 to 1,000,000 cases per year. The mortality rates due to tetanus are as high as 28 per 100,000 in developing countries.

Wounds, recognized or unrecognized, are the sites at which the organism multiplies and elaborates toxin. The Centers for Disease Control 2003 report lists acute trauma as the condition leading to tetanus in 73% of patients. No acute injury (i.e., patients with abscesses, ulcers, or gangrene) was reported in 26% of patients. Wounds do not need to be obviously contaminated for tetanus to develop, and in unvaccinated individuals or people with waning immunity, such as diabetics, intravenous drug users, and HIV-infected patients, even minor wounds can cause fatal disease. Neonatal tetanus is the most common form of tetanus in developing nations. The disease is caused by contamination of the umbilical stump, with spores following childbirth through cutting the cord with a non-sterile instrument or by application of animal dung or dirt to the cut cord.

Tetanus immunization and treatment become important in the setting of natural and mass casualty incidents, such as terrorist attacks. After the Oklahoma City terrorist bombing, the most common procedure performed on injury victims was wound care. Tetanus toxoid, antibiotics, and analgesics were the most common pharmaceuti-

*Department of Emergency Medicine, St. Luke's/Roosevelt Hospital Center, New York

cal agents used. Supplies of tetanus toxoid can be promptly depleted in the setting of a disaster.

PATHOGENESIS

Clostridium tetani is sensitive to heat and cannot survive in the presence of oxygen. The spores, in contrast, are very resistant to heat and the usual antiseptics. The spores are widely distributed in the soil and in the intestines and feces of many domestic animals. The organism usually enters the body through a wound. In the presence of anaerobic conditions the spores germinate and produce the toxin tetanospasmin.

Tetanospasmin is disseminated via blood and lymphatics and acts at several sites within the nervous system, including peripheral motor end plates, spinal cord, brain, and sympathetic nervous system. Tetanospasmin diffuses to the terminals of inhibitory cells and prevents glycine and GABA secretion. This leaves the motor neurons without inhibition, producing muscular rigidity. The autonomic nervous system is affected as well, predominantly manifested as a hypersympathetic state induced by failure to inhibit adrenal release of catecholamines. Toxin binding is irreversible and recovery depends on sprouting a new axon terminal at the neuromuscular junction.

PRESENTATION

Onset of the disease is gradual. The incubation period varies from 3 to 21 days, usually about 8 days, but can last months. In general, the further the injury site is from the central nervous system, the longer the incubation period. Shorter incubation periods have been associated with more heavily contaminated wounds, more severe disease, and a worse prognosis. Tetanus is classically subdivided into four clinical types: localized, cephalic, generalized, and neonatal. In neonatal tetanus, symptoms usually appear 4 to 14 days after birth, averaging about 7 days.

Localized tetanus manifests as local muscle spasms in areas contiguous to a wound. Local tetanus may precede the onset of generalized tetanus, but is generally milder and often resolves spontaneously.

Cephalic tetanus is a rare form of the disease, occasionally occurring with otitis media or following injuries to the head. It affects the cranial nerve musculature. It may also be seen preceding generalized tetanus.

Generalized tetanus is the most commonly recognized form. The disease usually presents with a descending pattern. It often begins with trismus (masseter rigidity or "lockjaw") and risus sardonicus (increased tone of the orbicularis oris). Rigidity of the abdominal muscles may also be present. The generalized spasm can resemble decorticate posturing and consists of opisthotonic posturing. Spasms are often triggered by sensory stimuli. During the spasm, the upper airway can be obstructed or the diaphragm may participate in the general muscle contraction, causing airway obstruction and respiratory compromise. Spasms continue for 3–4 weeks and complete recovery may take months. Autonomic dysfunction usually occurs after several days of symptoms with sweating, elevated blood pressure, and episodic rapid heart rate and, in the modern era of intensive care, is the leading cause of death.

Neonatal tetanus is the most common form of tetanus in developing countries. It occurs in infants born without protective passive immunity, because the mother is not immune. It usually manifests as generalized weakness and failure to nurse. Rigidity and spasms occur later. Convulsions occur with increasing frequency and intensity and its mortality rate exceeds 90%.

DIAGNOSIS

The diagnosis of tetanus is made clinically by excluding other causes of tetanic spasms. Tetanus is defined by the acute onset of hypertonia or by painful muscular contractions (usually of the muscles of the jaw and neck) and generalized muscle spasms without other apparent medical cause. *C. tetani* is recovered from the wound in only 30% of cases. A protective serum antitoxin concentration should not be used to exclude the diagnosis of tetanus.

Obtain blood samples in patients suspected of tetanus to test for antitoxin level, strychnine, electrolytes (including calcium), blood urea nitrogen, creatinine, creatinine kinase, and urinary myoglobin determination. These will help rule out other causes of tetanic spasms and determine the presence of complications from tetanus, such as rhabdomyolysis.

DIFFERENTIAL DIAGNOSIS

- Strychnine poisoning
- Dystonic reaction
- Hypocalcemia
- Dental infections causing trismus
- Rabies

TREATMENT

Treatment strategies involve three management principles: neutralizing tetanospasmin present in the body, removing the source of the toxin, and providing supportive care for muscles spasms, respirations, and autonomic instability.

Neutralizing Tetanospasmin

Tetanus immune globulin (TIG) is recommended for persons with tetanus. TIG can only help remove unbound tetanus and has no effect on toxin bound to nerve endings. A single total dose of 500 IU given IM is recommended for children and adults and has been found to be as effective as higher doses. Some authorities recommend infiltrating part of the dose around the wound if it can be identified. Intravenous immune globulin contains antibodies to tetanus and can be used if TIG is not available.

Removal of the Source of Toxin

All wounds should be cleaned and debrided of necrotic material. To prevent ongoing production of toxin, antibiotics are administered. Metronidazole is the drug of choice. It is superior to penicillin in recovery time and mortality. Begin 30 mg/kg/day (maximum of 4 g/day) of metronidazole intravenously divided every 6 hours for 10 to 14 days.

Supportive Care

Attention to the airway and to ventilation is paramount at the time of presentation. In the acute phase, death results from acute respiratory failure caused by diaphragmatic paralysis or laryngeal spasms. Administration of a benzodiazepine intravenously such as diazepam or lorazepam will help to control spasm and decrease rigidity. When benzodiazepines fail, other treatments that have been used with varying success include dantrolene, intrathecal baclofen, and propofol. Ultimately, in severe cases, long-acting non-depolarizing paralytics may be needed.

With patients surviving beyond the acute phase, autonomic instability becomes the major cause of death. It occurs several days after the onset of spasms and manifests as labile hypertension, tachycardia, and pyrexia. No therapeutic regimen has proven to be universally effective. Labetalol provides alpha and beta blockade and is recommended for blood pressure control. Morphine can be beneficial, as it can provide cardiovascular stability without cardiac compromise. Other agents that modulate sympathetic output have been tried with variable success. Clonidine and magnesium have given mixed results. Alpha adrenergic blocking agents, such as phentolamine, have been successfully used with propranolol in some studies.

Supportive care should include placing the patient in a quiet, dark environment and minimizing patient manipulation. Complications such as rhabdomyolysis, weight loss, and infections should be monitored and treated. It is important that all survivors receive a tetanus immunization series as the amount of tetanospasmin produced in clinical tetanus is small and an immune response does not occur.

PROGNOSIS

Prognosis of tetanus depends on the facilities available. In developing countries without facilities for prolonged intensive care, the case-fatality ratio can increase to over 50%, with more than half of the deaths occurring in neonates.

With patients surviving the initial acute phase of the illness, autonomic dysfunction and hospital-acquired pneumonias become the most common causes of death. Other complications of tetanus include weight loss, gastrointestinal hemorrhage, pressure sores, and thromboembolism. Mortality varies with patient. In the United States, 75% of tetanus patients who died between 1998 and 2000 were aged greater than 60.

PREVENTION

- Immunization
- Proper wound toilet

REFERENCES

Alson R, Alexander D, Leonard RB, Stringer LW. 1993. Analysis of medical treatment at a field hospital following Hurricane Andrew, 1992. *Ann Emerg Med* **22**(11):1721–1728.

American Academy of Pediatrics. 2003. Tetanus. In *Red book 2003: report of the committee of infectious diseases*, 26th ed., pp. 611–616. Elk Grove Village, IL: American Academy of Pediatrics.

Bunch TJ, Thalji MK, Pellikka PA, Aksamit TR. 2002. Respiratory failure in tetanus: case report and review of a 25-year experience. *Chest* **122**(4):1488–1492.

Centers for Disease Control. 2004. Tetanus. *Epidemiology and prevention of vaccine-preventable diseases: "the pink book"*, 8th ed., pp. chap. 6. Atlanta: Centers for Disease Control and Prevention. http://www.cdc.gov/nip/publications/pink/def_pink_text.ht.

Centers for Disease Control. 2003. *Facts about strychnine*. 14 May 2003. http://www.bt.cdc.gov/agent/strychnine/basics/facts.asp.

Cook TM, Protheroe RT, Handel JM. 2001 Tetanus: a review of the literature. *Br J Anaesthiol* **87**(3):477–487.

Hogan DE, Waeckerle JF, Dire DJ, Lillibridge SR. 1999. Emergency department impact of the Oklahoma City terrorist bombing. *Ann Emerg Med* **34**(2):160–167.

Hsu SS, Groleau G. 2001. Tetanus in the emergency department: a current review. *J Emerg Med* **20**(4):357–365.

Nagachinta TCM, Roper MH, Pascual FB, Murphy T. 2002. Tetanus. In *Manual for the surveillance of vaccine-presentable diseases*, 3rd ed., chap. 13. Ed MHH Wharton, M Reilly. Atlanta: Centers for Disease Control and Prevention.

Pascual FB, McGinley EL, Zanardi, LR, Cortese MM, Murphy TV. 2003. Tetanus surveillance—United States, 1998–2000. *MMWR Surveill Summ* **52**(3):1–8.

Thwaites CL, Farrar JJ. 2003. Preventing and treating tetanus. *Br Med J* **326**(7381):117–118.

von Behring E, Kitasato S. 1991. The mechanism of diphtheria immunity and tetanus immunity in animals [1890]. *Mol Immunol* **28**(12):1317, 1319–1320..

World Health Organization. 2003. WHO vaccine-preventable diseases: monitoring system 2003. In *Global summary: vaccine assessment and monitoring team of the department of vaccines and biologicals*. Geneva; World Health Organization.

60

BITE WOUNDS AND RABIES

Mischa Mirin, MD*

OVERVIEW

Humans can be injured by the bites and stings of many animals, including mammals, snakes, spiders, and insects. The most common wounds are those from larger companion animals, most frequently dog, cat, and human bites.

MAMMALS

Overview

Bites from dogs, cats, other mammals, and humans are a common problem seen in the developed and developing world. Most bites are of low severity.

Presentation

Dog bites may contain a large amount of crushing force. Tissue may be crushed, torn, or lacerated. Resultant infections will likely be polymicrobial. It is estimated that most bites worldwide are from domestic dogs.

Cat bites are often puncture wounds on the extremities. Needle-like teeth penetrate more deeply to tendon and bone. Such wounds are more likely to present a few days after with infection.

Human bites are usually on fingers, but may be on arms, breasts, genitals, or other regions. Secondary bites can occur from a closed clenched fist, also known as a fist-to-mouth injury.

*Department of Emergency Medicine, Allegheny General Hospital, Pittsburgh

MICROBIOLOGY

Dogs

- Usually polymicrobial oral flora, including staph, strep, and *eikenella*.

Cats

- Similar to dogs, but frequent *Pasturella* bacteria.

Humans

- All of the above; considered more infectious, also Hepatitis B and C, and HIV.

DIAGNOSIS

For all bites, get circumstances surrounding the bite wound: where, when, appearance, and medical status of biting animal, and current location of animal if known. Evaluate wound with attention to tendon, nerve, and vascular supply. Consider x-ray if available to look for underlying fractures or retained foreign bodies/teeth fragments. There is a high risk of tendon injury/tenosynovitis with cat bites to the hand and also a very high risk of tendon infection with clenched fist bites.

DIFFERENTIAL DIAGNOSIS

Human

- In any laceration to the hand, especially knuckles, strongly consider the possibility that the patient acquired it in a fight.
- Consider empiric treatment of lacerations over the 4th and 5th knuckles.
- Consider possibility of abuse in patients with human bites.

TREATMENT

General

- Control bleeding with direct pressure.
- Irrigate all wounds copiously with sterile water if possible; tap water otherwise.
- Anesthetize wound if able.
- Mechanically cleanse wound with removal of foreign debris.
- Consider debridement of dead or damaged tissue.
- Update tetanus prophylaxis.
- Consider rabies vaccine; most domestic animals are not immunized in the third world and any bite by domestic or wild animals there should be considered high risk of rabies transmission (see next section).

- Suturing is controversial. Unless the wound is gaping or the face is involved, wounds are left to heal by secondary intention.
- Bite wounds to the hand should not be closed primarily.
- All wounds should be rechecked in 1–2 days.
- Antibiotic choice is usually a penicillin, penicillase-resistant penicillin, a cephalosporin, or amoxicillin clavulanate.
- Quinolones or bactrim/clindamycin combination may be used in penicillin allergic patients.

Dogs

Treatment as above.

Cats

- Scratches require no treatment unless already infected or immunocompromised.
- Always leave wounds open.
- Cover *pasteurella* with antibiotic choice (amoxicillin clavulanate).

Humans

- If the joint space or tendon is involved strongly consider at least 24 hrs of IV antibiotics.
- If wound is >24 hours old strongly consider above and exposure and drainage.

Other Mammals

- For bites by other species, follow the general guidelines as listed above.
- Bites by large herbivores will involve more crushing injury and should prompt concern about underlying tissue.
- Monkey bites should be treated as human bites, and every attempt made to capture the biting animal. Old world monkeys may carry Herpes B in the oropharynx and bitten individuals are at risk of acquiring infection. Chemoprophylaxis for Herpes B should be started.
- Large cats (lions, tigers, leopards) and wild canines should be treated as above with the caveat that bites by larger animals will involve much more force, and associated injuries should be assessed as well.

SPIDERS

Overview

While there are many types of spiders that may bite, not all are venomous. Actual spider bites are rare occurrences. There are the forms of spider envenomations: neurotoxic and cytotoxic.

Diagnosis

Spider bites are hard to identify definitively. Every attempt should be made to identify the biting spider. Usually a white area appears around the lesion.

Treatment

- Apply ice to area for short periods of time.
- Local wound care.
- Update tetanus.
- Consider antibiotics.
- Antihistamines for local irritation.
- Antivenin is available for bites by spiders of the *Loxosceles* and *Latrodectus* genera and is somewhat effective if given soon after the bite. Spider antivenin is rarely available.
- Consider benzodiazepines for severe muscle cramps.
- Pain management as necessary.

SNAKES

Overview

Although most snakes are not venomous, any snakebite should be evaluated thoroughly.

Diagnosis

Most patients will be able to relate the history of snakebite. Every attempt should be made to identify the type of snake involved.

Treatment

- Local wound care: wash the wound with soap and water.
- Bandage firmly.
- Keep the injured area still and lower than the heart.
- Monitor the patient's condition and watch for signs of shock or airway compromise.
- Support ABCs.
- Consider antibiotics, similar to cat bites.
- If evidence of systemic envenomation (bleeding, DIC or neuromuscular involvement) antivenom should be given. Ideally, monovalent if the species of snake is known. The dose is the same in adults and children. A test dose is given first.
- Pain management as necessary.
- Do not apply tourniquet, apply electricity to the bite, or attempt to suck out the venom!

RABIES

Overview

Rabies is an acute, progressive, incurable viral encephalitis, caused by the bite of a rabid animal. The World Health Organization (WHO) reports that more deaths occur worldwide from rabies than from other common infections such as dengue fever, polio, meningococcal meningitis, or Japanese encephalitis. Of the 50,000 human rabies deaths reported annually, more than half occur in the Indian subcontinent, with most of the remaining cases occurring in Southeast Asia, Africa and Latin America.

In developed countries, rabies is mostly in wild animals, while in Africa, Asia, and Latin America infected dogs are directly responsible for most of the rabies deaths.

Presentation

- Incubation period may range from 20 to 90 days.
- Incubation longer for more distal sites of inoculation (hands, feet).
- Initial symptoms are nonspecific: fever, fatigue, chills, headache, flu-like symptoms.
- Acute symptoms follow in 5–10 days, one of two types.
- Furious rabies: anxiety, confusion, insomnia, agitation, psychosis and hyperactivity, throat spasms, hypersalivation.
- Dumb rabies: depression, intermittent periods of arousal, coma.
- Acute symptoms are followed in 2–10 days by paralysis and death.

Diagnosis

- Direct fluorescent antibody test of brain tissue (postmortem).
- PCR tests on serum, spinal fluid, skin biopsy and saliva.

Differential Diagnosis

Differential diagnosis should include multiple other forms of encephalitis, including bacterial encephalitis or meningitis, hysterical reaction to animal bites (pseudohydrophobia), polio, allergic reaction to rabies vaccine, Guillain-Barré syndrome, psychotic break, lupus, or stroke.

Treatment

There is no treatment once the disease has developed except supportive care. The disease is almost always fatal.

Prevention

The primary method of prevention in humans is post-exposure prophylaxis. In many developing countries, immunization of domestic animals plays a large part in rabies prevention.

Post-exposure prophylaxis consists of two components:

1. Passive immunization with antirabies antiserum (either 20 units/kg human rabies immune globulin (HRIG) or 40 units/kg equine antiserum).

- Infiltrate up to 50% of the total dose locally to the bite wound.
- The rest administered IM gluteally.

2. Antirabies vaccine should be administered.
    - Multiple types of vaccine, multiple methods of administration.
    - Classic: one dose of 1 ml IM (deltoid) vaccine on days 0, 3, 7, 14, and 28.
    - There are also alternative intradermal methods in areas where vaccine is scarce.
    - Additionally, initial local wound care including irrigation may lessen the risk of rabies.
    - WHO recommends disinfection of wound with iodine or alcohol.

Special Considerations

Who should receive rabies vaccination?

- Any bite wound by a dog in an endemic or third world country.
- Any bite wound in a developed country by wild animals.
- Any bite wound in any country by an unknown or unobservable animal.
- May defer vaccine in species unlikely to be infected with rabies or dog bites where the dog is observable and has a record of receiving two rabies vaccines within its first year.
- Bats: in the United States it is recommended to empirically vaccinate if patient is in close proximity to bats while asleep or debilitated.
- Occupational risk or potential exposure.

RESOURCES

www.cdc.gov/ncidod/dvrd/rabies/
www.emedicine.com
http://www.vh.org/adult/provider/familymedicine/FPHandbook/Chapter15/01-15.html
http://www.health.state.mn.us/divs/idepc/diseases/rabies/human.html
http://www.nyerrn.com/er/epa.htm

REFERENCES

Bleck TP, Wilde H. 2003. Management of rabies in humans. *Clin Infect Dis* **36**:60–63.

Brinker D, Hancox JD, Bernardon SO. 2003. Assessment and initial treatment of lacerations, mammalian bites, and insect stings. *J Am Acad Physician Asst* **16**:28–32.

Brook I. 1987. Microbiology of human and animal bite wounds in children. *Pediatr Infect Dis J* **6**:29–32.

CDC. 1999. Human rabies prevention—United States, 1999: recommendations of the advisory committee on immunization practices (ACIP). *MMWR* **48**, no. RR-1.

Chin J, ed. 2000. Rabies. *Control of communicable diseases manual*, pp. 411–419, 17th ed. Washington, DC: American Public Health Association.

Fleisher GR. 1999. The management of bite wounds. *N Engl J Med* **340**(2):138–140.

Messenger SL, Smith JS, Rupprecht CE. 2002. Emerging epidemiology of bat-associated cryptic cases of rabies in humans in the United States. *Clin Infect Dis* **35**:738–747.

Moran GJ, Talan DA, Mower W, Newdow M, Ong S, Nakase JY, Pinner RW, Childs JE. 2000. Appropriateness of rabies post-exposure prophylaxis treatment for animal exposures. *JAMA* **284**:1001–1007.

Sacks JJ, Kresnow M, Houston B. 1996. Dog Bites: how big a problem? *Inj Prev* **3**:52–54.

Weiss HB, Friedman DI, Coben JH. 1998. Incidence of dog bite injuries treated in emergency departments. *JAMA* **279**:51–53.

61 TICK-BORNE DISEASES

Megan Fix, MD*

OVERVIEW

Ticks are excellent vectors for disease transmission, and more than 800 species of these obligate blood-sucking creatures inhabit the planet. They are second only to mosquitoes in worldwide transmission as vectors of human disease, both infectious and toxic. In the United States, ticks are the most common vectors of vector-borne diseases. Ticks can carry and transmit a vast number of pathogens, including bacteria, spirochetes, rickettsiae, protozoa, viruses, nematodes, and toxins. A single tick bite can transmit multiple pathogens, which can also lead to atypical presentations of some classic tick-borne diseases; additionally, secondary infections and allergic reactions to proteins in tick saliva are also possible. It is especially important to discuss prevention of tick-borne diseases for relief workers and others at risk. Clinicians should be aware of the signs and symptoms of tick-borne illness because increased morbidity and mortality are associated with delay in treatment.

Ticks are arthropods of the class Arachnida. Of the three families of ticks, only the hard ticks (*Ixodidae*) and soft ticks (*Argasidae*) have medical importance. Hard ticks have a hard shell or scutum. Ticks have two main body parts: the capitulum (sucking structure) and the body. When a tick attaches to a host, it digs a barbed structure called a hypostome into the skin of the host, and release several substances including: a cement to anchor the attachment; enzymes; vasodilators; and antiinflammatory, antihemostatic, and immunosuppressive substances. These facilitate feeding, and an anesthetic in the saliva makes the bite relatively painless. In addition, the saliva also contains neurotoxins that can lead to tick paralysis.

The life cycle of most ticks lasts between 6 months and 6 years and includes three stages (larvae, lymph, and adult). Hard ticks usually attach for long periods of time but only feed one time at each stage. After its meal, the tick detaches, drops from the host, finds a resting place where it can digest its blood meal and molts to the next feed-

*Harvard-Affiliated Emergency Medicine Residency; Brigham and Women's Hospital/Massachusetts General Hospital, Boston

Table 1. Tick-Borne Diseases

Disease	Pathogen	Vector	Geography
BACTERIA			
Lyme	*Borrelia burgdorferi*	*Ixodes scapularis*	NE US
Tularemia	*Francisella tularensis* *Amblyomma americanum*	*Dermacentor variabilis*	SE US
Relapsing fever	*Borrelia* species	*Ornithodoros hemsii*	Western US, Africa, Asia
Rocky Mountain spotted fever	*Rickettsia rickettsii*	*D. andersoni* *D. variabilis*	SE US Eastern hemisphere
Q Fever	*Coxiella burnetti*	*D. andersoni*	Worldwide
Ehrlichiosis	*Ehrlichia canis*	*Rhipicephalus sanguineus*	South and Eastern US
Mediterranean spotted fever	*Rickettsia conorii*	*Rhipicephalus sanguineus*	Europe, Africa
PARASITIC			
Babesiosis	*Babesia microti*	*Ixodes scapularis*	Coastal New England
VIRAL			
Colorado tick fever	*Orbivirus*	*D. andersoni*	Rocky Mountains

ing stage. In contrast, soft ticks can feed much more rapidly and many times on the same host.

An overview of tick-borne diseases is summarized in Table 1.

LYME DISEASE

Lyme disease, named after the town Old Lyme, Connecticut, where the disease was recognized in 1975, is the most common vector-borne disease in the United States. It is caused by the spirochete *Borrelia burgdorferi*. It is most common in children, but also effects adults. It occurs worldwide but is endemic in three US areas: the coastal Northeast (MA to MD), Midwest (MN, WI), and West (CA, OR, UT, NV). The vector is the *Ixodes scapularis* (Northeast) and *I. pacificus* (West).

Presentation

Less than a third of infected patients recall a tick bite. This is likely due to the small size (1–2 mm) of the nymph tick that usually causes transmission. The nymph stage is most active from May to August. After a tick attaches, transmission does not usually occur until 2 days later during the blood feeding. This is important because ticks that are noted can be removed soon after attachment, resulting in a much lower transmission rate. If transmission of *B. burgdorferi* occurs, the incubation takes between 1–36 days. During this time, *Borrelia* spirochetes migrate hematogenously to synovial tissue, skin, and nervous system tissue.

Signs and Symptoms

There are three described stages of Lyme disease. During stage one, a "bull's-eye" rash (erythema migrans) at the site of the bite may develop. Constitutional symptoms that may develop include: low grade fever, lymphadenopathy, splenomegaly, myalgias, and headache. During the second stage when hematological spread occurs, neurologic (seventh cranial nerve palsy), joint (monoarticular arthritis with the knee being most commonly involved), and cardiac symptoms (AV block) predominate. During stage three, chronic arthritic and neurologic abnormalities (including encephalopathy) may manifest.

Diagnosis

Primarily based on clinical and epidemiologic features with serologic testing (ELISA confirmed by western blot). Although bacteria can be seen in body fluids, arthrocentesis and CSF analysis are generally non-diagnostic. The classic rash known as erythema migrans is present in most patients, but only a third report tick bite.

Treatment

Oral antibiotics are the treatment of choice for most cases of Lyme. Recommended dose is Doxycycline 200 mg/day x 21–30 days for men, nonpregnant woman, and children greater than 8. Amoxicillin is used for pregnant or lactating women and children less than 8. It is important to know that a Jarish-Herxheimer type reaction can occur in the first 24 hours of treatment. Treatment is generally extended to 30 days for associated mild neurologic symptoms. However, prednisone is not currently recommended for facial nerve palsy.

IV antibiotics are recommended if cardiac or neurological abnormalities such as meningitis, encephalitis, or peripheral neuropathies occur. The antibiotic of choice is Ceftriaxone for up to 4 weeks.

Prevention

In the United States a commercial vaccine is no longer available. Measures to avoid tick bites is the best means of protection: proper clothing, DEET repellant, and permethrin-treated clothes. Although debatable, an empiric dose of Doxycycline may decrease transmission if the bite is noted within 72 hours.

TICK-BORNE RELAPSING FEVER

Tick-borne relapsing fever is a spirochete disease caused by at least 13 different *Borrelia* species and is present worldwide. The vector is the soft tick *Ornithodoros*, and rodents are commonly infected. The soft tick bite is usually painless. The incubation period is 4–18 days. Relapsing fever presents as a viral-like illness with high fever, myalgias, chills, and headache, and many patients have an eschar at the bite site. The clinical course will usually involve the initial syndrome for 3 days followed by an asymptomatic period of 7 days then another relapse. Neurologic symptoms are common. Diagnosis is made by demonstration of *borreliae* in peripheral blood during a febrile episode (thick and thin smear preparation, Wright or Giemsa stain can be used). Treatment is with Doxycycline, Penicillin, Erythromycin, or Ceftriaxone.

TULAREMIA

Please see chapter 25 on Tularemia.

ROCKY MOUNTAIN SPOTTED FEVER (RMSF)

RMSF is an acute febrile systemic tick illness with significant mortality caused by the organism *Rickettsia rickettsii*. The infection is most commonly seen in the southeast United States. The incubation period is between 2 and 14 days. The symptoms are nonspecific, with fever, severe headache, myalgias, prostration, and nausea/vomiting. The characteristic maculopapular rash usually appears on the fourth febrile day on the wrists, ankles, palms, soles, and forearms. A vasculitis may develop that can cause hypotension, edema, and petechiae. Specific organ involvement includes: cardiac (cardiomegaly, myocarditis, EKG changes), pulmonary involvement (interstitial pneumonitis), and neurologic (mild headache to lethargy, seizures, coma, transient deafness, tremor, rigidity, paralysis, ataxia, aphasia, blindness). The initial diagnosis is often made clinically. Confirmation is obtained by: serology, skin biopsy, or direct isolation and identification of the organism. Treatment is with Doxycycline or Chloramphenicol.

Q FEVER

Please see chapter 28 on Q fever.

EHRLICHIOSIS

There are two forms of human ehrlichioses: HME (human monocytic ehrlichiosis) and HGE (human granulocytic ehrlichiosis). The organism is a rickettsia-like coccobacilli called *Ehrlichiosis*. There are multiple species that cause disease and are transmitted by different ticks, including the brown dog tick. The organisms invade monocytes in HME and neutrophils in HGE. Both are identified as emerging diseases by the Centers for Control and Prevention (CDC). Infection peaks from June through August, and those at risk are similar to those at risk for Lyme. HME is found in the south central and southeast United States, while HGE is found in the upper Midwest and Northeast. Reservoirs include the white tailed deer and white-footed mouse.

The incubation period ranges from a week to a month. Common symptoms are fever, headache, and myalgias. Leukopenia, thrombocytopenia, and elevated liver function tests can be seen in anywhere from 50 to 90% of patients. Rashes occur in approximately a third of patients with HME but in only 2–11% of those with HGE. Other findings such as ARDS, meningitis, pancarditis, renal failure, and DIC have been reported. Fatality rates have been reported at 2.7% for HME and 0.7% for HGE.

Diagnosis is usually clinical with serologic analysis. Most test results are retrospective. Sometimes microscopic identification of mulberry-like clusters, called morulae, inside leukocytes on peripheral blood smears can be visualized. The most common mode of diagnosis is confirmation of IgG antibodies with IFA. Treatment is with Doxycycline or Tetracycline for 7–14 days and is curative.

BABESIOSIS

Babesiosis is a tick-borne, malaria-like, acute febrile illness caused by the intra-erythrocytic protozoan parasite *Babesia*. Since the late 1960s, more than 200 cases have been documented in the United States. Almost all of these cases were caused by *B. microti* and occurred in the coastal regions of southern New England (Cape Cod, Nantucket, Martha's Vineyard, Block Island). Babesiosis has also been reported in Maryland, Virginia, Georgia, Wisconsin, Minnesota, California, and Washington. The mammalian reservoirs are deer and mice and the tick vector is the same as Lyme, *Ixodes dammini*. the Highest incidence is from May to August.

After an incubation period of 1 to 4 weeks the clinical presentation is with nonspecific flu-like symptoms, including fever, chills, headache, fatigue, and anorexia. Other less common symptoms are nausea, diaphoresis, depression, photophobia, myalgias, arthralgias, dark urine, emotional lability, and hyperesthesias. Unlike Lyme disease, rash is not a feature of the illness. Splenomegaly is present on exam in patients. More severe disease occurs in splenectomized patients. The diagnosis is established by examination of thick and thin Giemsa-stained blood smears. Characteristic intra-erythrocytic forms may be present.

Recovery without specific therapy is the rule for otherwise healthy patients. Antibiotic therapy is recommended only for patients with severe disease and those who have had splenectomies. Treatment with the combination quinine and clindamycin is the treatment of choice.

COLORADO TICK FEVER

Endemic to the Rocky Mountain area, Colorado tick fever (CTF) is an acute tick-borne viral infection characterized by headache, back pain, biphasic febrile course, an occasional maculopapular rash (around 10%), and leukopenia. The etiologic agent of CTF is an arbovirus in the genus *Orbivirus*. CTF occurs in altitudes from 4,000 to more than 10,000 feet, in the Canadian provinces of British Columbia and Alberta and the western parts of the United States. The tick vector is *Dermacentor andersoni*, the same vector as RMSF. It is important to contrast CTF and RMSF because the treatments are different. Even though RMSF was described in the Rockies, it is actually less common than CTF, which is twenty-fold more common in Colorado.

Diagnosis is clinical suspicion confirmed by serologic testing. Leukopenia and thrombocytopenia may be seen. The diagnosis can be confirmed by serologic testing. Treatment for CTF is entirely supportive and generally has a good prognosis. Most patients do not require hospitalization, but if RMSF remains a diagnostic possibility, initial treatment with Doxycycline or Chloramphenicol and a period of observation are necessary until the diagnosis of RMSF can be ruled out.

TICK PARALYSIS

Tick paralysis is a condition that occurs when an adult female tick attaches and releases a neurotoxin that can produce cerebellar dysfunction or an ascending paralysis in the host. It occurs worldwide, but most cases occur in the southeastern and northwestern regions of the United States, western Canada, and Australia. Both hard ticks and soft ticks have been implicated. Tick paralysis usually occurs in the spring and summer months, and most cases occur in children.

Onset of symptoms occurs 4 to 7 days after the tick attaches. Symptoms include weakness in the lower extremities, which ascends within hours or days to involve the trunk musculature, upper extremities, and head. Patients may present with ataxia or respiratory distress, and mortality rates of up to 10% have been reported. Analysis of CSF samples usually reveals no abnormalities, and the diagnosis is clinical and depends on a history of tick bite or finding a tick on the body of the patient. The differential diagnosis includes Guillain-Barré, Eaton-Lambert syndrome, myasthenia gravis, poliomyelitis, botulism, diphtheritic polyneuropathy, or any disease with an ascending flaccid paralysis or acute ataxia.

Treatment consists simply of removing the tick and supportive therapy; improvement is generally seen within a few hours and complete recovery within 48 hours. Supportive care, including mechanical ventilation, may be necessary. The mortality rate is approximately 10%; nearly all those who die are children. Tick paralysis in Australia is often more severe than in the United States. Hyperimmune serum is available in Australia and is often needed because symptoms may worsen up to 48 hours after removal.

PREVENTION OF TICK-BORNE DISEASES

Personal prevention of tick-borne disease involves removal of ticks from the body, prophylactic antibiotics, and prevention of tick bites. Ticks prefer to attach to the head, neck, and groin of humans, although they can be found anywhere. Removal of ticks is described below.

Second, there is the question of prophylactic antibiotics after finding a tick. If the tick has not been attached for 24 hours, the likelihood of disease transmission is low. Third, prevention of tick attachment is important, especially in those people traveling in endemic areas. Strategies to prevent tick exposure include wearing appropriate clothing and applying tick "repellant." Both topical DEET and clothing impregnated with permethrin have been shown to be effective in field trials when used alone. Wearing protective clothing treated with permethrin, in addition to using DEET on exposed skin, provides the greatest degree of protection against tick bites.

RECOMMENDED METHOD FOR TICK REMOVAL

1. Remove an embedded tick by grasping it with blunt forceps or tweezers as close to the point of attachment as possible and applying gradual but firm steady upward traction.
2. Do not use bare fingers to remove ticks from animals or humans; when tweezers are unavailable, fingers should be shielded with a tissue, paper towel, or rubber glove.
3. Do not handle the tick with bare hands. After removing the tick, thoroughly disinfect the bite site and wash hands with soap and water.
4. Dispose of ticks by placing them in a container of alcohol or flushing them down the toilet.

REFERENCES

Bolgiano E, Sexton J. 2002. Tick-borne illnesses. In *Rosen's emergency medicine: concepts and clinical practice*, 5th ed., chap. 128, St. Louis: Mosby.

Needham GR. 1985. Evaluation of five popular methods for tick removal. *Pediatrics* **75**(6):997–1002.

Parola P, Raoult D. 2001, Ticks and tick-borne bacterial diseases in humans: an emerging infectious threat. *Clin Infect Dis* **32**(6):897–928.

62 LEPTOSPIROSIS

Rishi Malhotra, MD*

OVERVIEW

Leptospirosis is a zoonotic disease caused by pathogenic spirochetes from the genus *Leptospira*. This febrile illness occurs worldwide, with the majority of cases occurring in underdeveloped tropical regions. Leptospirosis is likely the most common zoonosis worldwide. Exact incidence rates are difficult to determine due to the nonspecific nature of most leptospiral infections; however, lifetime prevalence as ascertained by seropositivity can be as high as 40% in certain subpopulations.

Leptospirosis was first described in 1886 by Adolf Weil, who observed four cases of "acute infectious illness with spleen tumor, jaundice, and nephritis." Over 200 serovars of pathogenic *Leptospira* have been identified. Recently the genus *Leptospira* has been subdivided into several species based on DNA-relatedness. However, for clinical purposes it is more useful to divide *Leptospira* based on serologies, so the serovar and serogroup designations continue to be used.

At-risk populations include those who have direct contact with the urine of carrier animals or contact with contaminated materials, such as fresh water or soil. Occupational risk includes: farm workers, veterinarians, adventure seekers, butchers, sewer workers, soldiers, hunters, hikers, miners, dog owners, inner-city dwellers, disaster survivors, and lab workers.

PATHOGENESIS

Leptospires are carried by a wide variety of wild and domesticated animals, most commonly rodents, dogs, cows, pigs, sheep, goat, and horses. Animals may experience active infection or be asymptomatic carriers, in which case the organism resides in the proximal tubule of nephrons and is shed in the urine. Humans contract the disease through direct contact with infected urine, or indirectly via infected urine deposited in the environment. Environments where exposure typically takes place

*Department of Medicine, St. Luke's/Roosevelt Hospital Center, New York

include freshwater bodies, swamps, floodwaters, cane fields, rice fields, farms, mines, and the inner-city. Leptospires can persist in warm water, moist soil, or mud for many months. Leptospires enter the human body via lacerated or abraded skin, and intact mucous membranes. It is uncertain whether they can enter via intact skin. Once inside, *Leptospira* diffusely disrupt the cell membranes of small-vessel endothelial cells, which explains the varying clinical manifestations that can encompass nearly all organ systems.

PRESENTATION AND CLINICAL COURSE

The presentation and clinical course of leptospirosis can be highly variable, ranging from asymptomatic infection to the extreme of hemorrhagic fever with hepatorenal failure, cardiac conduction abnormalities, and cardiovascular collapse. Broadly, leptospirosis may be split into two syndromes.

Anicteric Form

After an incubation period of 2–20 days (10 days on average), patients typically experience the sudden onset of fever, chills, nausea, vomiting, headache, and myalgia. This corresponds to the septicemic phase, which lasts 3–7 days. Physical exam findings at this time are relatively nonspecific, and include maculopapular skin rash, pharyngeal injection, lymphadenopathy, organomegaly, and muscle tenderness. The presence of conjunctival suffusion or muscle tenderness involving the calves and lumbar region should raise the suspicion of leptospirosis.

The illness may progress to a second stage, after a 1- to 4-day asymptomatic period, resulting in a biphasic illness. This immune phase, characterized by the appearance of IgM antibodies, is again difficult to distinguish from other febrile illnesses, and is thought to result from the host immune response rather than the pathogen itself. Fever is generally lower than in the septicemic phase. Signs and symptoms of meningitis are often present, including severe headache, nausea, vomiting, photophobia, neck stiffness, and mental status changes. Even in those with no signs or symptoms of meningitis, CSF examination reveals aseptic meningitis. In addition, patients may develop ocular manifestations 3–8 weeks after initial onset of symptoms, including iritis, iridocyclitis, or chorioretinitis. Ocular manifestations, which can be unilateral or bilateral, may resolve or become chronic.

Icteric Form (Weil's Disease)

Weil's disease is the most severe form of leptospirosis, occurring in approximately 5–10% of symptomatic infections. It is usually a progressive monophasic illness, although it can sometimes present as a biphasic illness. Initially, Weil's disease is indistinguishable from the anicteric form of the disease, but around 3–9 days after the onset of symptoms, jaundice, renal failure, and bleeding diathesis may become apparent.

In addition to the signs and symptoms present in the anicteric form, severe and persistent fever, abdominal tenderness in the right upper quadrant, organomegaly, cough, chest pain, hemoptysis, epistaxis, petechiae, and ecchymoses commonly occur. Renal failure may occur. Adult respiratory distress syndrome, and multiple organ system failure can also occur in severe cases.

DIAGNOSIS

General Laboratory Tests

The general laboratory values cannot make the diagnosis of leptospirosis, but they can help raise the suspicion.

- White blood cell (WBC) counts may be normal or slightly elevated in mild disease, with marked elevation in severe disease.
- Creatine phospokinase (CPK) is elevated in approximately 50% of patients.
- Acute renal failure (ARF) may result in elevated blood urea nitrogen (BUN) and creatinine.
- In Weil's disease serum bilirubin is elevated, infrequently reaching 60–80 mg/dl. Alkaline phosphatase and hepatic transaminases are also slightly elevated, with the transaminases rarely exceeding 200 U/L.
- Urine may show proteinuria, pyuria, microscopic hematuria and hyaline or granular casts.
- Cerebrospinal fluid (CSF) shows normal glucose and normal or elevated protein levels. Total CSF WBCs are generally <500/μl.

Diagnostic Tests

A definitive diagnosis of leptospirosis can be made through direct detection of the organism or serological tests that detect antibodies to the organism. If suspicion is high, treatment should not be delayed pending definitive diagnosis.

Direct Detection

- Leptospires can be cultured, although this test is slow and insensitive. The organisms grow best at a neutral pH at 28-30°C on selective media: Elinghausen-McCullough-Johnson-Harris (EMJH), Korthof's, and Fletcher's. Growth is typically observed in 2–6 weeks. During the first 10 days of illness, CSF and blood are more likely to yield positive cultures. Blood samples should be collected in heparin or oxalate, as citrate is inhibitory to the organism's growth. Leptospires can be cultured from the urine from week 1–3.
- Polymerase chain reaction (PCR) is extremely sensitive and can give a very early diagnosis, even when the patient has already been started on antibiotics.
- Dark-field microscopy and staining should be avoided as there are many false-positives and false-negatives with these tests.

Indirect detection

- Serologic tests for leptospires require clotted blood or serum. Regardless of the specific test, either a fourfold increase in titer or seroconversion in paired samples makes the diagnosis. A high IgM titer can also be diagnostic, but in endemic areas the cutoff needs to be adjusted based on local population studies.
- The microscopic agglutination test (MAT) is the gold standard serologic test.
- IgM ELISA is also sensitive and specific, but less so than MAT. It is positive earlier than the MAT. ELISA makes an excellent screening test, and many commercial kits are available.
- Numerous other serologic methods exist. Among those that are commercially available in some form, LEPTO Dip-S-Tick (an IgM-detecting enzyme-linked dot immunoassay) and the indirect hemagglutination test (IHA) have the highest sensitivity and specificity.

DIFFERENTIAL DIAGNOSIS

- Influenza
- Malaria
- Primary HIV infection
- Infectious mononucleosis
- Rickettsiosis
- Borreliosis
- Brucellosis
- Hantavirus
- Dengue fever
- Yellow fever
- Viral hepatitis
- Viral meningitis

TREATMENT

Some controversy exists as to the effectiveness of antimicrobial treatment in leptospirosis as very few randomized controlled trials exist, some with contradictory results. Jarisch-Herxheimer reactions have rarely been reported. Besides antibiotics, supportive care may be necessary.

Mild

- Doxycycline 100 mg PO BID for 7 days

Severe

- Penicillin G 1.5 million U IV QID for 7 days
- Ceftriaxone 1 g IV or IM QD for 7 days

Chemoprophylaxis

- Doxycycline 200 mg PO once weekly for duration of exposure

PROGNOSIS

Anicteric leptospirosis has an excellent prognosis. The mortality of Weil's disease is estimated to be 5–15%. Leptospirosis during pregnancy is associated with high fetal mortality.

PREVENTION

- Identification of reservoir species in a particular environment
- For domestic animals, antibiotics, vaccination and isolation can be used
- Improvements in sanitary conditions and sealed storage of food, so as not to attract reservoir animals

Preventing contact with infected urine can decrease transmission. Important measures include:

- Wearing protective clothing in high risk environments, such as fresh water bodies and floodwaters, or when contact with known carrier animals is anticipated
- Improving sanitation and hygienic measures
- Providing access to clean water

At the level of the human host:

- Chemoprophylaxis with doxycycline, for short-term heavy exposure
- Limited quantities of inactivated vaccines are available in Italy, France, Spain, Japan and China; several trials have shown various inactivated vaccines to have a limited efficacy: however, no long-term efficacy studies exist
- Dissemination of outbreak control information after disasters to the public via the press, and to physicians via public health agencies

RESOURCES

http://www.cdc.gov/ncidod/dbmd/diseaseinfo/leptospirosis_g.htm
http://www.cdc.gov/travel/diseases/lepto.htm
http://www.med.monash.edu.au/microbiology/staff/adler/ilspage.html
http://www.who.int/vaccine_research/diseases/leptospirosis/en/

REFERENCES

Bajani MD, Ashford DA, Bragg SL, Woods CW, Aye T, Spiegel RA, Plikaytis BD, Perkins BA, Phelan M, Levett PN, Weyant RS. 2003. Evaluation of four commercially available rapid serologic tests for diagnosis of leptospirosis. *J Clin Microbiol* **41**:803–809.

Bharti AR, Nally JE, Ricaldi JN, Matthias MA, Diaz MM, Lovett MA, Levett PN, Gilman RH, Willig MR, Gotuzzo E, Vinetz JM. 2003. Leptospirosis: a zoonotic disease of global importance. *Lancet Infect Dis* **3**:757–771.

Dupont H, Dupont-Perdrizet D, Perie JL, Zehner-Hansen S, Jarrige B, Daijardin JB. 1997. Leptospirosis: prognostic factors associated with mortality. *Clin Infect Dis* **25**:720–724.

Effler PV, Bogard AK, Domen HY, Katz AR, Higa HY, Sasaki DM. 2002. Evaluation of eight rapid screening tests for acute leptospirosis in Hawaii. *J Clin Microbiol* **40**:1464–1469.

Gsell O. 1984. The history of leptospirosis: 100 years. *Zentralblatt für Bakteriologie, Mikrobiologie und Hygiene, Series A: Medical Microbiology, Infectious Diseases, Virology, Parasitology.* **257**:473–8.

Guidugli F, Castro AA, Atallah AN. 2000. Antibiotics for preventing leptospirosis. *Cochrane Database Syst Rev* **4**:CD001305.

Katz AR, Ansdell VE, Effler PV, Middleton CR, Sasaki DM. 2001. Assessment of the clinical presentation and treatment of 353 cases of laboratory–confirmed leptospirosis in Hawaii, 1974-1998. *Clin Infect Dis* **33**:1834.

McClain JBL, Ballou WR, Harrison SM, Steinweg DL. 1984. Doxycycline therapy for leptospirosis. *Ann Intern Med* **100**:696–698.

Panaphut T, Domrongkitchaiporn S, Vibhagool A, Thinkamrop B, Susaengrat W. Ceftriaxone compared with sodium penicillin g for treatment of severe leptospirosis. *Clin Infect Dis* **36**:1507–1513.

Rathinam SR, Rathnam S, Selvaraj S, Dean D, Nozik RA, Namperumalsamy P. 1997. Uveitis associated with an epidemic outbreak of leptospirosis. *Am J Ophthalmol* **124**:71–79.

Sambasiva RR, Naveen G, Bhalla P, Agarwal SK. 2003. Leptospirosis in India and the rest of the world. *Braz J Infect Dis* **7**:178–193.

Watt G, Padre LP, Tuazon ML, Calubaquib C, Santiago E, Ranoa CP, Laughlin LW. 1988. Placebo-controlled trial of intravenous penicillin for severe and late leptospirosis. *Lancet* **1**:433–435.

World Health Organization. 2003. *Human leptospirosis: guidance for surveillance, diagnosis and control*. Geneva: WHO. http://www.who.int/csr/don/en/WHO_CDS_CSR_EPH_2002.23.pdf.

PART IVC

Basic Trauma Management

63 WOUND CARE MANAGEMENT

Neha Parikh MD, MS,* and George J. Raukar, MD**

OVERVIEW

Historically, wounds are a significant cause of mortality and morbidity during war. Most are caused by either blunt or penetrating trauma. Acutely, wounds may present with pain, bleeding, and direct visualization of soft tissue injury. Late presentation includes erythema, warmth, pain, swelling, purulent drainage, and ascending lymphangitis.

DIAGNOSIS

History

- AMPLE history: allergies, medications, PMHX (past medical history), last meal, events leading to injury
- Inquire about tetanus immunization status
- Ask about remote injuries

Physical Exam

- Physical exam
- Primary survey: assess airway, breathing, circulation
- Secondary survey including evaluation of the wound; determine integrity of underlying major blood vessels, major internal organs, nerves, tendons, and joints as appropriate
- Assess motor and sensory function and pulses distal to the injury before and after wound management

*Department of Sports Medicine/Emergency Medicine, Allegheny General Hospital, Pittsburgh
**Department of Orthopedics, West Virginia University, Morgantown

GENERAL WOUND MANAGEMENT

The goals of wound care are to: control bleeding, prevent infection: even trivial wounds are at risk for infection, and promote healing. Control of severe bleeding is a higher priority than wound cleaning.

Direct Pressure

The best method for the control of bleeding. Use the heel of your hand and the most sterile material available. Large wounds, in which your hands cannot cover the injury site, require that the wound first be packed with an absorbent material. Most blood loss will slow appreciably within 10 to 20 minutes.

Pressure Bandage

If >20 minutes of bleeding with direct pressure, apply a pressure dressing. Use a bulky dressing on the wound, and an elastic wrap or a clean strip of cloth wrapped securely around the extremity and tied with the knot over the wound. Blood flow should be assessed regularly by checking distal pulses and sensation. Do not remove even if the dressing becomes blood soaked.

Pressure Points

Use digital pressure on a pressure point to slow arterial bleeding. Maintain pressure points by placing a round stick in the joint, bending the joint over the stick, and then keeping it tightly bent. Elevation: whenever possible the wound should be immediately elevated above the patient's heart.

Tourniquet

Use a tourniquet only when all other methods do not control the bleeding. A tourniquet left in place too long can damage the tissues and progress to gangrene, with eventual loss of the limb. Never place a tourniquet directly over the wound or a fracture. Use a blood pressure cuff or a stick to tighten the tourniquet; tighten only enough to stop blood flow. After securing the tourniquet, identify the location of the torn vessels. A pressure dressing should be applied in this location. Release the tourniquet every 10 to 15 minutes for 1 or 2 minutes so blood can flow to the rest of the extremity and prevent limb loss.

Infection Prevention

All wounds should be regarded as contaminated. If the area is hairy, clip the hair adjacent to the wound with a pair of scissors. Shaving may increase the chance of infection and is not recommended. Disinfectants (alcohol, hydrogen peroxide, and soaps) should be used to wash the area around a wound and should not be poured into wounds, where they damage viable tissue and may increase the incidence of wound infection. Use a high-pressure irrigation syringe to clean the wound. Simply rinsing or soaking a wound is inadequate to remove bacteria. Irrigate with at least 100 ml of water per inch. Wound irrigation is the single most important factor in preventing infection. Deeply imbedded, visible debris not removed by irrigation may be removed carefully with sterile forceps. Motor and sensory function and pulses distal to the injury should be checked after wound management.

SPECIFIC WOUND MANAGEMENT

Contusions

Only large bruises require emergency care.

Abrasions

1. Irrigate and scrub using a sterile gauze pad to remove residual debris and prevent tattooing of the skin. Keep moist with antibiotic ointment.
2. Dress with sterile gauze.
3. Change the dressing twice a day and any time the gauze gets wet.

Lacerations

Superficial

1. For small lacerations, adhesive strips (or whatever tape is available) may be applied perpendicular to the wound.
2. Can use benzoin or cyanoacrylate glue to aid in adhesion.
3. Suture.

Heavily Contaminated

1. Clean thoroughly.
2. Suturing a heavily contaminated wound may lead to a higher risk of infection.
3. Use wet to dry dressings by loosely packing the wound with moistened gauze and cover with dry dressing. Change every 12 hours.
4. Antibiotic use may be considered.

Amputations/Avulsions

1. Control bleeding
2. Irrigate and bandage the stump and detached body part.
3. Wrap in moistened sterile gauze.
4. Place in a plastic bag.
5. Place the plastic bag in a bucket of ice or the coldest water possible. Do not apply ice directly to the body part or frostbite may ensue.
6. Treat an avulsion as a laceration without completing the separation.

Puncture Wounds

- Particularly high risk of infection
- Uncontaminated
  1. Irrigate
  2. Dress
  3. Monitor for infection

- Contaminated
  1. Irrigate thoroughly
  2. Start antibiotics since infection is almost certain: make sure to cover for *Pseudomonas*

Impaled Wounds

- Large objects: leave in place and transport to a medical facility. Before transport stabilize object with padding as high as the object to prevent movement during transport. Remember that metal objects that are impaled can conduct heat out of a cold patient.
- When removing an impaled object, remove it slowly and gently, but firmly, pulling out along the line the object entered. Stop if resistance or pain is encountered.
- If the object endangers the airway, remove it.
- If the object is in the eye, protect the object against movement, cover both eyes, place the patient at 45°, and carry the patient out.

RESOURCES

Emergency Preparedness Information: http://epix.hazard.net/topics/medical.html
For wound care algorithms and protocols: Exchange.http://www.hollister.com/us/resource_center/wound_care/

REFERENCES

Auerbach P, Weiss, EA, Donner H. 2001. *Field guide to wilderness medicine*, 4th ed. St. Louis: Mosby.
Landon BA. 1994. *An atlas of trauma management: the first hour*. London: Parthenon.
Trott ATT. 1997. *Wounds and lacerations: emergency care & closure*, 2nd ed. St. Louis: Mosby.

64

ABDOMINAL TRAUMA

Michael Levine, MD, and Charles N. Pozner, MD*

BACKGROUND

The accurate and timely assessment of abdominal trauma is paramount to reduce patient morbidity and mortality. Patients with abdominal trauma are generally divided into two classes: blunt and penetrating. While attention is often easily drawn to a penetrating wound of the abdomen, blunt abdominal trauma can be subtler. Abdominal pain may be absent in the setting of intoxication or other distracting injuries. Furthermore, patients may lose a significant amount of blood into the abdominal cavity before a change in the appearance of the abdomen occurs. The diagnostic challenge of blunt injuries, along with the higher likelihood of multi-organ involvement, results in a higher mortality compared with penetrating injuries.

ANATOMY

On inspection, the abdomen is divided into three regions: the anterior abdomen, flank, and back. The anterior abdomen is bounded by the anterior axillary line laterally, the symphysis pubis inferiorly, and the trans-nipple line superiorly. The anterior and posterior axillary lines make up the lateral borders of the flank. The sixth intercostal space defines the superior border, and the iliac crests define the inferior border. The back contains the entire space between the two posterior axillary lines, bordered inferiorly by the iliac crests and superiorly by the tips of the scapulae. Upon exhalation, the diaphragm may rise to the level of the fourth intercostal space, increasing the risk of associated abdominal injury if penetration occurs below the nipple line.

The internal anatomy of the abdomen is also divided into three regions; the peritoneal, retroperitoneal, and pelvic cavities. The peritoneum, bordered superiorly by the diaphragm, contains the liver, spleen, stomach, most of the small bowel, as well as

*Harvard-Affiliated Emergency Medicine Residency, Brigham and Women's Hospital/Massachusetts General Hospital, Boston

**Department of Emergency Medicine, Harvard Medical School, Boston

the transverse and sigmoid colon. Organs of the retroperitoneum include the kidneys, ureters, much of the duodenum, and the ascending and descending colon. The abdominal aorta and the inferior vena cava are also located within the retroperitoneum. Enclosed by the pelvic bones, the pelvic cavity contains the rectum and bladder, and in women the internal reproductive organs.

PATHOPHYSIOLOGY

Blunt trauma injuries result from compression, crushing, or shearing forces often occurring at the junction of fixed and mobile structures. Penetrating injuries result from cutting or lacerating forces. The most commonly injured organs in blunt abdominal trauma are the spleen and liver. Stab wounds and other impalement injuries most often injure the liver, followed by the small bowel, diaphragm, and colon. Gunshot wounds and other missile injuries most often injure the small bowel, followed by the colon, liver, and abdominal vasculature.

HISTORY

Depending on the condition or level of impairment of the patient, the history may be either unobtainable or unreliable; however, when possible, it should be obtained, as it may facilitate the assessment of injury patterns. Pertinent information to obtain following a motor vehicle crash includes the type of impact (e.g., frontal, roll-over), vehicular speed, the patient's location within the vehicle, the use or deployment of passenger restraints, the presence of passenger-space intrusion, and the condition of other passengers in the vehicle. In falls it is important to inquire about the height of the fall, the surface that the victim landed on, and if the fall was broken by any objects (i.e., trees).

For impalement injuries, it is helpful to know the length of the object (i.e., knife). In gunshot injuries, the patient or witnesses should be asked about how many shots were heard, the type of weapon used, and the approximate distance between the victim and the assailant. It is important to ascertain from pre-hospital providers or witnesses the amount of extracorporeal blood loss at the scene.

PHYSICAL EXAM

After the patient has been fully disrobed, examination of the abdomen should proceed in an organized fashion as part of a comprehensive secondary assessment. Unexplained hypotension and/or tachycardia must be assumed to emanate from intrathoracic or intraabdominal hemorrhage, until proven otherwise.

The abdomen should be inspected for abrasions, ecchymosis, distention, lacerations, and puncture wounds. It is imperative to log-roll the patient and examine both the back and perineum. While decreased or absent bowel sounds are common with intraperitoneal injuries, their presence does not rule out significant intraperitoneal injury. Abdominal tenderness is frequently elicited in the presence of intraabdominal visceral injury, but may be absent with retroperitoneal injuries. The presence of rebound tenderness on exam suggests peritoneal irritation; however, its absence does not exclude significant injury. The abdomen should also be palpated for a mass, which could represent a ventral wall hernia or a hematoma. Serial examinations facilitate the early discovery of occult intraabdominal injury.

A rectal examination is mandatory, looking for gross blood, subcutaneous emphysema, and rectal tone. The likelihood that the rectal exam will detect these is low, but their presence is highly specific for significant intraabdominal pathology. Urethral catheterization is standard; however, if upon inspection of the urethral meatus blood is found, or a high-riding prostate is elicited on the rectal examination of a male, urethral catheterization should be preceded by a retrograde urethrogram.

IMAGING

Various radiographic imaging studies—including plain film, ultrasound, and computerized tomography (CT)—may be used to evaluate the trauma patient. It is important, however, that imaging not take precedence over initial resuscitation and stabilization.

Ultrasound is rapidly becoming customary in the initial evaluation of abdominal trauma. The FAST exam can provide valuable information regarding the presence of free fluid in the abdomen. It is quick, noninvasive, and highly sensitive. Some shortcomings include an inadequate evaluation of the retroperitoneal space, poor sensitivity for the detection of bowel injury, and the failure to detect a bleeding source.

The use of CT is noninvasive and can provide a myriad of information. In addition to being highly sensitive for intraperitoneal blood, CT can also evaluate the retroperitoneal space, identify the organ injured or source of bleeding, and determine the extent of injury. It is invaluable for defining injuries that may be treated conservatively, without operative intervention. Furthermore, CT can accurately detect injuries to the bony structures of the pelvis and vertebral column. Among the limitations of CT are its poor sensitivity for detecting bowel, pancreatic, or diaphragmatic injuries. The major disadvantage of CT relates to the logistics of moving a critically ill patient from the resuscitation area. Therefore, CT is usually contraindicated in hemodynamically unstable patients.

Plain films of the abdomen are rarely useful in the evaluation of abdominal trauma. In penetrating trauma, they may be used to search for foreign bodies or missile tracks; however, CT is the preferred imaging modality. The chest x-ray, aside from being essential for identification of potential intrathoracic injury, may help to demonstrate free air. A pelvic x-ray may identify pelvic fractures, which could be a source of significant occult blood loss.

DIAGNOSTIC PROCEDURES

Diagnostic peritoneal lavage (DPL), once the standard of care in the pre-CT era, is a rapidly performed, invasive procedure to detect intraabdominal injuries. Similar to ultrasound, DPL screens for intraperitoneal blood but cannot identify the source of bleeding. It is now generally reserved for patients in whom there is unexplained hemodynamic instability, and ultrasound is unavailable or the results equivocal.

Local wound exploration can be performed in patients who have sustained a penetrating wound and have no evidence of hemodynamic instability or peritoneal signs.

Following local wound exploration, if the wound tract does not violate the peritoneum, the patient may be managed conservatively. If there is penetration, a DPL may be performed or the patient, most often, is taken for celiotomy.

MANAGEMENT

The fundamental principles of emergency care apply in the management of abdominal trauma; the ABCs are the first priority. Once all identified threats to life are managed, patients should have two large-bore Ivs initiated. Routine trauma labs should be obtained at this time. While hemodynamically unstable patients often require prompt operative intervention, one must never overlook other potential life-threats. For example, patients with upper abdominal penetrating trauma may be hypotensive due to intrathoracic emergencies, such as a tension pneumothorax or cardiac tamponade.

Blunt trauma patients are rarely operative candidates based solely on clinical grounds. These patients typically require CT or other diagnostic modalities prior to defining management and disposition options. The absolute indications for celiotomy in blunt trauma are listed in Table 1. Relative indications in the hemodynamically stable patient include solid visceral organ injury, and a positive FAST/DPL or hemoperitoneum on CT with no clear etiology. While the blood may ultimately be from a minor liver or spleen laceration that is not seen on CT, it could represent a perforated hollow viscous. A completely asymptomatic blunt-trauma patient with normal studies may be discharged home or kept for serial examinations.

Table 1. Absolute Indications for Celiotomy

Blunt	Penetrating (stab wounds)
Hemodynamic instability with anterior abdominal injury	Evisceration
Findings consistent with pneumoperitoneum on x-ray or CT	Positive DPL
CT-diagnosed injury necessitating surgical repair	CT-diagnosed injury necessitating surgical repair
Abdominal wall disruption	Diffuse abdominal tenderness (+/– peritoneal signs)

Except for long-distance shotgun blast wounds, all patients with a gunshot to the anterior abdomen require celiotomy. All hemodynamically unstable stab wounds require operative management. In the hemodynamically stable patient, indications for celiotomy are also listed in Table 1. All other patients can be observed with serial exams for 24 hours.

The hemodynamically stable patient with penetrating trauma to the back or flank may require double or triple contrast CT, if wound exploration is non-diagnostic. If the patient becomes unstable, or there is high suspicion for diaphragmatic injury, surgical intervention is indicated.

REFERENCES

Marx JA. 2002. Abdominal trauma. In *Rosen's emergency medicine: concepts and clinical practice,* 5th ed., pp. 415–436.

Ed JA Marx, RS Hockberger, RM Walls. St. Louis: Mosby.

Scalea TM, Boswell SA. 2002. Abdominal injuries. In *Emergency medicine: a comprehensive study guide,* 5th ed., pp. 1699–1708. Ed JE Tintinalli, GD Kelen, JS Stapcynski. New York: McGraw-Hill.

65 THORACIC TRAUMA

Liudvikas Jagminas, MD, FACEP*

OVERVIEW

Of all trauma-related deaths, approximately one quarter are attributed to thoracic injury. Less than 10% of blunt chest injuries and up to 30% of penetrating injuries require thoracotomy. The majority of patients with thoracic trauma can be managed by simple maneuvers and do not require surgical treatment. Immediate deaths are essentially due to either major disruption of the heart or great vessels. Early deaths due to thoracic trauma are as a result of hypoxia, hypercarbia and acidosis secondary to airway obstruction, pulmonary contusion, cardiac tamponade, exsanguination, or aspiration.

The extent of internal injuries cannot be judged by the appearance of a skin wound. Blunt forces applied to the chest wall cause injury by three mechanisms: rapid deceleration, direct impact, and compression. The degree of external trauma may not fully predict the severity of internal injuries, and clinical suspicion of cardiac and vascular trauma should be heightened. Direct impact by a blunt object can cause localized fractures of the ribs, sternum, or scapula with underlying lung parenchyma injury, cardiac contusion, or pneumothorax. Compression of the chest by a very heavy object, which prevents respiration and causes marked increases in blood pressure within veins of the upper thorax, may result in traumatic asphyxia. Anterior–posterior compression forces place indirect pressure on the ribs, causing lateral mid-shaft fractures.

More than respiratory insufficiency, thorax trauma can cause hemorrhagic shock due to hemothorax. Hemothorax is common in both penetrating and non-penetrating injures to the chest. If the hemorrhage is severe, it may not only cause hypovolemic shock but also dangerously reduces vital capacity by compressing the lung on the involved side. Persistent hemorrhage usually arises from an intercostal or internal thoracic (internal mammary) artery and less frequently from the major hilar vessels. Bleeding from the lung generally stops within a few minutes, although initially it may be profuse. In some cases hemothorax may come from a wound of the heart or from abdominal structures such as the liver or spleen if the diaphragm has been lacerated.

*Department of Emergency Medicine, Memorial Hospital, Pawtucket, Rhode Island

Hypovolemic shock and hemomediastinum can derive from a thoracic great vessel injury that may be the result of penetrating or blunt trauma. The most common etiology is penetrating trauma; however, the descending thoracic aorta, the innominate artery, the pulmonary veins, and the vena cava are susceptible to rupture from blunt trauma.

CLINICAL ENTITIES

Causes of Respiratory Distress

- Rib fractures/flail chest
- Pneumothorax
- Tension pneumothorax
- Hemothorax
- Pulmonary contusion
- Open pneumothorax
- Aspiration

Causes of Hemorrhagic Shock

- Hemothorax
- Hemomediastinum

Rib Fractures

Fractured ribs generally occur at the point of impact. Their presence indicates a need for examining the underlying lung for pulmonary contusion, laceration, hemo- or pneumothorax. Multiple or anterior and posterior rib fractures may cause a flail segment. Fracture of the relatively protected first through third ribs indicates severe impact and mandates careful search for associated vascular injury. In the elderly patient, fractured ribs may result from simple trauma; while in the young significant forces can be applied to the thoracic cage without a resulting fracture.

Flail Chest

A flail chest occurs when a segment of chest wall does not have continuity with the rest of the thoracic cage. This condition is present when two or more contiguous ribs are fractured in two or more places. The resulting flail segment causes severe disruption of normal chest wall movement contributing to serious respiratory distress. The unstable segment wall moves separately in a paradoxical manner to the rest of the chest cage during the respiratory cycle.

The pathophysiologic effects of flail chest are evidenced by a decrease in vital capacity, reduction in functional residual capacity, and hypoxia due to the underlying pulmonary contusion. Often patients exhibit ventilation-perfusion imbalance, decreased compliance, increased airway resistance, and increased breathing effort. Initial therapy includes adequate ventilation, administration of humidified oxygen, analgesia, and fluid resuscitation. The injured lung is sensitive to both under-resuscitation of shock as well as fluid overload.

Appropriate patient management involves selective use of endotracheal intubation and mechanical ventilation. The primary indication for endotracheal intubation and mechanical ventilation is respiratory decompensation. Aggressive pulmonary physiotherapy with suctioning, incentive spirometry, early mobilization, and humidification of air is appropriate for all patients. Intermittent positive pressure breathing, postural drainage, and therapeutic fiberoptic bronchoscopy to suction retained secretions and treat atelectasis are often necessary. Stabilization of the chest wall rarely requires external surgical fixation.

Pneumothorax

A high index of suspicion for the presence of a pneumothorax must be maintained in all blunt trauma victims. Pneumothorax usually results from a penetrating wound of the chest that creates a communication between the pleural space and external environment. As the size of this defect approaches two-thirds the size of the tracheal diameter, air passes preferentially through the lower-resistance injury tract rather than through the normal airways. This severely compromises oxygenation and ventilation and is immediately life threatening. In an open or "sucking" wound of the chest wall, the lung on the affected side is exposed to atmospheric pressure, which results in the lung's collapse and a shift of the mediastinum to the uninvolved side. Because of the profound ventilation-perfusion inequality, the patient becomes cyanotic and has serious respiratory distress. The open pneumothorax must be treated rapidly using one of two approaches. In the spontaneously ventilating patient, application of a sterile occlusive dressing with vaseline gauze large enough to cover the wound entirely taped on three sides is the treatment of choice. Tube thoracostomy at a remote site to the injury should be placed.

If the chest wall defect is relatively small, the pleura may soon seal and no further intervention is necessary. A second approach is to simply intubate the patient and initiate positive pressure ventilation. Often surgical repair is required.

Tension Pneumothorax

Tension pneumothorax develops when air enters the pleural space via a penetrating chest wound with a valve-like opening but cannot exit. This leads to progressively increasing intrathoracic pressure in the affected hemithorax, resulting in impaired central venous return and mediastinal shift to the opposite side. Clinically the patient exhibits dyspnea, tachycardia, hypotension, tracheal deviation, unilateral absence of breath sounds, neck vein distention, and cyanosis, and may complain of chest pain. The hemodynamic instability is secondary to decreased venous return due to endopleural hypertension. The presence of hyperresonance and the absence of breath sounds are useful in differentiating a tension pneumothorax from cardiac tamponade. Tension pneumothorax is an emergency requiring immediate decompression using a large-bore needle placed into the second intercostal space in the midclavicular line of the affected hemithorax. This converts the injury into a simple pneumothorax. Definitive treatment requires the insertion of a thoracostomy tube with underwater-seal drainage. If the lung does not fully re-expand after tube thoracostomy and there is a large ongoing air leak, the airways should be evaluated bronchoscopically to exclude a major bronchial injury. However, in most cases, no further treatment for tension pneumothorax will be required after thoracostomy tube insertion.

Hemothorax

Hemothorax is more common in penetrating than in non-penetrating injures to the chest. If the hemorrhage is severe, hypovolemic shock will occur as well as respiratory distress due to compression of the lung on the involved side. Patients who sustain acute hemothorax are at risk for hemodynamic instability due to loss of intravascular volume and compromised central venous return due to increased intrathoracic pressure. Lung compression due to massive blood accumulation may also cause respiratory compromise. Sources of hemothorax are: lung, intercostal vessels, internal mammary artery, thoracoacromial artery, lateral thoracic artery, mediastinal great vessels, heart, and abdominal structures (liver, spleen) with an associated diaphragmatic hernia. The diagnosis is readily made from the clinical picture and x-ray evidence of fluid in the pleural space. Optimal therapy consists of the placement of a large (36 french) thoracostomy tube. A moderate size hemothorax (500–1500 ml) that stops bleeding after thoracostomy can generally be treated by closed drainage alone. However, a hemothorax of greater than 1500 to 2000 ml, as with continued bleeding of more than 100 to 200 ml, per hour is an indication for emergency thoracotomy or thoracoscopy.

Pulmonary Contusion

Pulmonary contusion is common after any form of blunt chest trauma and frequently manifests itself as hypoxemia. The goals for treatment are oxygen therapy, positive pressure either with a Continuous Positive Airway Pressure (CPAP) mask or by intubation and mechanical ventilation with Positive End Expiratory Pressure (PEEP). Splinting from the pain associated with rib fractures requires adequate pain management. The contused lung is prone to capillary leak, and therefore careful fluid management is paramount. It is a potentially life-threatening condition unless recognized early and treated aggressively. The onset of symptoms may be slow and may progress over 24 hours post injury.

Open Chest Wounds

In open or "sucking" wounds of the chest wall, the lung on the affected side is exposed to atmospheric pressure, resulting in lung collapse and a shift of the mediastinum to the uninvolved side. This clinical entity must be treated rapidly. A non-occlusive seal taped on three sides and applied over the wound is sufficient, and can be applied until reaching definitive care. In compromised patients, thoracostomy tube placement, intubation, and positive pressure ventilation are often required.

Rupture of Trachea or Major Bronchi

The trachea and major bronchi because of their similar anatomic position are subject to the same mechanisms of injury for either blunt or penetrating trauma. It is a serious injury with an estimated mortality of 30%. More than 80% of the ruptures of bronchi are within 2.5 cm of the carina. Injuries to the main bronchi and intrathoracic trachea are more prevalent than those to the cervical trachea because the latter is protected by the mandible and sternum anteriorly and by vertebrae posteriorly. The intimate anatomical relationship of the trachea to the great vessels, lungs, and heart explain the high incidence of serious associated injuries in blunt and penetrating trauma. The clinical picture appears in two patterns, depending on whether or not there is free communication between the rupture of the trachea-bronchial tree and the pleural cavity. If there is free communication, a large pneumothorax results. The usual signs of tracheobronchial disruption are the following: hemoptysis, dyspnea, subcutaneous, and/or mediastinal emphysema, and occasionally cyanosis. Tube thoracostomy shows continuous bubbling of air in the water seal, and suction fails to re-expand the lung. The chest x-ray may demonstrate pneumothorax, pleural effusion, pneumomediastinum, or subcutaneous air. Overall, 90% of these patients will have an abnormal chest x-ray.

Bronchoscopy should be carried out promptly when tracheobronchial rupture is suspected, since it is the most reliable means of establishing the diagnosis. If it indicates that the bronchial tear involves less than one-third of the lumen, the patient is stable, and if the thoracostomy tube underwater-seal drainage results in complete expansion of the lung, treatment may be conservative. However, in all other types of tracheobronchial injury, thoracotomy should be performed as soon as possible.

Myocardial Contusion

Myocardial contusion in blunt chest trauma may be associated with fractures of the sternum or ribs. The diagnosis is supported by abnormalities on ECG, frequently sinus tachycardia or frequent PVCs (premature ventricular contractions), along with potentially elevated cardiac enzymes, and wall motion abnormalities on echocardiogram. Cardiac contusion can simulate a myocardial infarction. The patient suspected of cardiac contusion must be admitted for cardiac monitoring. This type of injury is more common than generally realized and may be a cause of sudden death within 24 to 48 hours after the incident.

Pericardial Tamponade

Penetrating cardiac injuries are a leading cause of death in trauma. It is rare to have pericardial tamponade with blunt trauma. Echocardiography or pericardiocentesis must be undertaken early if this injury is considered likely. Suspect it in patients with: shock/hypotension, distended neck veins, muffled heart sounds, cool extremities, and no pneumothorax Initial treatment is pericardiocentesis. Removal of as little as 15 to 20 ml of blood will result in immediate hemodynamic improvement. All patients with this entity will require thoracotomy or median sternotomy for pericardiography, inspection, and repair of the heart.

Thoracic Great Vessel Injuries

Injury to the pulmonary veins and arteries is often fatal, and is one of the major causes of on-site death and accounts of 8–9% of vascular injuries seen in trauma centers. It may be the result of penetrating or blunt trauma. The patient with chest trauma may present with respiratory distress due to hemothorax. An initial "rush" of a large volume of blood after tube thoracostomy may indicate great vessels injury. The classic sign of pericardial tamponade may be present. Suggestive radiological signs include presence of a hemothorax, pneumothorax, widening of the superior mediastinum more than 8 cm, widened paratracheal stripe, apical cap, and depression of the left main-stem bronchus.

CT angiography or aortography should be performed in the patient with moderate to severe injuries. The patient with signs of respiratory distress, hemodynamic instability and suspected pneumothorax should undergo immediate tube thoracostomy. If blood loss is greater than 1 liter, with continued bleeding along with hemodynamic instability, a thoracotomy must be performed in an attempt to repair the ruptured vessel.

Trauma to the Esophagus

Trauma to the esophagus is rare in patients following blunt trauma injury. Perforation of the esophagus is more frequently caused by penetrating injury. It is lethal if unrecognized because of mediastinitis. Patients often complain of sudden sharp pain in the epigastrium and chest with radiation to the back. Dyspnea, cyanosis, and shock occur, but these may be late symptoms.

Diaphragmatic Injuries

Diaphragmatic injuries occur more frequently in blunt chest trauma, and almost exclusively on the left side. They are frequently missed since rarely does the chest x-ray show any abnormality like an elevated hemidiaphragm or nasogastric tube in the left chest. Operation for other abdominal injuries often reveals diaphragmatic tears which require direct repair.

REFERENCES

Cachecho R, Grindlinger GA, Lee VW. 1992. The clinical significance of myocardial contusion. *J Trauma* **33**(1):68–73.

Calhoon JH, Grover FL, Trinkle JK. 1992. Chest trauma: approach and management. *Clin Chest Med* **13**(1):55–67.

Feghali NT, Prisant LM. 1995. Blunt myocardial injury. *Chest* **108**(6):1673–1677.

Mattox KL, Wall MJ. 1997. Newer diagnostic measures and emergency management. *Chest Surg Clin North Am* **2**:213–226.

Perchinsky MJ, Long WB, Hill JG. 1995. Blunt cardiac rupture. *Arch Surg* **130**:852–857.

Pezzella AT, Silva WE, Lancey RA. 1998. Cardiothoracic trauma. *Curr Prob Surgery* **35**(8):649–650.

Rosenthal MA, Ellis JI. 1995. Cardiac and mediastinal trauma. *Emerg Med Clin North Am* **13**(4):887–902.

Shorr RM, Crittenden M, Indeck M, Hartunian SL, Rodriguez A. 1987. Blunt thoracic trauma: analysis of 515 patients. *Ann Surg* **206**:200–205.

66 NEUROTRAUMA

Robert E. Antosia, MD, MPH*

HEAD INJURY

Head injuries account for 50% of all trauma-related deaths. Traumatic brain injury (TBI) results from either direct or indirect forces to the brain and may occur both as an immediate consequence and from complications, e.g., hematomas (subdural, epidural, intraparenchymal) or cerebral swelling with herniation syndromes.

Initial Evaluation

The ABCs of trauma apply to the head-injured patient. If intubation is required, the orotracheal route with in-line C-spine stabilization should be used. A rapid sequence technique is preferred to help blunt an increase in intracranial pressure (ICP) seen during intubation. Cervical spine precautions should be maintained until injury is ruled out clinically or by x-ray. Important aspects of the history include: witnesses concerning onset and mechanism of injury, lucid intervals, seizure activity, past medical history including medication(s), and any recreational drug history. Physical exam should focus on the primary survey, followed by determination of the level of consciousness using the Glasgow Coma Scale (GCS). If the GCS is 8, the patient is considered unable to protect the airway and should be intubated. The initial neurological assessment should include: cranial nerves (including pupil size and reactivity), sensorimotor exam, and reflexes. Beware of a unilateral dilated pupil in the unresponsive patient, which may indicate increased ICP and impending herniation. Evaluate lacerations of the face or scalp and deep wounds and palpate with a sterile glove to check for any "step-off" deformities. Document any periorbital (raccoon sign), or postauricular (Battle sign) ecchymosis. Also, check for CSF leak, clear fluid from ear (otorrhea) or nose (rhinorrhea), and look for blood behind the tympanic membrane (hemotympanum). These three signs suggest a basilar skull fracture and mandate a CT scan. Palpate the neck posteriorly for C-spine tenderness or deformity. Finally, complete the

*Department of Emergency Medicine, Beth Israel Deaconess Medical Center, Harvard Medical School, Boston

rest of the physical examination. For those patients who cannot respond, it is imperative to obtain radiographs of the complete axial skeleton from the base of the skull to the sacrum in at least two views. A head CT should be performed on all patients with acute head injuries and a history of loss of consciousness or focal neurological deficits.

Pathological Conditions and Management

Skull Fractures

May be obvious or subtle. Isolated linear non-displaced fractures with an intact scalp require no specific treatment and may be discharged with appropriate analgesic and head injury precautions. Open or depressed fractures require urgent neurosurgery consultation and admission, and may require operative debridement and/or elevation. Basilar skull fractures require admission for neurologic observation; if CSF leak, monitor for meningitis.

Epidural Hematomas

Are usually associated with temporal bone fracture and tear of the middle meningeal artery. They may have a "classic presentation" of head trauma and loss of consciousness followed by lucid interval with a typical hyperdense lens (biconvex) shape appearance on CT. They are less common than subdural hematomas, but require emergent neurosurgical evacuation.

Subdural Hematomas

Usually result from tears of cortical bridging veins. Alcoholic and elderly patients are at increased risk. Acutely, there is typical hyperdense crescent appearance on CT; however, in the subacute phase (2 day to 2 weeks) they may be difficult to visualize. Neurosurgical consultation is mandated since evacuation may be necessary (evidence of increased ICP, >5 mm midline shift, focal neurologic findings, posterior fossa location).

Intraparenchymal Hemorrhages

Often occur in the frontal or temporal lobes when brain strikes bone during deceleration. Clinical findings depend on the size and location of the hematoma, which can be seen on CT as a hyperdense focal area. Edema can result in rapid increased ICP. Treatment includes admission, control of ICP, and possible neurosurgical evacuation.

Diffuse Axonal Injury

Is a result of a shearing force causing microscopic hemorrhages, which may not be visible on CT and are best seen on MRI. Clinical findings range from mild neurologic impairment to coma. Treatment includes admission, control of increased ICP if necessary, and expectant management.

Subarachnoid Hemorrhages

May present with severe headache and nuchal rigidity. CT reveals blood within the ventricles, cisterns, or sulci. Treatment includes prompt neurosurgical consultation, admission, seizure prophylaxis with Phenytoin (load 20 mg/kg IV) and possible shunt placement.

Concussion

Is a diffuse head injury that may occur following blunt trauma to the head. It is associated with brief altered mental status or transient loss of consciousness. Initial symptoms of headache, dizziness, nausea, amnesia, and confusion are usually present but complete recovery is the rule.

Classification of TBI based on the GCS

The best score from each of the categories is used as a method to judge severity (Table 1). An overall score is made by summing the score from the 3 areas assessed. The total score may range from 3 to 15, and severe injury, GCS = 8; moderate injury, GCS 9-12; minor injury GCS 13-15.

Table 1. Glasgow Coma Scale (GCS)

	6	5	4	3	2	1
Eye-opening	–	–	Spontaneous	To voice	To pain	None
Verbal	oriented	Full but conversant	Confused	Inappropriate	Sounds only	None
Motor	Follows commands	Localizes pain	Withdraws to painful stimuli	Decorticate posturing	Decerebrate posturing	None

SPINAL TRAUMA

Cervical spine (C-spine) injuries are present in around 1–2% of all blunt trauma patients and 5–10% of patients with head trauma. It is important to maintain C-spine precautions, document a complete neurologic exam, and assess the respiratory status frequently since high spinal injuries can impair breathing.

Evaluation

The patient may be cleared clinically if there is no C-spine pain, a full range of motion, no tenderness to palpation, no intoxication or altered mental status, no distracting injury, and no neurologic deficits. In all other cases, C-spine x-rays must be obtained and the full cervical spine seen, including C7-T1. In patients with a fracture on plain films or those with a neurologic deficit, neurosurgery should be called immediately. Extensive diagnostic investigations, including CT or MRI, may be required.

Spinal Cord Injury (SCI) Syndromes

Anterior Cord Syndrome

Compression of the cord or spinal artery occlusion results in loss of all motor and sensory function below the lesion other than position sense which is preserved.

Posterior Cord Syndrome

Rarely traumatic; usually related to vitamin deficiencies and infections (e.g., syphilis); results in loss of position and vibratory sense.

Central Cord Syndrome

Typically seen in elderly patients following hyperextension injuries to the neck, often without x-ray abnormality; weakness in hands, arms greater than legs; with loss of pain and temperature sensation.

Brown-Sequard Syndrome

Hemisection of the cord producing ipsilateral paralysis and loss of proprioception below the injury, with contralateral loss of pain and temperature; typically results from penetrating trauma.

SCIWORA (Spinal Cord Injury Without Radiographic Abnormality) Syndrome

Typically seen in pediatric trauma; neurologic deficits may be subtle, transient, and/or delayed (mean 1.2 days); MRI is normal in up to 50%, with atrophy of cord evident 1–3 months post-injury; the vast majority (83%) involve the cervical cord.

Complete Cord Injury

Flaccid below injury level and distal areflexia; vasomotor instability from loss of sympathetic vascular tone results in peripheral vasodilation with hypotension, warm/dry extremities and paradoxical bradycardia; decreased anal tone on rectal exam; and priapism.

Spinal Shock

In contrast, is defined as a temporary loss of spinal reflex activity below a total or near-total SCI.

Management

There are three priorities in the care of patients with potential SCI:

1. Airway management involves in-line stabilization (not traction), cricoid pressure, and rapid sequence intubation (RSI) for patients unable to ventilate adequately or protect their airway. Fluid resuscitation also is important; obvious bleeding must be controlled and occult hemorrhage ruled out.

2. Patients must have constant full spine immobilization, including C-spine stabilization with a hard collar and sandbags or other similar devices to prevent further spinal injury.
3. Aside from fluid resuscitation and oxygenation, neurogenic shock usually responds to low-dose Dopamine at 2.5–10 µg/kg/min. However, in the trauma patient, this diagnosis should be one of exclusion. Closed SCIs with neurologic deficits should be treated with IV high-dose Methprednisolone, 30 mg/kg IV bolus followed by an infusion at 5.4 mg/kg/h for 24 hours, which may improve neurologic recovery.

REFERENCES

Antosia RE. 1999. Emergencies. In *Oxford handbook of clinical medicine*. New York: Oxford UP.

Bracken MB, Shepard MJ, Holford TR. 1997. Administration of methylprednisolone for 24 or 48 hours or tirilazad mesylate for 48 hours in the treatment of acute spinal cord injury, results of the third national acute spinal cord injury randomized controlled trial. *JAMA* **277**:1597–1604.

Scarletta TA, Schaider JJ. 2001. *Emergent management of trauma*, 2nd ed., pp. 73–83. New York: McGraw-Hill.

67

BLAST INJURIES

David Riley, MD,* and John D. Cahill, MD**

In the past, blast injuries were usually associated with conventional warfare or unintentional accidents occurring in the workplace or at home. Over the last several decades, terrorism and landmines have increasingly contributed to the amount of injuries seen. Currently, worldwide there are over 120 million active landmines, with 25,000 serious injuries or death occurring annually. Proximity to an explosion and where it occurs (inside versus outside) both impact the extent of injury that occurs. The physical effects of blast injuries may be divided into primary, secondary, tertiary, or miscellaneous injuries.

PRIMARY BLAST INJURY

Results as a direct effect of changes in atmospheric pressure caused by a blast wave. Air-filled organ systems are mostly infected and include the ear, lung, and bowel. Injuries seen include: tympanic membrane rupture, pulmonary contusions, bronchopleural fistulas, arterial air embolism, pneumothorax, hemothorax, ARDS, and hemorrhage/perforation of the bowel. The physician must have a high index of suspicion and be able to identify the unique three "killers" of primary blast injury: pulmonary barotrauma (the most common), acute arterial or venous gas embolism, and intestinal barotraumas (a major source of delayed mortality).

SECONDARY BLAST INJURY

Results when objects accelerated by the energy of the explosion strike a victim, causing either blunt or penetrating ballistic trauma. These may include total body disruption and traumatic amputations. Head injuries are a common cause of death in this as well as in tertiary injuries.

*Columbia University College of Physicians and Surgeons, New York

**Department of Emergency Medicine and Division of Infectious Diseases, St. Luke's/Roosevelt Hospital Center, New York

TERTIARY BLAST INJURY

Results from a victim's body being displaced by expanding gases and high winds; trauma then occurs from tumbling and impacting objects. Common injuries include abrasions, contusions, lacerations, and miscellaneous blunt trauma. Children are especially prone to tertiary blast injury.

MISCELLANEOUS INJURY

Miscellaneous blast-related injuries include: inhalations and exposures of toxic substances such as asbestos dust, carbon monoxide, cyanide, white phosphorus, and phosgene gas; burns from direct flashes and burning buildings; and crush injuries from the collapse of buildings. Oxygen therapy is the main treatment for most of the miscellaneous blast-related injuries. Patients exposed to cyanide would be expected to have an anion gap metabolic acidosis, and sodium thiosulfate therapy would be indicated as it causes less hypotension compared to sodium nitrite.

Phosgene gas is a unique exposure because it may cause severe delayed pulmonary edema. It was the most lethal of the World War I gases. Phosgene is currently used in the manufacture of dyestuffs, pharmaceuticals, polyurethanes, and metallurgic applications, with an estimated worldwide production of five billion pounds. Treatment is mainly supportive, with oxygen, steroids, and inhaled beta-2 agonists. The key point is to first suspect phosgene gas exposure and then admit the patient for close monitoring for 24 hours.

White phosphorus is also a unique chemical exposure because it is found in munitions, industrial accidents, and fireworks. White phosphorus ignites on contact with air, creating heat and releasing phosphorus pentoxide, a pulmonary irritant. In addition, it can cause severe hypocalcemia and hyperphosphatemia. Treatment involves copious lavage of any exposed areas and placing any raw particles in water to prevent further combustion. Additionally, a 1% copper sulfate solution should be applied to the skin to neutralize the white phosphorus.

INITIAL ASSESSMENT

Important aspects of the history include: where the patient was in relation to the explosion; was it indoors, outdoors, or underwater; and was the explosion industrial related, accidental, or from a terrorist event? One should also get an idea of the number injured, so an appropriate disaster plan can be activated if needed. If necessary, proper decontamination measures should be taken by the staff, before a patient potentially exposes others or contaminates an area of the hospital. Physical exam should start with checking the vital signs and the ABCs. Aside from obvious physical exam findings, careful attention should be placed on the pulmonary and abdominal exam. The tympanic membranes should always be examined, for perforation indicates the presence of a high-pressure wave (greater than 40 kilopascals, 6 psi) and may correlate with other significant organ injury. Any individual with suspicion of significant injury or abnormal vital signs should have venous access established with a large bore intravenous catheter.

MANAGEMENT

After initial assessment, injuries should be treated appropriately. As mentioned before, a high index of suspicion must be held for pulmonary and abdominal injuries. Laboratory tests that may be helpful include a complete blood count, type, and screen or crossmatch for transfusion, basic electrolytes, creatine kinase (in crush injuries) carboxyhemoglobin and/or cyanide level (if indoors), arterial blood gas, urinalysis, and chest x-ray. Other tests may be ordered based upon injuries noted. Pulse oximetry can be helpful, but it needs to be remembered that readings can be reassuringly normal in carbon monoxide poisoning. In managing pulmonary injuries, oxygen, bronchodilators, and ventilators should be available. Obvious acute abdominal injuries require acute surgical care; otherwise, further radiological studies for evaluation or serial exams may be warranted. Portable emergency department ultrasound use can detect blood in the abdomen or intraabdominal fluid using the focused assessment with sonography for trauma (FAST) examination, and it can improve outcomes in penetrating cardiac injury. Based upon the pattern of injuries seen, the attention of a pulmonologist, general surgeon, orthopedist, neurosurgeon, or burn specialist may be required.

REFERENCE

Borak J, Diller WF. 2001. Phosgene exposure: mechanisms of injury and treatment strategies. *J Occup Environ Med* **43**(2):110–119.

Cahill J, ed. 2002. *Updates in emergency medicine*. New York: Kluwer Academic.

Chou TD, Lee TW, Chen SL, Tung YM, Dai NT, Chen SG, Lee CH, Chen TM, Wang HJ. 2001. The management of white phosphorus burns. *Burns* **27**(5):492–497.

Ma O, Mateer J, Ogata M, Kefer MP, Wittmann D, Aprahamian C. 1995. Prospective analysis of a rapid trauma ultrasound examination performed by emergency physicians. *J Trauma* **38:** 879–885.

Plummer D, Brunette D, Asinger R, Ruiz E. 1992. Emergency department echocardiography improves outcome in penetrating cardiac injury. *Ann Emerg Med* **21**:709–712.

Quintana DA, Parker JR, Jordan FB. 1997. The spectrum of pediatric injuries after a bomb blast. *J Pediatr Surg* **32**(2):307–10; disc. 310–311.

68

CRUSH INJURIES

Tommy Y.S. Wong, MD*

CRUSH INJURY/CRUSH SYNDROME

Earthquakes and manmade disasters are the leading causes of crush injuries and an increased incidence of crush syndrome. The estimated incidence are ~20% and ~2–5%, respectively. However, given the global climate of war and acts of terrorism, we should anticipate a rise in manmade disasters in the future. Bywaters and Beall offered the first classic description of crush syndrome in Londoners treated during the German Blitz in 1940–41. Zhi-Yong described its devastation in one of history's worst natural catastrophes, the 1973 Tangshan earthquake in China, where the death toll was 242,769 and the additional injured 164,851. The mechanism of injury is entrapment of victims under collapsed structures for periods of 4 hours or longer. In crush-injured victims, deaths within the first hours are caused by shock and hyperkalemia, while deaths days later are from myoglobinuric acute renal failure.

The pathogenesis of all crush injuries begins with rhabdomyolysis, whereby increased and prolonged pressure on skeletal muscle leads to cellular death and the release of its intracellular contents. While generally resistant to ischemia, muscle tissue is very sensitive to pressure. It impairs the cellular Na^+,K^+-ATPase pump and calcium transport, resulting in a rise in intracellular free calcium, which in turn activates neutral proteases that disrupt myofibrils and leads to cellular damage and death. This cascade of events leads to the clinical features of myoglobinemia, hyperphosphatemia, hyperkalemia, hyperuricemia, hypocalcemia, metabolic acidosis, DIC, and hypovolemic and hemodynamic shock, the hallmark of crush syndrome.

Hyperkalemia with acute renal failure is the most immediate and life-threatening complication, occurring hours to days after a patient's extrication. An oxygen-binding heme protein found in skeletal and cardiac muscle, myoglobin is rapidly cleared from plasma primarily through renal excretion. With massive muscle destruction, the release of myoglobin surpasses its clearance, resulting in the typical discoloration of pink spun plasma and reddish brown urine. The urine dipstick will test positive as it reacts with the heme-containing myoglobin. To differentiate between heme and myo-

*Department of Emergency Medicine, St. Luke's/Roosevelt Hospital Center, New York

globin as opposed to hemoglobin, a microscopic examination of the brown urine will reveal an absence of red blood cells. The direct renal toxic effect of myoglobin and its secondary obstructive effects as it precipitates in the renal tubules play a critical role in the development of acute renal failure. An estimated 50% of the crush-injured patients with severe rhabdomyolysis will develop acute renal failure secondary to myoglobinemia. It is important to note that the degree of creatine phosphokinase elevation and the presence of myoglobinemia do not predict those who will go on to develop ARF. Other important factors include hypovolemia, metabolic acidosis, and age.

Presentation

Patients with crush injury will typically present with flaccid paralysis and sensory loss in the affected limbs. While they can appear like victims of spinal cord injury, their deficits do not correspond to a nerve distribution. On neurologic examination, their rectal tone and urinary-bladder function will also be preserved. Initially, extricated patients appear relatively well and without systemic signs metabolic derangement. The compressive force that entrapped the limbs in effect acts as a tourniquet, preventing systemic return of metabolic byproducts of cellular ischemia and necrosis. With rescue and decompression, a paradoxical acceleration to shock and hemoconcentration may develop. This may account for reports of victims dying immediately after extrication from collapsed structures.

Management

Anticipating and preventing the systemic and renal complications of crush syndrome is essential. Aggressive fluid resuscitation should begin during patient rescue, since a delay of 12 hours or more is associated with up to 100% incidence of acute renal failure. A large-bore intravenous line should be established as soon as a free limb is available and normal saline infused at a rate of 1.5 liters per hour. It is generally expected that 4 to 8 hours are needed to fully free an entrapped victim and remove them to the medical treatment area. Postponement of full extrication has been suggested until adequate fluid resuscitation has been achieved.

With stabilized blood pressure and urine flow, forced mannitol alkaline diuresis should be initiated to prevent hyperkalemia and acute renal failure. This therapy generally occurs in the medical facilities, where input and output are strictly monitored. Alkaline urine prevents the precipitation of myoglobin in the renal tubules while mannitol aids in the osmotic diuresis of myoglobin. The fluid of choice is D5 0.5NS, with each liter containing 10 g of mannitol as a 20% solution and 40 mmol of bicarbonate. The goal is to maintain a urine output of ~300 ml/h and urine pH >6.5 until myoglobinuria resolves. This aggressive fluid management usually leads to a positive fluid balance of 4 liters per day. While well tolerated in young adults, this therapy must be tailored to the elderly. If the patient becomes oliguric, a bolus of 20 g of mannitol along with 120 mg of furosemide may be used. The theoretical disadvantage of urine acidification by loop diuretics is outweighed by its benefits. It is important to note that mannitol in excess of 200 g/d may produce acute renal failure and thus should be avoided. If anuria and renal failure develops despite treatment, daily hemodialysis must be instituted.

COMPARTMENT SYNDROME

The mechanism of crush with entrapment is the ideal setting for compartment syndrome. It is defined as elevated pressure within a closed tissue space that impairs neurovascular function, leading to tissue death. Compartment pressure can rise either from external compression or from internal volume expansion (hematoma or third spaced fluid). Normal tissue pressure is usually less than 10 mm Hg. At 20 mm Hg, capillary blood flow diminishes. Above 30–40 mm Hg, tissue will be at risk for ischemic necrosis, with nerve being more susceptible than muscle. Since all skeletal muscle groups are invested in fascia, compartment syndrome can occur anywhere in the body. The compartments most frequently involved by this syndrome are those in the forearm and the lower leg.

The classic presentation of those with compartment syndrome will be muscle weakness and pain that is out of proportion to their injury or examination. On inspection, there might be swelling, ecchymosis, and deformity suggesting an underlying fracture. On palpation of the muscle, severe pain will be elicited. Active contraction or passive stretching of muscle within the compartment will also worsen the pain. Hypoesthesia in the distribution of the nerves that traverse the involved compartment can occur. Do not wait for the classic description of pain, pallor, paresthesia, pulselessness, and paralysis (the 5Ps), as they are late findings and suggest irreversible damage. To confirm the diagnosis, compartment pressures must be measured.

Controversy exists regarding absolute criteria that mandates fasciotomy, a surgical procedure that carries high morbidity of bleeding, infection, and loss of limb. Pressures that exceed 40 mm Hg are generally accepted as indications for surgery. Some authors recommend a trial of intravenous hypertonic mannitol first to decompress compartment pressures. When effective, relief of symptoms, size of swollen limb, and compartment pressures are expected within approximately 40 minutes of treatment. Should conservative management fail, emergent fasciotomy is needed. This entails longitudinal incisions over the skin, and then the fascia of the affected compartment to release the swollen and injured muscle. In a disaster setting where the crush victim might be neurologically impaired, a high index of suspicion in needed. Early and multiple repeat compartment pressures might be needed to make the diagnosis. Treatment initiated within 4 hours of the onset of symptoms has an excellent prognosis to full recovery of function.

REFERENCES

Better OS. 1999. Rescue and salvage of casualties suffering from the crush syndrome after mass disasters. *Mil Med* **164**:366–369.

Better OS, Stein JH. 1990. Early management of shock and prophylaxis of acute renal failure in traumatic rhabdomyolysis. *N Engl J Med* **322**:825–829.

Bywaters EGL. 1990. 50 years on: the crush syndrome. *Br Med J* **301**:22–29.

Bywaters EGL, Beal D. 1941. Crush injuries and renal function. *Br Med J* **1**:427–432.

Counselman FL. 2000. Rhabdomyolysis. In *Emergency medicine: a comprehensive study guide*, 5th ed., pp. 1841–1845. Ed JE Tintinalli, GD Kelen, JS Stapczynski. New York: McGraw-Hill.

Gans L, Kennedy T. 1996. Management of unique clinical entities in disaster medicine. *Emerg Med Clin North Am* **14**(2):312–317.

Ruiz E. 2000. Compartment syndromes. In *Emergency medicine: a comprehensive study guide*, 5th ed., pp. 1838–1841. Ed JE Tintinalli, GD Kelen, JS Stapczynski. New York: McGraw-Hill.
Sheng ZY. 1987. Medical support in the Tangshan earthquake: a review of the management of mass casualties and certain major injuries. *J Trauma* **27**:1130–1135.

69

MISSILE INJURIES

Liudvikas Jagminas, MD, FACEP*

OVERVIEW

Many authors previously devoted considerable effort to differentiating between the magnitude of injury caused by "ordinary" versus "high-velocity" missile wounds. As a result of experience gained in recent conflicts and to a greater extent based on wound ballistic research performed over the past decade, new and somewhat different concepts are evolving. One very fundamental concept is that the high-velocity wound is not necessarily a totally different entity, as had been previously thought.

From a military perspective, the switch to high-velocity rounds is based on a practical standpoint. The automatic weapon, with its increased requirement for ammunition, necessitated lighter-weight ammunition. To compensate for the loss in missile mass, if wounding power was to be maintained, it was necessary to increase missile velocity. The lighter cartridge allowed the individual infantryman to carry the increase in basic load of ammunition (more rounds, same weight) and allowed for greater and more sustained firepower.

The penetrating missile or fragment destroys tissue by crushing it as it punches a hole through the tissue. This hole or missile track represents the so-called permanent cavity. The cross-sectional area of the missile track is comparable to the presenting area of the missile, and its dimensions are roughly the same for all soft tissues.

After passage of the projectile, the walls of the permanent cavity are temporarily stretched radially outward. The maximum lateral tissue displacement delineates the temporary cavity. Any damage resulting from temporary cavitation is due to stretching of the tissue. Resistance or vulnerability to stretch damage depends mostly on tissue elasticity. The same stretch that causes only moderate contusion and minor functional changes in relatively elastic skeletal muscle can cause devastating disruption of the liver. The result of temporary displacement of tissue is analogous to a localized area of blunt trauma surrounding the permanent cavity left by the projectile's passage. If one presented at the average large city hospital with a gunshot wound in the thigh (entrance and exit holes of less than 1 cm in diameter) and gave the history of being

*Department of Emergency Medicine, Memorial Hospital, Pawtucket, Rhode Island

shot with a 22 Long Rifle bullet, the surgical treatment rendered would be minimal. The same would probably apply if the history were of a wound from a 38 Special or a 45 Automatic. If, however, the history was given that the wound had been made by an M-16, the victim would most likely be subjected to an excision of the entire bullet track and possibly even several cm of tissue on all sides of the track. Comparing the first 12 cm of penetration on the M-16 wound profile with that of the other examples shows that in such a wound the M-16 is unlikely to cause any more tissue disruption than the 22 Long Rifle. The reason for this is that the M-16 round does not fragment or yaw in the first 12 cm of soft tissue it traverses, nor does it develop its very significant temporary cavitation effects prior to 12 cm of penetration. The widespread belief that each and every wound caused by "high-velocity" projectiles must be treated by "radical debridement" is incorrect and results from failure to recognize the role of other variables, such as bullet mass and construction, in the projectile-tissue interaction.

PHYSICAL PROPERTIES

Penetrating missiles include both munition fragments and bullets (which are often divided into "high" and "low" velocity). Velocity is not as important as the amount of kinetic energy transferred to tissues. Kinetic energy transfer depends on: velocity, presenting area of fragment, and the mechanical properties of tissue.

FRAGMENT INJURIES

Fragments are usually small and numerous. They are of low velocity (100–500 m/s) and low energy (10–100 J), and have poor tissue penetration. Although injuries are often numerous, they are usually limited to the fragment track.

BULLET WOUNDS

Hand-gun bullets are of low velocity (<250 m/s) and low energy (200–300 J). Rifle bullets are of high velocity (750–1000 m/s) and high energy (2–3 kJ). Physiological effects depend on degree of energy transfer. High-velocity bullets can result in low-energy transfer wounds.

PATHOPHYSIOLOGY

The effects of bullets can result from both direct and indirect effects. In low-energy transfer wounds, injury results from direct effects along the bullet track. In high-energy transfer wounds, indirect effects are more important: radial forces perpendicular to the track may result in cavitation, which in turn may generate contusions and lacerations away from the track, and negative pressure within the cavity can suck in environmental contaminants. Rifle bullets also tumble (yaw) within the wound, which may increase the presenting area and increase energy transfer, which in turn can result in small entry and exit wounds but a large wound cavity. Radial-energy transfer can also cause indirect fractures. Bullet and bone fragmentation can cause secondary tracks and further unpredictable damage

TREATMENT

Low-Velocity Injuries

- Debride the wounds superficially.
- Lavage the wound with sterile fluid.
- Do not close the skin.
- Administer intravenous antibiotics such as Penicillin for 1–3 days.
- Give tetanus prophylaxis.
- Treat fractures by closed means with a cast, traction or external fixation.
- If bullet fragments remain in a joint cavity, arrange to have them removed within a few weeks.

High-Velocity Injuries

- Debride the wounds in the operating theater, using adequate anaesthesia.
- Lavage each wound after removing all dead tissue and foreign material.
- Lavage between the entrance and exit wounds, passing gauze through the track if necessary.
- Do not close the wound. Re-debride in 2–5 days and close or skin graft when clean.
- Administer antibiotics such as Penicillin and Gentamicin along with tetanus prophylaxis.
- Treat fractures with a cast or, preferably, external fixation or traction.

Wound Debridement/Excision

Debridement should be rational rather than radical. The recommendation is not to excise the wound to the extent that viable muscle is intentionally excised circumferentially, but rather to open the wound such that drainage is assured, while at the same time excising that muscle which is severely damaged or disrupted and therefore devitalized. The physician must aggressively incise the wound, but should not empirically excise tissue more widely than clinical judgment would normally dictate. The majority of combat surgeons continue to utilize the 4 Cs for identifying nonviable muscle: Color—dark; Consistency—"mushy"; Contraction—lack of failure when pinched with forceps; and the Cut—noted is the absence of brisk bleeding from the cut surface.

The single most important principle in the management of battle wounds is their nonclosure following debridement. The physician must not give in to the temptation to primarily close certain "very clean appearing" war wounds. Such closure is ill advised and inappropriate and can only be condemned. All wounds must be left widely open with the following exceptions: sucking chest wounds, joint capsules, wounds of the dura, and some head and neck wounds; however, with severe contamination it may be safer to leave these open.

In some circumstances, delayed primary wound closure may be performed 4–10 days after debridement. The indication for delayed primary closure is the clinically clean appearance of the wound. Whereas most wounds are closed in the operating room utilizing the interrupted wire technique and local or general anesthesia, some may be very amenable to tape closure.

REFERENCES

Amato JJ, Amato JL, Billy LJ, Lawson NS, Rich NM. 1974. High-velocity missile injury. *Am J Surg* **127**:454–459.

Charters AC, Charters AC. 1976. Wounding mechanism of very high velocity projectiles. *J Trauma* **16**:464–470.

Dimond FC Jr, Rich NM. 1967. M-16 rifle wounds in Vietnam. *J Trauma* **7**:619–625.

Dziemian AJ, Mendelson JA, Lindsey D. 1961. Comparison of the wounding characteristics of some commonly encountered bullets. *J Trauma* **1**:341–353.

Hampton OP. 1961. The indications for debridement of gunshot (bullet) wounds of the extremities in civilian practice. *J Trauma* **1**:368–372.

Hopkinson DAW, Marshall TK. 1967. Firearm injuries. *Br J Surg* **54**:344–353.

Morgan NM, Spencer AD, Hershey FB. 1961. Debridement of civilian gunshot wounds of soft tissue. *J Trauma* **1**:354–360.

Schwach RP, Parks RD. 1979. Gunshot fractures of extremities: Classification, management, and complications. *Vet Surg* **8**:57–62.

Silliphant WM, Beyer JC. 1955. Wound ballistics. *Mil Med* **117**:238–246.

Thoresby FP, Darlow HM. 1967. The mechanism of primary infection of bullet wounds. *Br J Surg* **54**:359–361.

Ziperman HH. 1961. The management of soft tissue missile wounds in war and peace. *J Trauma* **1**:361–367.

70 BURN MANAGEMENT

Liudvikas Jagminas, MD, FACEP*

An evaluation of the Airway, Breathing, and Circulation (the ABCs) should receive first priority. The history should include the time, location, and circumstances of the injury, where the patient was found, and their condition. Past medical and social history, current medication usage, drug allergies, and tetanus status should be rapidly determined.

Smoke inhalation causes more than 50% of fire-related deaths. Patients sustaining an inhalation injury may require aggressive airway intervention. Most injuries result from the inhalation of toxic smoke; however, superheated air may rarely cause direct thermal injury to the upper respiratory tract.

Patients who are breathing spontaneously and at risk for inhalation injury should be placed on high-flow humidified oxygen. Patients trapped in buildings or those caught in an explosion are at higher risk for inhalation injury. These patients may have facial burns, singeing of the eyebrows and nasal hair, pharyngeal burns, carbonaceous sputum, or impaired mentation. A change in voice quality, stridorous respirations, or wheezing may be noted. The upper airway may be visualized by laryngoscopy, and the tracheobronchial tree should be evaluated by bronchoscopy. Chest radiography is not sensitive for detecting inhalation injury.

FIRST AID AT SCENE

1. Stop the burning process and remove the patient to a safe area.
2. Place patient in a supine position and initiate CPR if indicated. The same general principles of cardiopulmonary resuscitation apply, and are a priority.
3. Cover patient (clean sheet and/or "space blanket").
4. If possible, start large-bore (16 ga) IV with lactated Ringer's solution (LR).
5. Oxygen: intubate if necessary. Carbon monoxide poisoning is the most frequent cause of death in the first hours after a fire.

*Department of Emergency Medicine, Memorial Hospital, Pawtucket, Rhode Island

ADDITIONAL CONSIDERATIONS

- Rapidly remove burning clothing.
- Electrical burns: ensure patient is clear of electrical source prior to rescue.
- Chemical burns: remove soaked clothing, and irrigate with copious amounts of water.
- Ensure that the patient and the medical team are completely clear of the fire area for their protection and to avoid interference in fire fighting efforts.

EMERGENCY DEPARTMENT TREATMENT

1. Reassess ABCs of Basic Life Support. Begin fluid resuscitation per the Parkland formula (see below).
2. Oxygen by high-flow mask, nasogastric tube, and Foley for all serious burns. Intubation if indicated.
3. Assess extent and severity of burns (rule of 9s or mapping; patients hand = 1% body surface).
4. IV analgesics titrated to reduce pain to tolerable levels during initial cleaning and debridement.
5. Gently clean and debride wounds; cover wounds with Silvadene or Sulfamylon. Keep patient warm; clean and re-cover wounds daily.
6. Evaluate the eyes using fluorescent instrumentation.

SPECIAL SITUATIONS

Chemical Burns

- Alkali powder (lime): brush the powder from the skin before lavage is begun.
- Phenol: instead of lavage and in any case after lavage as well, the skin should be washed with a solvent such as polyethylene glycol, propylene glycol (anti-freeze), or glycerol to remove residual phenol.
- White phosphorous: must be kept moist to prevent ignition of the retained phosphorous particles. Wash the involved area with an 0.5 or 1.0% solution of copper sulfate. This will cause formation of a blue-black film of cupric phosphide on the surface of the retained particles. Debride the particles and keep them moist or you will have another fire.

ESTIMATING SURFACE AREA WITH THE RULE OF 9s

Child

- Head: 18%
- Torso back: 18%

- Torso front: 18%
- Leg left: 14%
- Leg right: 14%
- Arm left: 9%
- Arm right: 9%

Adult

- Torso front: 18%
- Torso back: 18%
- Leg left: 18%
- Leg right: 18%
- Head: 9%
- Arm left: 9%
- Arm right: 9%
- Genitalia: 1%
- Size of patient's palm: 1%

BURN ASSESSMENT

After completion of the primary survey, a secondary survey should assess the depth and total body surface area (TBSA) burned.

First-Degree Burns

First-degree burns involve the epidermis layer of the skin, but not the dermal layer. These injuries are characterized by pain, erythema, and lack of blisters. These burns heal without scar formation. First-degree burns are not considered in calculation of the TBSA burned.

Second-Degree Burns

Second-degree burns are subdivided into superficial and deep partial-thickness burns.

Superficial Partial-Thickness Burn Injury

Superficial partial-thickness burn injury involves the papillary dermis, containing pain-sensitive nerve endings. Burn management, burns, burn blisters, or bullae may be present, and the burns usually appear pink and moist. These burn management, burns, and burn injuries heal with little or no scarring.

Deep Partial-Thickness Burn Injury

Deep partial-thickness burn injury damages both the papillary and reticular dermis. These injuries may not be burn management, burns, or burn painful, and often appear white or mottled pink. Deep partial-thickness burns can produce burn management, burns, and burn with significant scarring.

Full-Thickness or Third-Degree Burns

Full-thickness or third-degree burns involve all layers of the epidermis and dermis and may destroy subcutaneous structures. They appear white or charred. These burns are usually insensate because of destruction of nerve endings, but the surrounding areas are extremely painful. Third-degree burns are best treated with skin grafting to limit scarring.

Fourth-Degree Burns

Fourth-degree burns involve structures beneath the subcutaneous fat, including muscle and bone.

Note circumferential, or near-circumferential, burn wounds because they may cause progressive extremity ischemia or interfere with ventilation as burn wound swelling increases. In such situations, timely escharotomy is essential. Perform extremity escharotomies as soon as peripheral perfusion is threatened. Do not wait until the extremity is overtly ischemic. Perform torso escharotomies as soon as ventilation appears compromised.

MANAGEMENT OF MODERATE TO SEVERE BURNS

Initial Fluid Resuscitation: The Parkland Formula

Initiation of fluid resuscitation should precede initial wound care. In adults, IV fluid resuscitation is usually necessary in second- or third-degree burns involving greater than 20% TBSA. In pediatric patients, fluid resuscitation should be initiated in all infants with burns with 10% or greater TBSA and in older children with burns with greater than 15% TBSA.

Two large-bore IV lines should be placed. Lactated Ringer's solution is the most commonly used fluid for burn resuscitation.

The Parkland formula is used to guide initial fluid resuscitation during the first 24 hours. The formula calls for 4 cc/kg/TBSA burn (second- and third-degree) of lactated Ringer's solution over the first 24 hours. Half of the fluid should be administered over the first 8 hours post-burn, and the remaining half should be administered over the next 16 hours. The volume of fluid given is based on the time elapsed since the burn.

Urine output should be used as a measure of renal perfusion and to assess fluid balance. In adults, a urine output of 0.5–1.0 ml/kg/h should be maintained. Patients with significant burns should have a Foley catheter inserted in order to monitor urine output.

A nasogastric (NG) tube should be placed in patients with burns involving 20% or more TBSA in order to prevent gastric distention and emesis associated.

Second 24 Hours

- 5% albumin in LR @ 0.5 ml/kg/%burn (200 cc of salt-poor albumin placed in 800 cc of LR).

Plus

- D5W (or 1/4 normal saline (1/4 NS) primarily for children) to yield the same hourly infusion rate as the first 24 hours.
- Adjust D5W or the 1/4 NS rate, not the 5% albumin solution, in order to maintain urine output of 30–50 ml/hr.

GENERAL CONSIDERATIONS

1. ALL medications must be given IV during the resuscitation because of the dramatic changes in capillary permeability. Otherwise, the patient can receive an overdose when fluid mobilization occurs.
2. Sodium shifts can cause serious hyponatremia. The rate of fall of serum sodium levels is very important, especially in young patients. Serum sodium must be carefully monitored when giving large volumes of IV fluids.
3. Transfusion is indicated for hematocrit under 30. Packed RBCs are preferred.
4. Insulin infusion may be instituted for serum glucose over 200 mg%.
5. Histamine (H2) blockers and antacids should be used to keep the gastric pH at 7.0.

AMERICAN BURN ASSOCIATION BURN CENTER TRANSFER CRITERIA

- Second- or third-degree burns greater than 10% TBSA in patients younger than 10 years or older than 50 years.
- Second- or third-degree burns greater than 20% TBSA in persons of other age groups.
- Second- or third-degree burns that involve the face, hands, feet, genitalia, perineum, or major joints.
- Third-degree burns greater than 5% TBSA in persons of any age group.
- Electrical burns, including lightening injury.
- Chemical burns.
- Inhalational injury.
- Burn injury in patients with preexisting medical disorders that could complicate management, prolong recovery, or affect mortality.
- Any patients with burns or concomitant trauma (e.g., fracture) in which the burn injury poses the greatest risk of morbidity or mortality. In such cases, if the trauma poses the greater immediate risk, the patient may be treated initially in a trauma center until stable before being transferred to a burn center. Physician judgment is necessary in such situations and should be in concert with the regional medical control plan and triage protocols.
- A lack of qualified personnel or equipment for the care of children (transfer to facility with these qualities).
- Burn injury in patients who require special social/emotional and/or long-term rehabilitative support, including cases involving suspected child abuse or substance abuse

REFERENCES

American Burn Association. 1990. Hospital and pre-hospital resources for optimal care of patients with burn injury: guidelines for development and operation of burn centers. *J Burn Care Rehabil* **11**:98–104.

Anantharaman V. 1992. Burns mass disasters: aetiology, predisposing situations and initial management. *Ann Acad Med Singapore* **21**(5):635–639.

Brigham PA, McLoughlin E. 1996. Burn incidence and medical care use in the United States: estimates, trends, and data sources. *J Burn Care Rehabil* **17**:95–107.

Deitch EA, Wheelahan TM, Rose MP, Clothier J, Cotter J. 1983. Hypertrophic burn scars: analysis of variables. *J Trauma* **23**:895–398.

Diamond AW, Piggott RW, Townsend PL. 1975. Immediate care of burns. *Anaesthesia* **30**(6):791–802.

Gordon M, Goodwin CW. 1997. Burn management. Initial assessment, management, and stabilization. *Nurs Clin North Am* **32**(2):237–249.

Griglak MJ. 1992. Thermal injury. *Emerg Med Clin North Am* **10**(2):369–383.

Hartford CE. 1996. Care of outpatient burns. In *Total burn care*, pp. 71–80. Ed DN Herndon. Philadelphia: Saunders.

Heimbach D, Mann R, Engrav L. 1996. Evaluation of the burn wound: management decisions. In *Total burn care*, pp. 81–87. Ed DN Herndon. Philadelphia: Saunders.

Lund C, Browder N. 1944. The estimation of areas of burns. *Surg Gynecol Obstet* **79**:352–358.

Milner SM, Hodgetts TJ, Rylah LT. 1993. The Burns calculator: a simple proposed guide for fluid resuscitation. *Lancet* **342**(8879):1089–1091.

Monafo WW. 1996. Initial management of burns. *New Engl J Med* **335**:1581–1586.

Moncrief JA. 1979. Burns, I: assessment. *JAMA* **242**(1):72–74.

Muller MJ, Herndon DN. 1994. The challenge of burns. *Lancet* **343**:216–220.

Northeastern Ohio trauma study: v: burn injury. 1986. *J Trauma* **26**(9):844–847.

Sheridan RL. 1998. The seriously burned child: resuscitation through reintegration—2. *Curr Probl Pediatr* **28**(5):139–167.

PART V

Pediatric Considerations and Disasters

71

PEDIATRIC PROBLEMS IN DEVELOPING COUNTRIES

Ramona Sunderworth, MD*

At the turn of the 21st century, the number of children in developing countries will account for greater than 50% of the world's population. A mind-shattering thought indeed, for all of us in the medical profession. Recent reports from WHO, UNICEF, and several international conferences have emphasized the need for a stronger focus on the issue of the well-being of children, and taking the necessary steps to prevent potential disasters.

The widening economic disparity between the rich and poor counties contributes to social inequity and worsens the poverty responsible for diseases claiming children's lives. Infant mortality rates are approximately five times higher in less developed nations than in the more developed nations. At present, between 11 and 12 million children under 5 die each year (99% of these in developing nations). About 70% of these deaths are caused by five largely preventable illnesses: acute respiratory illness (ARI), diarrhea (dehydration), measles, malaria, and perinatal causes. Malnutrition (protein/caloric and micronutrient) is a factor contributing to 60% of these deaths. One third of African children are underweight. Poverty is a major cause of malnutrition combined with inadequate health services, care and support for women and children.

The link between infant, child, and maternal health is one of the most powerful. Half of infant deaths are due to inadequate maternal and newborn care. A mother's death doubles the death rate among surviving sons and quadruples the death rate among surviving daughters. Most programs addressing infant/child survival include interventions directed at maternal health.

Wars have killed greater than 2 million children in the past 10 years and left millions more physically and mentally disabled. Recruitment of child soldiers continues to be a serious problem worldwide, especially in developing countries. Availability of arms and landmines manufactured by the northern hemisphere contribute to the death and disability of thousands of children long after active conflicts cease. Increasing numbers of children are displaced at any one time due to disasters (natural

*Department of Emergency Medicine, St. Luke's/Roosevelt Hospital Center, New York

and manmade), 20 million from 1990 to 2000 (more than half of the total displaced population). These children are exposed to an increased risk of malnutrition, infectious diseases, violence, and mental illnesses, as well as delays in education, with long-term consequences.

Urbanization has brought both advantages and disadvantages. In developing nations it has often been uncontrolled and has led to environmental degradation and the breakdown of traditional family life, values, and culture. This has resulted in increased numbers of children living in slums and poverty, victims of violence, motor vehicle accidents, abandonment (street children, institutionalization), exposure to pollutants (lead, dioxins, etc), alcohol, tobacco, drugs, prostitution, child abuse, mental illness, and suicide. Many of these children suffer from infectious diseases (TB, STDs, AIDS, etc.) and serious psychological trauma.

The AIDS epidemic is a major pediatric threat not only from infection but with regard to the risk of orphanhood. AIDS kills more than 1 million children per year. Over 10 million children have already been orphaned and many forced into the streets, victims of abusive child labor entrapment, deprived of the most basic health care, societal support, and rudimentary education. By 2010 it is predicted that more than 40 million children will have become orphans from the AIDS pandemic.

Degradation of the environment and increases in pollution claims more than 3 million children's lives each year. The negative consequences of industrialization, urbanization, and globalization spiral out of control, due to the lack of regulation and enforcement policies, leading to a deterioration of basic hygiene and sanitation and increases in respiratory and diarrheal diseases, cancers, poisonings, injuries, and congenital malformations. Poor pesticide control also contributes greatly to unnecessary deaths due to environmental hazards.

Climate changes, global warming, desertification, and the El Niño phenomenon have resulted in floods and droughts, thus contributing to poverty, malnutrition, and the resurgence of vector-borne diseases (dengue fever, tick-borne diseases, malaria), infectious diseases, poverty, and ill health.

The population explosion in developing countries stresses already inadequate systems and services, not only for health but for education, social, and sanitation/water, and sources of energy.

The gender gap, while narrowing in the past 20 years, is still responsible for harmful traditional practices affecting girls: infanticide, female genital mutilation, and unequal access to education, health care, and psychosocial stimulation.

While new technology has improved the quality of health and healthcare systems, the digital divide has widened the gap between the "haves and have nots" in terms of access to sophisticated imaging and diagnostic tests and treatments. The promise of new health technologies has to be balanced against the costly inappropriateness of its introduction in certain settings.

Improved survival without improvement in the levels of poverty or other physical, social, mental, and emotional stressors has led to large numbers of impaired children. Learning disabilities are estimated to be present in a third of the children under 15 years of age in developing countries. Resources are still scarce for children with chronic illnesses, malignancies, head traumas, physically disabilities, congenital disorders, and metabolic disorders. An increased number of children growing up with physical, mental, and educational disabilities with no available or appropriate rehabilitative or educational resources will have dire consequences on national/international development.

In addition, the historical contributors to child morbidity and mortality have not been completely conquered. In 2000 almost 25% of the developing world's total population still lacked improved drinking water sources, and only about 50% had adequate sanitation facilities. Immunization rates for the complete EPI (Expanded Program on Immunization) averaged 73% among 1-year-old children, leaving millions of children susceptible to preventable deaths and disability (e.g., diphtheria, pertussis, tetanus, polio, TB, measles). The availability and use of ORT (Oral Rehydration Therapy) worldwide stood at around 25%. Coverage for non-EPI vaccine for preventable diseases (Hepatitis B, *Hemophilus influenza b,* varicella, *Strep pneumococcus,* rubella, etc.) remains low or nonexistent in most developing countries.

As the determinants of ill health are multifactorial, so are the efforts to address them, as evidenced by the multitude of rights-based international initiatives aiming to protect children in general and benefit the families and communities in general. The WHO, UNICEF, USAID, CDC, the Rockefeller Foundation, UNDP, the World Bank, and the many national and international NGOs collaborate on a multitude of programs worldwide.

The EPI, the GOBI-FFF program (growth monitoring, oral rehydration, breastfeeding, immunization, food supplementation, female literacy and family planning), the Combating Childhood Communicable Diseases (focusing on immunization and treatment of diarrhea and malaria), the CVI (children's vaccine initiative), the Child Survival Campaign, the Mother and Baby Package, the Safe Motherhood Initiative, and numerous other child and maternal health projects have been launched. The Integrated Management of Childhood Illness strategy integrates elements of existing diarrheal disease and respiratory infection control, immunization, nutrition, maternal, and child health programs.

Various agencies have focused attention on public education, healthcare financing, and operational research, and training of health professionals in epidemiological, research, and computerization.

Great progress has been made by national and international efforts over the past 50 years. In 1955 there were 21 million deaths in children under 5 years of age and in 1997 about 10 million. This decrease can be mainly attributed to improvement in public health projects, improved water and sanitation, the EPI, ORT, and basic primary health projects.

Projected deaths of 5 million in the year 2025 seem optimistic given the slow reversal of projected deaths due to the growing epidemics, disasters (manmade and natural), increasing financial constraints on financing basic, and new immunization and primary health programs.

The child health issues in the developing world will continue along the lines of the epidemiological transition, with the double burden of infectious diseases and increasing numbers of children with noncommunicable diseases and injuries stemming mainly from violations of children's rights in large, poor, urban areas.

Increasingly, emerging and reemerging infections will contribute to mortality and morbidity, as seen with the present outbreaks of AIDS, tuberculosis, malaria, dengue, cholera, diphtheria, pertussis, and schistosomiasis.

72 NUTRITIONAL ASSESSMENT IN MALNUTRITION

Scott Cohen, MD*

OVERVIEW

Malnutrition remains one of the leading causes of pediatric morbidity and mortality in the developing world. It is an especially significant problem in disaster and refugee situations. Breastfeeding mothers and young infants and children are at the highest risk for malnutrition. This is because they require the highest amount of calories per kilogram of body weight.

PRESENTATION

Malnutrition will cause infections in the child by suppressing the immune system. In addition, some infections will lead to malnutrition in children. This sets up a cycle of increasing morbidity in the child. Severe viral illnesses, such as measles, consume nutrients at a faster rate of intake, and cause a disruption in the nitrogen balance in the body. Intestinal infections can cause a decreased absorption of nutrients from the gut, also leading to a malnourished state, especially if intake is compromised. In addition, helminthic infections such as hookworm, can cause blood loss and severe iron-deficiency anemia in infected children.

Initial pertinent history to obtain:

- Normal diet before presentation (i.e., breastfeeding history or solid food intake history)
- Volume of liquids consumed over past 24–48 hours
- Urinary output
- Other signs/symptoms of dehydration
- Recent vomiting and diarrhea (length of time and frequency of symptoms)
- Known weight loss

*Global Pediatric Alliance, Oakland, California

- Exposure to active TB or measles
- Recent family deaths
- Developmental milestones
- Immunization history

INITIAL EXAM

- Current weight and height
- General state of health
- State of current hydration
- Vital signs including temperature
- Signs of respiratory distress
- Skin turgor
- Edema
- Abdominal distention
- Hepatomegaly
- Jaundice
- Pallor
- Skin or mucous membrane infections

DIAGNOSIS

There are several ways to make the diagnosis of malnutrition in children. Infants and children with moderate to severe malnutrition will have obvious signs on history and exam.

Body mass index (BMI)

- Assesses body weight relative to the child's height
- BMI = body wt in kg/height^2 (height in meters)
- Normal values for children are: 20–26
- A BMI of less than 18 requires immediate treatment for malnutrition

Growth Charts

- Healthy children's weight should plot out between the 3rd and 97th percentile.
- A child below the 3rd percentile for age is probably malnourished.
- A child's weight should be measured at frequent intervals in time to determine if they are simply small for their population or are in fact falling off their growth curve and not maintaining the rate of growth expected.
- Any child who's growth curve is flat, or not following expected parameters, should be considered to be failing to thrive, and/or malnourished.

Mean Upper Arm Circumference (MUAC)

- Useful in children from 1 to 5 years of age
- Circumference measurement is made around the mid- to upper forearm on child.
- Values: less than 12.5 cm implies severe malnutrition; 12.5–13.5 cm implies moderate malnutrition

REFERENCES

Eddleston M, Pierini S. 1999. *Oxford handbook of tropical medicine*. New York: Oxford UP.

Behrman RE, Kliegman RM, Jenson HB, eds. 2000. *Nelson's textbook of pediatrics*, 16th ed. Philadelphia: Saunders.

73 TREATMENT OF MALNUTRITION IN CHILDREN

Scott Cohen, MD*

OVERVIEW

A child who presents with severe malnutrition is a medical emergency and should be treated as such. There are several concurrent issues that must be addressed upon presentation. Issues such as dehydration, electrolyte imbalance, infection, septic shock, hypoglycemia, and hypothermia all require immediate attention. This functions best with a well-established team approach to care.

Children with severe malnutrition should be admitted to a hospital for care and observation. Frequent vital signs should be monitored, as should daily weights, and strict measurements of intake and urinary output. These children should be kept clean, warm, and dry. IV hydration should be reserved only for cases of severe dehydration or shock. In addition, IM injections should be limited, and given only in the buttocks with small gauge needles and 0.5–1 cc max volume.

Sometimes children placed on appropriate treatment regimens will fail to respond and not grow adequately. In these circumstances, consider underlying infections such as TB, HIV, UTI, pneumonia, malaria, or intestinal infections.

PHASE 1: IMMEDIATE TREATMENT

Hypoglycemia

Severely hypoglycemic children will be confused, lethargic or obtunded.

1. Give 1 cc/kg 50% dextrose IV
2. Then, 50 cc of 10% glucose via NG tube
3. Begin feeding special diet (outlined below) when regains consciousness

*Global Pediatric Alliance, Oakland, California

Hypothermia

- Defined as rectal temperature less than 35.5°C or less than 96°F
- Wrap child in blanket and place under heat lamp
- Alternatively, mother may place child on her chest, and wrap both persons in her clothes and an outer blanket
- All hypothermic children should be assumed to have hypoglycemia and infection; they should be given prophylactic antibiotics and dextrose

Severe Dehydration and Septic Shock

Children with severe dehydration should be given IV fluids, 20–30 cc/kg boluses over 30–60 minutes. These boluses should be repeated until child begins to urinate and other clinical signs of dehydration improve. If the child is significantly dehydrated and lethargic or obtunded, septic shock should be the assumed diagnosis and IV antibiotics are indicated. If available, consider pressors (such as dopamine or epinephrine) if the child's blood pressure is abnormally low after two fluid bolus. These medications should only be given by somebody who is competent to administer them.

Moderate Dehydration

If the child is determined not to be severely dehydrated, then oral or NG fluids are the treatment of choice, and not Ivs. In the initial rehydration period, half-strength ORS should be used, that is, add 2 liters of purified water to the rehydration salt packet. Alternatively, one can prepare in 1 liter of water, a 3-finger pinch of salt, and 1 adult-sized palm full of sugar.

- Give 70–100 cc/kg over the first 12 hours.
- Begin slow feeds (see below) when tolerating oral fluids.
- Breast-feeding or formula feeding may be resumed when child's dehydration is corrected

Bacterial Infection

All children with severe malnutrition are at significant risk for bacterial infection and all of these children should be given antibiotics. Oftentimes, the malnourished child is unable to mount a fever response in the presence of infection.

Antibiotics can be administered as follows:

1. Bactrim (Cotrimoxazole) for malnourished children without overt signs of infection
2. Parenteral antibiotics for children in septic shock; these include IM or IV Penicillin and Gentamicin, or Cefotaxime
3. PO Chloramphenicol is an acceptable alternative if parenteral antibiotics are not available, or the child does not respond

Measles Infection

All malnourished children admitted to the hospital should be given a measles vaccine (MMR). There is a significant risk of measles death in this population of patients.

Vitamin and Nutrient Deficiencies

All children with malnutrition should be given Vitamin A, 200,000 IU PO upon admission. There is a high risk of blindness in this population from this deficiency. Also, folic acid, 5 mg PO along with a daily multivitamin should be given. Vitamin A deficiency with concurrent measles infection can cause blindness within 24–28 hours.

Falciparum Malaria

In geographic areas where *Plasmodium falciparum* exists, malnourished children should be given empiric therapy for this disease upon presentation.

Cardiac Care

During the initial fluid resuscitation phase, careful attention should be given to cardiac function. Severely malnourished children may not have cardiac output capabilities that normal children have, and can easily be put into congestive heart failure. During fluid resuscitation, if the child develops increased respiratory rate, distended neck veins, cold hands or feet, or enlarged liver, fluid administration should be stopped immediately. A dose of furosemide (1 mg/kg) IV should be given, and the child should be closely observed.

PHASE 2: DIETARY TREATMENT

After the malnourished child is admitted to the hospital, and all of the above issues are addressed and treated, a slow feeding program can be instituted. There are sensitive metabolic imbalances that can occur if the child receives more than 100 kcal/kg/day, and this amount should be avoided initially. However, malnourished children will require at least 70 kcal/kg/day to reverse the malnutrition.

Many different formula preparations for treating malnutrition are available in different parts of the world. Basic considerations are as follows:

- Initial phase, give 70–80 kcal/kg/day
- Build up to 100 kcal/kg/day, by days 4 to 7
- Small and frequent feeds with dilute formula
- Feed every 1 to 3 hours by PO or nasogastric (NG) tube
- Gradually increase volume and strength of formula, and decrease frequency over 5 days.
- By the time of discharge, the child should be eating 200 kcal/kg/day

The goal is to progress to a high-calorie/high-protein diet, but slowly. When introduced too rapidly, the liver engorges, abdominal distention is present, and the child can neither absorb nor utilize the new nutrients.

By the days 4–7, the child should be drinking all feeds on their own without an NG tube. At this point, the child will demonstrate hunger, and the caloric intake can be increased to 100–150 kcal/kg/day. When he is taking adequate amounts without problems or encouragement, the diet may be liberalized. At this point, the child should be given emotional and physical stimulation, and the mother should be prepared and educated to care for the child on her own.

For older children, when they are actively hungry and tolerating ~150 kcal/kg/day, the following foods may be introduced:

- Foods rich in potassium
- Protein-rich diet, such as eggs, beans, lentils, nuts, soy, fish, chicken, and beef
- Breast-feed if possible

It is normal for children to initially lose body weight during treatment. This is due to loss of edema and mobilization of third-spaced fluids.

Discharge Criteria

- Child eating well on his own
- Normal mental status/smiles/playful
- Developmentally normal motor skills (sits, crawls, walks)
- Normal temperature
- No vomiting or diarrhea
- No edema
- Child gains at least 5 g/kg body wt/day for 3 successive days
- Nighttime feed no longer necessary to maintain ~200 kcal/kg/day
- No medical problems requiring hospital care
- Immunizations up to date (especially MMR)
- Mother can demonstrate appropriate food preparation for the child
- Mother is emotionally bonded to the child and offers appropriate contact and stimulation
- Mother know how to prepare home ORS with purified water for diarrhea
- Follow-up for the mother–child pair is arranged

REFERENCES

Behrman RE, Kliegman RM, Jenson HB, eds. 2000. *Nelson's textbook of pediatrics*, 16th ed. Philadelphia: Saunders.

WHO. 1999. *Child health dialogue. children's health in emergencies: a practical approach*. Geneva: World Health Organization.

Eddleston M, Pierini S. 1999. *Oxford handbook of tropical medicine*. New York: Oxford UP.

74

EVALUATION AND MANAGEMENT OF PEDIATRIC DISASTER VICTIMS

Debra Weiner, MD, PhD, Lise Nigrovic, MD,
Shannon Manzi, PHARMD, and Michael W. Shannon, MD*

The general approach to the evaluation and management of pediatric patients is similar to that of adults; however, because of differences in their anatomy and physiology and differences in their pattern of illness and injury, pediatric-specific approaches are critical to the successful care of these patients. Evaluation of pediatric patients must be appropriate/modified for developmental age, especially for preverbal patients. Given greater capacity of children to compensate for organ dysfunction, initial appearance may not be indicative of severity of injury even with the greater likelihood that they have sustained multiple trauma. Frequent reevaluation and anticipation are essential because pediatric patients can deteriorate precipitously. Equipment, supplies, and dosing of fluids and pharmaceutical agents for pediatric patients is based on patient weight. A Broselow Pediatric Resuscitation Measuring Tape may be used to estimate weight based on length. The average American child weighs 3.5 kg at birth, birth weight triples by the end of the first year, and at age 5 years the average weight is 20 kg.

VITAL SIGNS IN PEDIATRIC PATIENTS

Vital signs are age dependent. Pulse and respiratory rate in children are greater than in adults and blood pressure is lower. Tachycardia and tachypnea are earlier and more pronounced compensatory mechanisms in pediatric patients, while hypotension in pediatric patients occurs relatively late.

PEDIATRIC TRAUMA SCORE

Pediatric trauma patients can be evaluated using the Pediatric Trauma Score (PTS), a modified Injury Severity Score, developed for the assessment of pediatric

*Harvard School of Medicine, Children's Hospital Boston

trauma patients. The PTS evaluates patients based on weight, airway function, blood pressure, neurologic status, open wounds, and skeletal wounds.

AIRWAY

Several anatomic features of the pediatric airway can make it challenging to establish and maintain a patent airway.

- Infants less than 4 months of age are obligate nasal breathers. Nasal obstruction due to trauma or illness may cause significant respiratory distress.
- The larger occiput of children places the head of the supine child in flexion, which results in buckling of the airway. Restoring the anatomic sniffing position of the pediatric airway is easily accomplished by placing a roll under the shoulder blades of the pediatric patient. In the patient with concern of C-spine injury, padding should be placed under the entire spine to maintain a neutral position of the spine. The C-spine should not be cleared clinically in children, usually less than age 5, in whom a reliable exam cannot be obtained. Anatomic position can also be established by the jaw thrust or chin lift maneuvers. The tongue and tonsils, particularly in children less than 2 years of age, are disproportionately large and may obstruct the airway in the obtunded patient. In the unconscious patient an oral airway may be inserted, but, unlike in the adult, the device should be inserted with the curve of the airway closest to the palate rather than inverting it to minimize the risk of inflicting oropharyngeal soft tissue injury.
- The larynx is more superior and anterior and the vocal cords are angled more anterocaudally. The Sellick maneuver in which pressure is applied to the cricoid, prevents the aspiration of gastric contents during aspiration and also displaces the vocal cords more posteriorly, often aiding in visualization and successful orotracheal intubation. Excessive cricoid pressure however may impede passing the endotracheal tube through the vocal cords. The anteriosuperior positioning of the larynx makes nasogastric intubation much more difficult than in adults and therefore is not recommended in children less than 9 years of age.
- The epiglottis is omega shaped, floppy, and angled. Unlike the stiff, flat, and relatively vertically positioned adult epiglottis that can be visualized by placing a curved laryngoscope blade in the vallecula, visualization of the epiglottis in children requires lifting the epiglottis which is best accomplished using a straight blade.
- The pediatric airway is narrower; therefore, it is more easily occluded by debris, foreign body, blood, secretions or edema. The airway is most narrow at the cricoid ring, therefore the endotracheal tube used should be uncuffed in children under 12 years of age to prevent airway injury including. The pediatric airway is also more prone to bronchospasm.
- The trachea is shorter, making intubation of the main-stem bronchus, particularly of the straighter right main stem, more common. In the neonate, the trachea averages 5 cm in length and by 18 months of age it is approximately 7 cm. The ETT tube should be inserted 2–3 cm beyond the vocal

cords, which usually corresponds to three times the ETT size. The ETT must be meticulously secured, and head position must be vigilantly maintained to prevent flexion that may result in main-stem bronchus intubation or extension that may result in extubation.

Oral airway, ETT, and laryngoscope blade size can be estimated based on age. In addition, oral airway size can be estimated as the length from the teeth to the angle of the jaw. ETT size can be estimated as the diameter of the child's external nares or 5th finger or can calculated as (16 + age in years)/4. Stylets are usually helpful in maintaining the rigidity of the smaller ETT used for children and in appropriately angling the tube. Laryngeal mask airways can be used in pediatric patients. Cricothyroidotomy is indicated for patients in whom endotracheal intubation is impossible or unsuccessful. For patients under 9 years of age, needle cricothyroidotomy is preferred to the surgical cricothyroidotomy performed in adults. Because of the limited capacity of jet insufflation to provide adequate ventilation, needle cricothyroidotomy is a temporizing measure until a tracheal airway can be surgically placed.

BREATHING

Increased metabolic demand for oxygen, lower functional residual capacity, and limited physiologic ability of pediatric patients to increase their respiratory effort predisposes pediatric patients to hypoxia and respiratory arrest. Tachypnea is compensatory; bradypnea is ominous. Respiratory arrest is the etiology of cardiac arrest in 95% of pediatric patients who sustain cardiopulmonary arrest. Establishing and maintaining adequate ventilation and tissue oxygenation is therefore critically important.

For patients receiving bag-valve mask ventilation, the mask should fit over the bridge of the nose and in the cleft of the chin to obtain a good seal. In the intubated patient, ETT placement is confirmed initially by auscultation. Breath sounds are easily transmitted throughout the small pediatric chest; therefore, auscultation at both axilla as well as over the stomach is performed to determine ETT placement. Because of high metabolic demand and lower functional residual capacity, 100% oxygen should be initiated in all critically injured and ill pediatric patients. Respiratory rate decreases with age from 40–60 in the neonate and infant to 20 in the child. Tidal volume is 7–10 ml/kg for infants and children compared to 15 ml/kg for adults. Appropriate rate at which breaths should be delivered and size of anesthesia bag are age dependent. Because of the relatively horizontal position of the ribs and immaturity of the intercostals muscles, pediatric patients are more dependent on diaphragmatic muscle activity for pulmonary function. An appropriately sized NG or OG tube should be placed in all patients receiving bag-valve-mask ventilation to avoid abdominal distension, which limits diaphragmatic excursion. Indications and technique for chest tube placement is similar in children and adults. Chest tube size is dependent on the size of the child. Inadequate ventilation may cause hypoxia and/or hypercarbia, which may make the patient unresponsive to resuscitation.

CIRCULATION

Cardiac output (CO = SV x HR) in infants and young children is modulated primarily by heart rate rather than stroke volume because the ventricles of children are relatively noncompliant. A compensatory increase in heart rate is one of the earliest indicators of circulatory compromise in pediatric patients. Bradycardia is a late indicator, usually secondary to hypoxia, acidosis, hypothermia, hypokalemia, and/or increased intracranial pressure, and heralds impending cardiopulmonary arrest. Other indicators of circulatory compromise include poor perfusion, manifest as skin mottling in very young children, cool extremities, capillary refill greater than 2 seconds, decreased responsiveness, and hypotension. Hypotension in pediatric patients is a late and extremely ominous finding. Pediatric patients usually do not exhibit signs of even minimal shock until they have lost 30% of their circulating blood volume loss, and do not become hypotensive until they have lost at least 45%. Minimum normal systolic blood pressure in pediatric patients is 70 + twice the age in years. A palpable peripheral pulse, carotid for children over 1 year of age, and brachial for children under 1 year of age, correlates with a systolic blood pressure of 80. If the pulse is only palpable centrally, systolic blood pressure is 50–60 mm Hg. Diastolic blood pressure is normally 2/rds of systolic blood pressure. A pulse pressure that exceeds 20 mm Hg over the expected difference is also a sign of hypovolemia. In a child with hypotensive shock associated with trauma, blood loss due to abdominal trauma is the presumed etiology until proven otherwise.

Chest Compressions

Chest compressions, using cardiopulmonary resuscitation techniques appropriate for pediatric patients, should be initiated in infants and children if the pulse is less than 60. Open thoracotomy is rarely indicated in pediatric patients.

Vascular Access, Fluid Resuscitation

Early volume resuscitation is essential to prevent or reverse circulatory compromise, and for the hypotensive patient very aggressive volume and pressure management is essential. As in adults, two IVs should be placed in critically injured and ill pediatric patients, preferentially in large peripheral veins using the largest-gauge IV possible, recognizing that may be a 20 or 22 gauge catheter. Site for vascular access in order of preference include: antecubital, saphenous, hand, and foot, and in neonates and infants up to 2 years of age, scalp vein, and in neonates up to 1 week, the umbilical vein. An intraosseus (IO) line in children up to 6 years of age should be placed after 90 seconds of unsuccessful attempts at peripheral vein access. The preferred site of placement is the tibia approximately 1–3 cm inferiomedially to the tibial tuberosity. The anteriormedial femur approximately 1–3 cm proximal to the superior aspect of the patella is an option if the lower legs are injured. Although an IO is not ideal in children greater than 6 years of age because the bony cortex is more difficult to penetrate and the marrow is more fatty and less vascular, if necessary an IO can be placed in the superior iliac crest. Initial fluid resuscitation using IO may restore intravascular volume sufficiently to allow peripheral vein cannulation. All drugs that can be administered intravenously can be given IO without delay in effect. For central lines the femoral vein is preferred. A venous cutdown of the saphenous vein may also be attempted. The landmarks are 1 cm anteriomedial to medial malleolus.

Normal saline or lactated Ringer's should be given as the initial resuscitation fluid; 10 cc/kg for neonates and 20 cc/kg for infants and children. If there has been blood loss and there is no response to 2 or 3 crystalloid boluses, 10 cc/kg blood type

O, Rh negative PRBCs or whole blood should be administered. If there has not been blood loss and/or there is inadequate response to repeated transfusion, pressors should be considered. Maintenance fluids—D5 0.25NS <10 g, D5 0.5NS >10 kg, with hourly rates of 10 ml/kg for the first 10 kg of body weight, 5 ml/kg for the next 10 kg, and 2 ml/kg for each additional kg above 20 kg given over 24 hours. Alternatively, hourly replacement can be calculated an 4, 2, and 1 ml/kg/hr, respectively, for the first 10 kg, next 10 kg, and each kg above 20 kg. Ongoing losses must also be replaced on an ml-for-ml basis. Hypovolemia must be corrected even in patients with head injury. Vital signs, exam, and urinary output should be monitored for response to therapy. Normal urine output is 1–2 ml/kg/hr in the newborn and infant, 1 ml/kg/hr in the toddler and school-age child, and 0.5 ml/kg/hr in children who have completed growth. kg, A Foley catheter without a balloon should be placed in children less than 15.

HEAD INJURY

Signs and symptoms of significant head injury are similar in children and adults and include loss of consciousness, decreased alertness, lethargy, sleepiness, irritability, memory loss with the exception of amnesia for the event, recurrent seizure activity, persistent vomiting, focal neurologic exam, and CSF leak. Seizure activity immediately following head trauma is more common in children than adults, and if self-limited is not necessarily a sign of severe head trauma. Scalp swelling, particularly nonfrontal, and/or palpable bony deformity, are concerning for skull fracture, especially in children under 2 years of age. In the first few months of life, skull fracture without clinical findings is not uncommon even after falls of only a few feet. Children with skull fractures are more likely to have intracranial injury. The expandable intracranial space in neonates and infants may become hypovolemic from intracranial bleeds and usually manifest signs and symptoms of increased intracranial pressure relatively late, at which point rapid deterioration may occur.

The Glasgow Coma Scale, with the verbal component modified for age, and the Pediatric Trauma Score are indicators of severity of neurologic injury or illness. Bulging of the fontanelle or widening of the sutures in neonates and infants can suggest severe intracranial injury. The pediatric brain is very sensitive to hypovolemia and acidosis, and these must be prevented/corrected to minimize secondary injury. C-spine injury is more common in patients with severe head trauma, particularly beyond infancy, and should not be ruled out clinically.

EXPOSURE

Hypothermia

Given the greater risk of pediatric patients for hypothermia and the detrimental effects of hypothermia, which include impaired circulation, arrhythmia, abnormal coagulation, increased metabolic demand, decreased CNS function, and poor response to resuscitation, every effort should be made to prevent/rapidly correct hypothermia. Options include radiant warmers, warmed IVF, gastric lavage with warmed fluids, and warmed blankets.

Burns

For burn victims, calculation of burn surface area must take into account the different body proportions of children. Pediatric patients with 20% BSA burns are at risk of shock compared to adults who usually tolerate up to 30% BSA involvement.

Newborn Delivery and Resuscitation

Teams must be prepared for and trained in the delivery and resuscitation of newborn infants. At least a two-person team is recommended to care for newborn resuscitation. This is in addition to the team required for maternal care and newborn delivery. Pre- and perinatal conditions that may complicate delivery include: maternal hypertension, maternal infection, gestational diabetes, chronic maternal illness, medications, tobacco, alcohol, drug use, premature or prolonged rupture of membranes, prematurity, breech presentation, nuchal cord, shoulder dystocia, multiple gestation, meconium, and postpartum hemorrhage. Additional complications that may complicate resuscitation include: respiratory depression, apnea, pneumothorax, asystole, bradycardia, hypothermia, hypovolemia, acidosis, anemia, infection, sepsis, fetal anomalies, and CNS depression. Neonatal resuscitation protocols developed by the American Heart Association should be followed. Providing warmth, suction, vitamin K to prevent hemorrhage of the newborn, and treatment to prevent GC and/or chlamydial ocular infection are minimum requirements. Airway, breathing, and circulatory support may be required.

PSYCHOSOCIAL

The immediate effects of a disaster are disruption of routine and possible loss of the social care support system. Reuniting children with relatives and not leaving them alone, providing basic needs, and attempting to address their fears is usually helpful. Recognize that they are at risk for long-term psychosocial sequelae. Inform families of possible signs of posttraumatic stress that may indicate that the child may benefit from counseling, such as decreased activity, social withdrawal, behavioral regression, decreased appetite, change in sleep pattern, fear of being alone, and wishing they were dead.

75 PEDIATRIC-SPECIFIC DISASTER-RELATED CONSIDERATIONS

Debra Weiner, MD, PhD, Lise Nigrovic, MD, Shannon Manzi, PHARMD, and Michael W Shannon, MD*

Because of their unique anatomy and physiology, children have increased vulnerability to the hazards of disasters and emergencies and have different patterns of injury and illness, psychosocial response.

VULNERABILITIES OF CHILDREN TO DISASTERS

The type, time, and site of a disaster will determine the number of children likely to be involved, the nature and severity of their injuries, and the secondary disaster-related events. Children may be disproportionately affected depending on whether the disaster site is one where youngsters are present. Worksites are likely to have no or relatively few children, while sites such as schools have relatively fewer adults. Manmade disasters often intentionally target particular segments of a population. Children may also be disproportionately affected based on their location a disaster site. A day care center within an office building may be relatively spared or more severely damaged, and may be more or less accessible for rescue efforts based on its location. The more broadly based the disaster, the more likely that the proportion of children affected will reflect the demographics of the population base.

Pediatric vulnerabilities based on mechanisms of injury and illness that may be encountered during a disaster include:

Blunt Trauma From Falls and Flying or Falling Debris

Young children are less likely to attempt to avoid flying debris and/or to position themselves to minimize the impact of debris. If trapped by debris, they may be less capable of extracting themselves and may be more easily overlooked in search and rescue efforts because they can be trapped in very small spaces. They are, however, able to crawl through smaller spaces to free themselves. In children with blunt trauma, multisystem organ injuries are the rule rather than the exception because their organs are proportionately larger and are in much closer proximity to each other.

*Harvard Medical School, Children's Hospital Boston, Boston

Blast Injury

Children are more likely to be propelled by the force of an explosion because they have less body mass. It is also more likely that projectile objects from a blast will penetrate their vital structures.

Fire

Children, particularly young children, are less likely able to avoid the hazards of smoke and fire because they require someone older to get them to safely. If children or their clothing are on fire, they are more likely to do nothing or run than to drop and roll. They are at greater risk of deeper burns because of thinner skin and at greater risk of circumferential burns because of their smaller size. Young children are also at increased risk of secondary infection because of their less competent immune system.

Flood

Children, particularly young children, are less likely to know how to swim or float and are at risk of drowning even in standing water. Even children who can swim are more likely than adults to drown in fast-moving waters because they have less mass, strength, and stamina.

Heat and Cold Exposure

Children are more vulnerable to heat illness because their larger body surface-to-mass ratio results in greater conduction of heat from the environment and greater fluid loss. Also, it may be difficult to get children to drink enough to maintain their hydration. Children are also more vulnerable to hypothermia due to greater radiation, convection, conduction, and evaporation heat loss because of a larger body surface-to-mass ratio, less subcutaneous tissue, and proportionately larger head size.

Electrical Injury

Children are less likely to recognize downed power lines as hazards and are therefore more likely to sustain electrical burns.

WEAPONS OF MASS DESTRUCTION

Biological Agents

The less fully developed immunologic system of children less than 2 years of age, particularly those less than 3 months of age, increases their risk of infection with biologic agents. If and when vaccination programs are initiated against biologic WMDs, young children may not be vaccine candidates.

Chemical Exposures

- *Inhalation*: Children are at risk of greater exposure to inhaled agents per unit mass than adults, because the concentration of many of the chemicals most likely to be used as WMDs (fast-acting nerve agents) are denser than oxygen, thus higher at the level where children breath, and because the normal respiratory rate of children is higher than that of adults.

- *Skin contamination*: Their thinner cutaneous layers and greater body surface-area-to mass ratio place children at greater risk of skin absorption of toxic chemicals.
- *GI*: Children may be more or less at risk depending on whether the agent is in something that the child is more or less likely to consume.

Radiation

Children are more sensitive in the short term to radiation sickness and in the long term to radiation-induced malignancy.

Social Issues

Less adult supervision of children during and after a disaster, and a more hazardous environment increases their risk of post-disaster injury, illness, and poisoning. Also, particularly in foreign countries where families have been given food and diapers that they are not used to, refusal to eat and diaper rash often become common problems. Because children, particularly young children, require an adult, or at the very least older child, to get them to a provider, children may not receive care if caregivers are themselves killed or incapacitated by the disaster. Parents who are able to seek care will often do so for their children before seeking care for themselves, and pediatric health care providers should make an effort to recognize when parents may also require care.

Newborn Delivery

In addition to births that would normally occur during this time, disasters may result in premature delivery because of preterm labor caused by the physical and emotional stresses associated with disasters and/or because of the need to deliver a child prematurely due to maternal injury.

UNIQUE ASPECTS OF PEDIATRIC INJURY AND ILLNESS

Differences in the anatomy and physiology of children predispose them to different patterns of and response to injury and illness. While differences in activities in which children and adults participate and the types of accidents they are involved in also contribute, during disasters the mechanisms of injury to which children and adults are exposed may be more similar.

Head Trauma

The disproportionately larger head size of a child's head increases the risk of head trauma due to airborne objects and falls. Compared to adults, brain injury in children is more likely to be diffuse than focal. Children, particularly young children, are more susceptible to acceleration–deceleration injury because the combination of large head size, less-developed neck musculature, higher water content and less myelinization of the brain increase the mobility of the brain within the calvarium, making it more susceptible to shearing of neuronal and vascular structures. Young children are more tolerant of intracranial hemorrhage, because the open fontanelles and mobile sutures in young children allow for expansion of the intracranial space. They are also able to tolerate direct impact because their open fontanelles, mobile sutures, and a more pliable skull help dissipate the force. The pediatric brain is much more susceptible to secondary injury and cerebral edema from hypovolemia, hypoxia, hyperthermia, and seizures because cerebral blood flow in children is greater than that in the adult, increasing between birth and 5 years of age to twice that of an adult, after which it decreases. Head trauma is the leading cause of trauma death in pediatric patients. In general, children with head trauma have a better outcome than adults, although children less than age 3 have a worse outcome than older children. The pediatric brain doubles in size in the first 6 months of life and is approximately 75% of adult brain size by age 2 years, 85% by 8 years, and 95% by adolescence. Because neuronal development is not complete, there is more plasticity in recovery, so that children even with severe injury may recover with little or no sequelae. In the child with multiple injuries, it is usually the severity of head injury that is the major determinant of outcome.

Cervical Spine Injury

Cervical spinal injuries are less common in children than in adults, and the specific types of C-spine injuries differ particularly in those less than 8 years of age because of anatomic differences. C-spine fractures are rare in pediatric patients. If they do occur, they are usually higher in the spine—C1, C2—than in the adult, because in children the fulcrum of movement is at C2–3 compared to C5–7 in older children and adults. Children are at greater risk for subluxation because their disproportionately large head size increases the force to the neck, and with flexion and extension vertebral bodies are more anteriorly wedged, the facet joints are flatter, the joint capsules and intraspinous ligaments are more flexible, and the paraspinal muscles are less well developed. Anterior pseudosubluxation up to 4 mm, usually of C2 or C3 and less commonly of C3 on C4, is a normal variant that is seen in 40% of children aged less than 7 years and 20% less than age 14 years. Children are also nearly uniquely at risk for spinal cord injury without radiologic abnormality (SCIWORA) because the incompletely calcified flexible spinal cord allows stretching and even transaction of the spinal cord and nerve roots without vertebral fracture. In most cases, neurologic deficits are transient. It is estimated that up to 40% of children with C-spine cord injury have SCIWORA. While C-spine injury must always be considered in children with head trauma, the combination of C-spine injury and head injury is less common than in adults.

Chest Trauma

The chest wall of pediatric patients is more compliant and mobile than that of adults. Much greater force is thus required to fracture children's ribs; therefore, patients without rib fractures or even signs of external trauma may have significant intrathoracic cardiopulmonary injury. Flail chest is less likely in pediatric patients than in adults, but is more likely to cause respiratory compromise because they are usually associated with severe pulmonary injury. The most common intrathoracic injuries in pediatric patients are pulmonary contusion, pneumothorax, and hemothorax. Tension pneumothorax when it occurs is more likely to result in cardiopulmonary compromise in pediatric patients because of the greater mobility of their mediastinal structures. Uncommon intrathoracic injuries in children include tracheobronchial tears, cardiac contusion, disruption of cardiac structures, great vessel injury including aortic transaction, and diaphragmatic rupture. More than two-thirds of patients who have thoracic injury have injury to other organ systems. Following head trauma, thoracic trauma is the most common cause of trauma related death in children.

Abdominal Trauma

Children are at increased risk of abdominal trauma. Intraabdominal injury in pediatric disaster patients is usually due to blunt trauma. An object striking the abdomen of a child imparts more force per unit body area because of their smaller, more pliable rib cage, less well-developed abdominal wall musculature, and relative paucity of abdominal cavity adipose tissue. The close proximity of intraabdominal organs predisposes children to increased likelihood of damage to more than one. The spleen is the most commonly injured intraabdominal structure, followed by the liver and then the kidney. Bladder injury is uncommon, but is still more common than in adults because the pediatric bladder is an intraabdominal organ relatively unprotected by the pelvis. Stomach, biliary tract, and pancreatic injuries are less common than in the adult. The most common hollow viscous injury in children is duodenal hematoma. Approximately 10% of pediatric trauma fatalities are due to intraabdominal injury. In 70% of pediatric deaths, patients have both severe head injury and intraabdominal trauma.

Orthopedic Injury

Anatomic differences in the pediatric bone—including decreased bone density due to incomplete calcification, increased deformability, open physes (growth plates), and a very active periosteum—make bony injury more likely than ligament or tendon injury in children, and result in fractures and healing patterns that are unique to children.

Physeal (Growth Plate, Salter Harris) Fractures

The growth plate or physis, a cartilaginous zone of provisional calcification, is more susceptible to injury than bone, ligament, or tendon. Physeal fractures account for 18–30% of fractures in pediatric patients and are more common in adolescents than younger children, with a peak age of occurrence of 11–12 years. Physeal fractures occur most frequently in the distal radius and ulna, followed by the distal tibia and fibula. They are most commonly classified based on the Salter-Harris classification scheme.

- SH I: through the physis with widening, separates the epiphysis from the metaphysis. Widening of the physis and/or swelling of soft tissue at the physis may or may not be appreciable on radiograph. A clinical exam that reveals pain localized to the physis is sufficient to make the diagnosis.
- SH II: physeal fracture extending into metaphysis, i.e., above the physis. This is the most common physeal fracture.

- SH III: horizontally through the physis, and vertically through the epiphysis, i.e., below the physis.
- SH IV: extends vertically through the epiphysis, physis, and metaphysis.
- SH V: compression injury of the physis. Narrowing of the physis may or may not be appreciable on x-ray, and the diagnosis may be clinical based on history and examination.

Torus (Buckle) Fracture

Compression injury that causes outward buckling of metaphyseal cortex adjacent to physis.

Toddler's Fracture

Hairline spiral fracture of the tibial metaphysis and diaphysis due to a torque of the lower leg.

Plastic Deformity (Bowing)

Bowing of the bone without cortical disruption.

Greenstick Fracture

Incomplete fracture at the metaphyseal, diaphyseal with disruption of cortex only on the side opposite the impact.

Avulsion Fracture

Avulsion of the apophysis, most commonly of the pelvis, hip, tibial tuberosity and phalanges

The most commonly fractured bones in pediatric patients are the clavicle, distal humerus (supracondylar), distal and midshaft radius, and the ulna. Pelvic fractures are unusual in children and may be associated with intraabdominal and/or genitourinary trauma. Subluxation of the radial head (nursemaid's elbow), in which the annular ligament partially detaches from the radial head, is also a common injury unique to children, usually less than 5 years of age. Shoulder dislocations are rare in children prior to physeal closure. Children have greater blood loss associated with long bone fractures, particularly femur fractures, with which they may lose up to two units of blood. Pediatric bones heal more quickly than adult bones, with greater capacity for remodeling and lower likelihood of nonunion but with risk of growth arrest, particularly following physeal fractures. Complications are highest in elbow fractures, particularly supracondylar fractures, which can result in long-term neurovascular and functional deficits.

76

PEDIATRIC SPECIALTY TEAM RESPONSE TO DISASTER

Debra Weiner, MD, PhD, Lise Nigrovic, MD, Shannon Manzi, PharmD, and Michael Shannon, MD*

Disaster Medical Assistance Teams (DMATs), which were developed as part of the United States Federal Response Plan, and are now part of the National Response Plan, provide medical resources in response to the consequences of disasters. In recognition of the unique vulnerabilities of children to the hazards of disasters, and their medical and psychosocial needs as a consequence of disasters, Pediatric Specialty Teams (PSTs), which are specialty DMATs, were created in 1995. PSTs, along with other specialty teams, including International Medical Surgical Response Teams (IMSuRTs) and Burn Specialty Teams (BSTs), are elements within the National Disaster Medical System (NDMS) administered by FEMA within the Department of Homeland Security (DHS). Meeting the needs of pediatric victims requires individuals trained in the care of these patients and pediatric-specific equipment, supplies, and pharmaceuticals. Presently, there are two operational PSTs: PST-1 in Boston and PST-2 in Atlanta. A third PST in Loma Linda, California, is under development.

PST MEMBER COMPOSITION

PST members, like DMAT and IMSuRT members, are volunteer medical professionals and paraprofessionals. Each PST is affiliated with and sponsored by a hospital with specialized pediatric expertise, and may in addition have other public- or private-sector sponsors. For efficient use of resources, PSTs are Type II teams that require external communications/logistics support personnel, equipment, supplies, and pharmaceuticals provided by fully operational Type I DMATs and IMSuRTs or other FEMA assets with which they deploy. The objectives of PSTs are the same as for DMATs, i.e., triage, medical stabilization, and patient evacuation, but with a focus on pediatric patients. PSTs ideally consist of physicians, nurses, respiratory therapists, and pharmacists trained in the care of critically ill and injured children. The most critical subspecialties to be represented are pediatric emergency medicine, critical care, general surgery, and general pediatrics. Anesthesia, orthopedic surgery, cardiac surgery, plastic surgery, and neonatology should also be considered. Individuals interest-

*Harvard Medical School, Children's Hospital Boston, Boston

ed in becoming team members must complete an NDMS application form, which can be found on the NDMS website given below.

TRAINING

The goal of training is to teach members about the role of the NDMS system and teams in disaster and emergency response, and to prepare members for deployment and field service. In addition to training appropriate for an individual's position—including BLS, PALS or APLS, and ATLS—yearly training specific to disaster medicine and deployment is required. Training consists of computer, classroom, and field exercises that focus on team structure, function, and objectives, and deployment-related issues, including personnel safety during travel and in the field, secure communication, constructing shelters and healthcare facilities, use and maintenance of equipment and supplies, disaster and mass casualty field medicine, patient aeromedical evacuation, and emergency team evacuation. Ideally, training of PST members is with DMAT/IMSuRT members to allow for cross-training and for individuals to work together as a team.

DEPLOYMENT

Deployment may be local, state, national, or international. When activated by the federal government, team members become temporary federal employees as FEMA assets under the Department of Homeland Security. Teams rotate alert status. While PSTs may be more likely to deploy with local DMATs, given the small number of PSTs and frequency with which they will be on alert, they may deploy with different DMATs/specialty teams.

EQUIPMENT, SUPPLIES, AND PHARMACEUTICALS

PSTs work with DMATs to assure that the team has appropriate pediatric-specific equipment, supplies, and pharmaceuticals, as well as adequate equipment, supplies, and pharmaceuticals that are not age-specific for use by the PST. Items should be packed separately from supplies and equipment used exclusively for adults but stored with the DMAT cache. The NDMS plan is that all DMATs/IMSuRTs have identical caches.

PEDIATRIC EQUIPMENT AND SUPPLIES

While the spectrum of injury and illness will vary with the type of disaster and the time to response in general, commonly used equipment and supplies include cardiopulmonary monitors, pulse oximeters, nebulizers, supplies for venipuncture, intravenous catheterization, and bladder catheterization, nasogastric tubes, chest tubes, laceration repair kits, and orthopedic supplies for casting and splinting. Equipment and supplies that are rarely used include intubation supplies, intraosseous needles and central lines for vascular access, kits for lumbar puncture. Pediatric-specific needs also include formula, baby bottles, baby food and diapers. (See Table 1.)

Table 1. Pediatric Equipment and Supplies

Airway/breathing
- Oxygen nasal cannula pediatric and adult
- Masks, aerosol (nebulizer) pediatric and adult
- Masks, oxygen, pediatric and adult
- Oxygen tubing, nebulizer, inline/handheld
- Peak flow meters
- Airways, oral, adult, child, infant
- Airways, nasopharyngeal, 24 and 32 french.
- Bags, anesthesia, 500, 1000, 1500 ml
- Emergency cricothyroidotomy kit pediatric and adult
- Forceps, Magill, pediatric and adult
- Intubation indicator kit pediatric and adult
- Intubation pouch
- Laryngoscope handle
- Laryngoscope Mac blades sizes 1, 2, 3, 4
- Laryngoscope Miller blades, sizes 0, 1, 2, 3, 4
- Masks, bag-valve, neonate, infant, child, adult
- Masks, face, anesthesia, neonate, infant, toddler, child, adult
- Stylets, intubation pediatric and adult
- Tubes, endotracheal, size: uncuffed 2.5, 3, 3.5, 4, 4.5, 5, 5.5; cuffed 6, 6.5, 7
- Tubes, oxygen supply
- Tubes, nasogastric, 6, 10, 12, 14, 16 fr
- Suction catheters, size 6, 8, 10, 12, 14 fr
- Suction units, portable (including canister, tubing and Yankauer tip)
- Airlife T-adaptors
- Ventilators
- Combined end-tidal CO_2 machine, adaptors, pediatric and adult
- Monitor O_2 sat.: portable, probes, pediatric and adult

Circulation: vascular access
- IV pressure infusors
- IV catheters 16, 18, 22, 24 g
- Heparin locks
- IV administration sets macro and micro
- IV starter sets
- Needles butterfly 23 g
- Needles, 21 g x 1.5 inch
- Needles 23 g x 1 inch
- Needles 25 g x 5/8 inch
- Needles, intraosseous (IO)
- Syringes Luer-Lok 1, 3, 5, 10 ml
- Sharps container
- Stop cocks, 3-way
- Tourniquets, disposable
- Arm boards, long and short
- Defibrillator, Life-Pak with pediatric paddles and all supplies

Bladder catheterization
- Catheters, foley, tray 16 fr
- Catheters, foley, 8,10,12,14 fr
- Catheters, kit, straight, 5,8 fr

Thoracentesis
- Tubes, drainage, thoracic, sizes 10,12,14,20,24 fr.
- Tubes, drainage, Heimlich
- Pleurovac chest tube drainage systems

Examination/monitoring equipment
- Sphygmomanometer, infant, child, adult
- Dynamapp, non-invasive BP monitor, infant, child, adult cuffs
- Stethoscopes
- Thermometers, electronic ear, with probes
- Monitor, blood glucose, with supplies
- Speculum, ear, pediatric and adult
- Ophthalmoscope, Welch Allyn
- Syringes, ear aspirator
- Tongue blades, sterile

Bandages/tapes
- Bandages, Kerlix, sterile, 2, 3, 4 inch
- Bandages, Kling, sterile, 2, 3, 4 inch
- Bandages, Tegaderm, IV Op Site
- Pads, ABD, sterile
- Pads, Gauze, Telfa, 3 x 4 inch
- Pads, alcohol, 2 x 2 inch sterile
- Pads, eye sterile
- Sponges, sterile 4 x 4 inch
- Sponges, unsterile, 4 x 4 inch
- Tape Durapore, 1/2, 1, 2, 3 inch
- Tape, Micropore, 1/2, 1, 2, 3 inch
- Gauze, vaseline 3 x 36 inch
- Razors, disposable

Wound care
- Bands, identification, pediatric size
- Band-aids
- Bandages, triangular
- Cotton tip, sterile applicators
- Packs, cold
- Surgical packs disposable, multipurpose

Laceration repair
- Irrigation kit, w/ syringe, Luer-Lok 60 ml, splash guards
- Sutures, nonabsorbable monofilament, 3-0, 4-0, 5-0, 6-0
- Sutures, synthetic absorbable, 4-0, 5-0
- Sutures, silk, 0-0, 1-0 straight and curved needle
- Suture removal kits
- Suture, surgical staplers
- Suture, staple removers
- Suture kits (laceration tray)
- Sterile fields, disposable
- Trays, incision and drainage

Orthopedic supplies
- Cervical collars
- Splinting materials
- Web roll
- Plaster casting material
- Ace bandages, 2, 3, 4 inch

Neonatal resuscitation
- Nasal suction bulbs
- $D_{10}W$
- Erythromycin eye ointment
- Vitamin K injectable
- Umbilical clamps, umbilical tape
- Stockingette for hats
- Bassinets, can be made from boxes

Universal precautions/sterile field
- Caps, surgeon
- Gloves, exam small, medium, large
- Gloves, sterile, size 6, 6.5, 7, 7.5, 8
- Gowns, isolation, protection
- Shields, full faceguard
- Face masks
- Masks, HEPA large and small
- Masks, surgical
- Surgical packs disposable, multipurpose
- Sterile fields, disposable

Miscellaneous
- Povidone iodine
- Warming lamp
- Flashlights, penlights, headlamps
- Batteries, (appropriate sizes)
- Chux
- Emesis basins
- Pens, black ball point
- Permanent markers, black
- Trauma shears
- Diapers

Table 2. Pediatric Pharmaceuticals (*injectable, +oral)

Resuscitation
- Epinephrine 1:1000, 1:10,000*
- Atropine*
- Dextrose 10%, 25%, 50%*
- Normal saline, D5 0.25NS, D5 0.5NS*
- Oxygen
- Sodium bicarbonate*
- Blood, O negative
- Calcium gluconate*
- Lidocaine 0:5%*
- Adenosine*
- Mannitol*

Antipyretics, analgesics
- Acetaminophen+
- Ibuprofen+
- Codeine+
- Morphine*+

Antibiotics
- Amoxicillin+
- Ampicillin+
- LA-Bicillin*[IM only]
- Augmentin+
- Unasyn*
- Bactrim+
- Cephalexin+
- Cefazolin*
- Ceftriaxone*
- Erythromycin+
- Gentamicin*

Antivirals
- Acyclovir*+
- Anesthetics
- Lidocaine 1%, 2%, w/ and w/o epinephrine*[IM only]

Narcotics and reversal agents
- Codeine+
- Fentanyl*
- Morphine*+
- Flumazenil*
- Naloxone*

Paralytics
- Succinylcholine*
- Rocuronium*
- Pancuronium*

Rapid sequence intubation/procedural sedation
- Etomidate*
- Fentanyl*
- Ketamaine*
- Midazolam*

Anticonvulsants
- Carbamazepine+
- Fosphenytoin*
- Lorazepam*
- Phenobarbital*

Anti-allergy, anaphylaxis
- Diphenhydramine*+
- Asthma, croup
- Albuterol nebulizer solution, MDI
- Ipatropium nebulizer solution, MDI
- Epinephrine 1:1000*[subcutaneous only] (can also nebulize)
- Normal saline 0.9% nebulizer bullets
- Dexamethasone*+
- Methylprednisolone*
- Prednisone+
- Racemic epinephrine nebulizer solution

Dermatological
- Hydrocortisone 1% topical ointment

Poisoning antidotes
- Charcoal, activated+
- Thiopental kit*

Ocular
- Erythromycin ophthalmic ointment
- Tetracaine ophthalmic drops

Miscellaneous
- Dextromethorphan hydrobromide+
- Heparin sodium*
- Tetanus DT, Td*[IM only]
- Insulin regular, NPH*

Medications for pediatric patients must be specific for the conditions that affect them, safe for pediatric use, and available in preparations that can be dosed based on weight and that pediatric patients can and will take. Commonly used pharmaceuticals include antipyretics, oral and intravenous rehydration solutions, antibiotics, bronchodilators, corticosteroids, analgesics, local anesthetics, and minor sedatives. Rarely used pharmaceuticals include cardiac resuscitation medications, diuretics, anticonvulsants, antidotes, muscle relaxants and major sedatives. (See Table 2.)

ACKNOWLEDGEMENT

We wish to thank Susan Briggs, MD, MPH, Massachusetts General Hospital, Harvard Medical School, Founder/Team Leader, MA-1 DMAT, IMSuRT-East, for discussion and review of this chapter.

RESOURCES

NDMS: http://www.ndms.dhhs.gov/
FEMA: www.fema.gov
Homeland Security: http://www.dhs.gov/dhspublic/

REFERENCES

Briggs SM, Brinsfield KH, eds. 2003. *Advanced disaster medical response: manual for providers.* Boston: Harvard Medical International Trauma and Disaster Institute.

PART VI

MEDICAL AND HUMANITARIAN DISASTERS

77 WATER, SANITATION, AND HYGIENE

John D. Cahill, MD*

The World Health Organization estimates that each year more than 1.1 billion individuals have no access to safe drinking water, which results in the death of 3900 children per day. Also, 4 out of every 10 people in the world do not have access to even a simple pit latrine. These numbers only increase during a disaster, where whole populations or regions may be affected. Water, sanitation, and hygiene are top priorities in almost all disasters and are directly related to one another other, and therefore will be considered together in this chapter.

WATER

Water is used for drinking, personal hygiene, cleaning of other essential items, and food production. In the initial response the quantity of water is more important than the quality. The absolute minimum requirement of water is 5 liters/person/day; this should be increased as soon as possible to reach a level of 20–40 liters/person/day. The quality of water should be free from biological and chemical contaminants. It should also be acceptable in terms of taste, color, and smell. An excellent source on water quality is the *WHO Guidelines on the Quality of Drinking Water* (2004), which may be downloaded for free (the link is in the resource section of the chapter).

Water can come from many acceptable sources: surface water, ground water, and rainfall. Surface water has the advantage of being easy to access, but it may be heavily contaminated in a disaster. Ground water is often of a better quality than surface water, but relies on equipment and expertise to access. Options include: springs, shallow wells (easier to install and can run on a hand pump), and deep wells. If rainfall is going to be collected, it needs to be collected and stored in a safe manner.

Storage and protection of water from contaminants (particularly human feces and animals) is important. Stored water should be in a secure place where distribution can be controlled. Other things to consider about water include: accessibility, location, and availability of carrying containers.

*Department of Emergency Medicine and Division of Infectious Diseases, St. Luke's/Roosevelt Hospital Center, New York

Table 1. Waterborne from Fecal/Oral Ingestion

Disease	Morbidity per annum	Mortality per annum
Diarrhea	1,000 million	3.3 million
Typhoid	12.5 million	>125,000
Cholera	>300,000	>3000
Ascaris	1 billion	

Depending on the source and the quality of the water, treatment may be necessary. Treatment options/combinations include: boiling (should be for at least 1 minute), flocculation and sedimentation, filtration, and disinfection with chlorine. Commercial kits for water treatment are available for individual use.

Testing of water should be done on a regular basis looking at physical, chemical, and biological properties. Physical parameters include: color (turbidity), taste, and smell. Chemical parameters include looking for evidence of: arsenic, iron, fluoride, phosphates, and nitrates. The main indicator of biological contamination is the presence of fecal coliforms at a rate greater than 10 coliforms/100 ml.

Water can be a source of disease on many different levels. Contaminated water as shown in Table 1 contributes significantly to global morbidity and mortality. Fresh water can act as a home for the intermediate hosts that cause schistosomiasis and guinea worm infection. These infections commonly occur when an individual stands in water as they are collecting it. Lack of water or contaminated water can also contribute to trachoma, which is a major cause of blindness or skin infections. Finally, water can act as the home to insect vectors that cause malaria, dengue fever, filariasis, onchocerciasis, and African trypanosomiasis.

SANITATION AND HYGIENE

Aside from water, sanitation and hygiene are of top priority in the emergency response. It should be remembered that these measures are the first barrier to preventing the spread of fecal/oral disease. On average, the human produces 0.25 liters of stool/day and 1.5 liters of urine/day. One can easily see how quickly proper disposal and management of this can become a problem. The principles of sanitation systems include:

- They should be safe, for example, impossible for a child to fall into.
- They should be built using hygienic and easy-to-clean materials.
- They should be accessible to all members of a community, old and young.
- They should be designed to minimize the proliferation of flies, mosquitoes, and vermin that can spread disease.
- They should afford privacy for the user.
- They should be away from local water sources.
- They should avoid the need to handle fresh feces.

When considering a sanitation system one needs to be culturally sensitive to the population that is being served. It is a futile effort to set up a sanitation system if no one is going to use it. It is not a bad idea to involve the locals in setting up your system, thus avoiding some of these problems. Environmental implications should be

Table 2. Sanitation Systems

Wet	Dry
Water seal latrines	Trench
Aquaprives	Pit latrines
Oxfam sanitation unit	VIP latrine
	Bore holed
	Composting

considered as well: what impact may it have, how long is it going to be used, and is there any potential to contaminate the water supply? Sanitation systems come in one of two forms, as listed in Table 2. Which type of system is chosen will depend on a number of factors: water availability, water table, soil type, skills available in the community, materials, and finances.

HYGIENE

Even during disasters, one should also remember the old adage that our mothers told us "wash your hands"! As soon as water is available, hand washing should be encouraged and promoted, particularly after going to the bathroom, handling food,

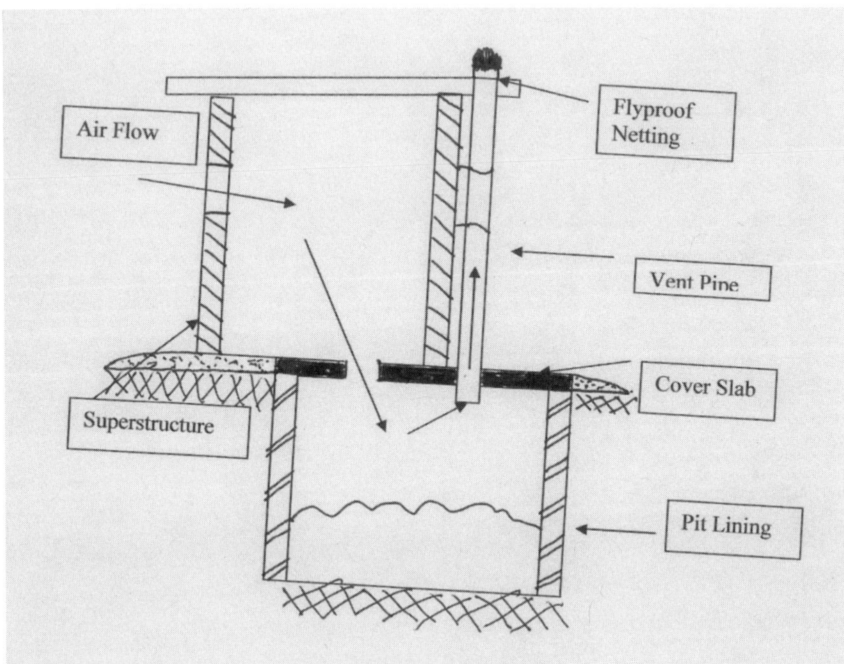

Figure 1. Ventilated improved pit latrine.

coming in contact with animals, or as a healthcare provider. Ideally, soap and water for hand washing should be available, especially adjacent to sanitation systems. An expensive alternative consists of commercially available antiseptic lotions.

RESOURCES

http://www.who.int/water_sanitation_health/en/
http://www.who.int/water_sanitation_health/dwq/gdwq3/en/
http://www.irc.nl/
http://www.collinsassoc.ca/water/resources.htm
http://www.who.int/docstore/water_sanitation_health/onsitesan/ch04.htm

REFERENCES

Cahill J, ed. 2002. *Updates in emergency medicine*, pp. 131–133. New York: Kluwer Academic.

Eade D, Williams S, eds. 1994. *The OXFAM handbook of development and relief*, 3 vols. Oxford: OXFAM.

http://www.who.int/docstore/water_sanitation_health/onsitesan/ch04.htm. Accessed on 6 April 2005.

World Health Organization. 2005. *Celebrating water for life: the international decade for action 2005–2015: an advocacy guide*. Geneva: WHO. http://www.who.int/water_sanitation_health/en/2005advocacyguide.pdf

78

SHELTER

Rashid F. Kysia, MD, MPH*

OVERVIEW

Shelter is a basic human right recognized universally by international law. Minimum adequate housing provides dignity for the displaced individual and protection from the extremes of climate and disease vectors. Médecins Sans Frontières estimates that 14 million refugees and up to 25 million internally displaced persons live in temporary shelters throughout the world. Shelter is among the highest priorities in the direct aftermath of a disaster, and shelter planning must be instituted as early as possible to avoid spontaneous overcrowding and further detriment to the health of disaster victims.

The planning of post-disaster emergency sheltering is largely dictated by the nature of the displacing event, the preexistent infrastructure, and local climate conditions. In the preparation of an emergency sheltering site, the three most salient concerns should be security, proximity to suitable water supply, and the ability to provide adequate sanitation. Substandard sheltering may compound multiple health morbidities, including transmission of infectious disease, degradation of immunity by exposure to extremes of the elements, exposure to ongoing causes of displacement, and morbidity.

OPTIONS

After displacement, the order of priority for sheltering should be (1) the return of individuals to their own housing, (2) the redistribution of displaced individuals within other local family or host households, and, if the former options are not possible, (3) the mass settlement of displaced persons in collective sheltering areas. Of highest priority, when possible, should be to assure the return of displaced persons to safe housing in the disaster-damaged area and provision of assistance to self-sheltering popu-

*Harvard-Affiliated Residency Program, Massachusetts General Hospital/Brigham and Women's Hospital, Boston

lations. Certain situations may preclude this option, including ongoing armed conflict, the presence of toxic exposure, and the possibility of recurrent natural or manmade disaster. Organizers should undertake an early assessment of the structural integrity of remaining buildings and discourage sheltering in structurally unsound units. Residents should be aided with provision of blankets, kerosene lamps, water purification kits, tarpaulins, and repair materials to establish minimum standards of safety when sheltering in existing housing. Water testing and establishment of locally safe sources of water should be provided. Programs can provide assistance in the local redistribution of refugees into other structurally sound housing units. One disadvantage of redistributing refugees within a host population is the loss of centralized access to the displaced persons for medical and relief efforts, and to allow monitoring of health status.

Collective settlement should be considered when the other options are not feasible. The advantage of collective housing lies in the ability for aid workers to provide asylum and security for large numbers of displaced persons. Camps and group sheltering expedite distribution of basic services like mass vaccinations, food distribution, water purification, and epidemic surveillance. However, if not properly planned, collective settlement may result in overcrowding, thereby increasing susceptibility to outbreaks of communicable diseases.

STANDARDS

Minimal standards of sheltering must be observed in the creation of refugee camps or sheltering compounds. In an urban setting, collective settlement can be provided in large public buildings like schools, sports facilities, community centers, and civic buildings. Utilization of spacious public buildings as evacuation centers provides the advantage of rapid short-term sheltering from the climate for large numbers of displaced persons. Such facilities, however, are often not appropriate for long-term sheltering due to crowding and health safety concerns.

Refugee vulnerability assessment should guide the establishment of de novo settlement efforts. Persisting risks should be evaluated in the post–natural disaster period to avoid threats of flooding, aftershocks, or recurrent high winds. In disasters involving hazardous materials or biologic agent exposures, site safety and isolation of exposure victims must be carefully considered.

Water quality and water management are key components of shelter planning. Sites, when possible, should be provided with basic equipment for filtering, boiling, disinfecting, and storing water in closed cisterns. The shelter perimeter should be surveyed for ditches, empty tires, and other potential vessels for pools of stagnant water. Such sites should be covered with a thin film of oil or backfilled with soil to prevent insect vector propagation. Inadequate spatial design may impact water tables and degrade existing water supplies in the camp. Multiple water points should be designed to provide for not more than 250 persons per point.

The United Nations High Commissioner for Refugees has established minimum standards for the spatial layout of shelters. Crowding is a common problem during acute displacement. Population density beyond certain limits will predispose a population to increased infectious disease morbidities. Refugee camps should contain no more than 10,000 individuals, and these persons should be divided into independent sub-camps of no more than 1,000 people per block. Housing must provide a minimum space of 3.5 m^2 per person in warm climates and 4.5 m^2 in cold climates, where stoves and heating elements must be employed. The inside space of each shelter should provide no less than 20 m^3 of fresh air per person per hour, necessitating mechanical ventilation if indicated. Individual beds inside the unit should be separated by a minimum of 0.75 meters from each other. Individual shelters ideally should house single families.

Units should be situated in groups of 10 to 12, arranged with roads on either side of the cluster. Individual shelters should be separated by a minimum of 8 meters from the next shelter unit, and roads should be offset a minimum of 2 meters from tent pegs. Roads should be a minimum of 10 meters wide to allow through-traffic and access for ambulances and aid distribution vehicles. A minimum of two large roads through the shelter site should be provided to allow for security, emergency access, or evacuation. Shelter sites should ideally be situated in proximity to local road infrastructure and airstrips, railways, or seaports for the supply of relief assistance.

Surveyors should assess surface topography to avoid both water-impermeable rocky grounds that will be unforgiving with flooding and lowland positions that may fill with floodwaters. If toilet pits are to be the primary method of sanitation, site topography must not be too rocky so as to prohibit sufficient evacuation of pit latrines. The site should be situated above flood level and should ideally be not more than 500 meters from a clean water source. Areas with excessively dense brush should be avoided or cleared, as the brush may provide cover for insects, rodents, and other disease vectors. Particularly in sites at risk of flooding, trenches should be dug around tents or temporary shelters. Site design should lead water away from shelters and latrines. Latrines should be built to accommodate not more than 20 individuals per latrine, and should be situated at least 100 meters from the camps water source.

Emergency sheltering efforts should include a controlled plan for handling of the dead. Shelter areas must have spatial distance from areas where the dead are handled and buried to avoid transmission of infectious disease. Gravesites should be at least 30 meters from sources of the camp's potable groundwater. The bottom of any grave must be at least 1.5 meters above the level of the groundwater table.

Temporary housing, due to crowding and use of scrap materials in construction, is at increased risk of fire hazard. Shelter site administrators should discourage the use of indoor stoves or smoking in makeshift housing. Spatial design should include adequate access roads to allow for fire control. Residents should be educated to store lamp oils and other combustibles outside of housing blocks. Lamps with oil should be suspended when in use, and should be clear of flammable shelter materials. Camp administrators should designate volunteers for fire preparedness. If electrical supply is available, care must be taken to avoid overloading of circuits. Buildings should have a spatial layout that includes fire lines that are bare of building or flammable brush. Such firebreaks should permit 30 meters width between blocks of buildings to allow for control of spreading flames. Roads may be situated along such fire lines.

Refugees have usually fled their homes with little or no preparation. On arrival to a mass shelter site, they find themselves completely reliant on outside resources for food and basic maintenance. Sheltering programs should give camp inhabitants an active role in planning and implementation of the site development. Programs should seek community participation in regular camp maintenance, assignment of work duties, site hygiene, and aid distribution. Recruitment of community members empowers individuals to become involved in decision-making and implementation of camp projects, helping to alleviate helplessness and passive dependence that may develop among the displaced.

REFERENCES

Doctors Without Borders/Médecins Sans Frontières. 1994. *Public health engineering in emergency situations.* Paris: MSF.

Doctors Without Borders/Médecins Sans Frontières. 1997. *Refugee health: an approach to emergency situations.* London: Macmillan.

The Sphere Project. 2004. *The sphere handbook: humanitarian charter and minimum standards in disaster response.* Geneva: The Sphere Project. http://www.sphereproject.org/handbook//

United Nations High Commission for Refugees. 1982. *Handbook for emergencies.* Geneva: UNHCR.

Wisner B, Adams J. 2002. *Environmental health in emergencies and disasters: a practical guide.* Geneva: World Health Organization.

79

REFUGEES AND INTERNALLY DISPLACED POPULATIONS

Philip D. Anderson, MD*

The global dimensions of the international refugee crisis are enormous. According to the Office of the United Nations High Commissioner for Refugees (UNHCR), there were just over 17 million refugees, asylum seekers, and internally displaced persons worldwide in 2004. This represents about 1 out of every 350 human beings on the planet displaced from their homes. This chapter outlines some of the conditions that have led to this humanitarian crisis, the characteristics of displaced populations, their emergency health needs, and the humanitarian aid priorities for addressing them.

DISASTERS AND COMPLEX HUMANITARIAN EMERGENCIES

Disasters, whether they are natural or manmade, are inherently disruptive to the environmental, social, economic, and political infrastructures of human societies. The degree and type of disruptive effects varies depending on the nature of the specific disaster. Prior to the end of the Cold War era, international humanitarian relief efforts focused primarily on responding to natural disasters, such as earthquakes, floods, and famine. However, since the end of the Cold War in the early 1990s, the focus of humanitarian relief efforts has shifted in response to an increasing number of regional conflicts that have resulted in refugee populations of greater magnitude than those associated with natural disasters in past years. The locations of these regional conflicts include Sub-Saharan Africa, the Middle East, the Caucasus region, Central Asia, Southern Asia, and Southeast Asia. In many cases, longstanding ethnic, religious, or communal hostilities lay at the root of these conflicts. During the time of the Cold War, these tensions were suppressed by superpower domination in these regions. Following the decline of the Soviet Union, interest and involvement in these regions has declined, thereby creating a climate where these old hostilities have resurfaced.

This new type of regional conflict differs in substantive ways from traditional wars of the past and has come to be referred to as a "complex humanitarian emergency" (CHE). Traditional wars tended to be waged between nation states, and although civilian casualties did occur, they were in most cases not intentional targets of military operations. The casualties of war were predominantly combatants. Mo-

*Department of Medicine, Harvard Medical School, Boston

dern-day CHEs tend to be conflicts between warring factions within national boundaries. The civilian constituencies of the opposing groups are often the intentional targets of attacks, resulting in a disproportionately large ratio of civilian to combatant casualties. CHEs are characterized by organized violence directed against the civilian population that is often motivated by "identity politics" and associated with widespread human rights abuses ranging from rape, torture, "ethnic cleansing," and genocide. The combatants in a CHE are often poorly trained, irregular forces with erratic leadership and chains of command rather than standing, professional military units. There is typically an ignorance or disregard for the principles of international humanitarian law. International aid organizations often have difficulty reaching civilians in need and establishing neutral safe zones for provision of medical care. The resulting human suffering and widespread insecurity among the local population leads to mass population dislocations as affected individuals flee seeking refuge.

CHARACTERISTICS OF DISPLACED POPULATIONS

In discussing the human consequences of disasters, the affected populations can be grouped into several categories depending on the degree to which they have been displaced from their communities: (1) refugees and asylum seekers, (2) internally displaced persons, and (3) locally entrapped persons.

Refugees and Asylum Seekers

Refugees and Asylum Seekers represent the most significantly displaced individuals affected by disasters. These groups are forced to flee their country of origin due to fear of persecution and seek asylum in other countries. Individuals apply for asylum in order to be recognized as bona fide refugees and receive legal protection and material assistance. The majority of the world's refugees come from developing countries and seek asylum in neighboring developing countries. The leading countries of origin of refugees in 2004 included Afghanistan, Somalia, Burundi, the Democratic Republic of Congo, Palestinians, Somalia, Iraq, Vietnam, Liberia, and Angola. Many refugees are forced to walk long distances in order to reach the country or region of asylum. They may have sustained injuries as a result of the conflict and may have limited access to food, water, shelter, and health care during their journey. As a result, many refugees are already ill and/or malnourished on arrival. Refugees arriving in large numbers from neighboring countries tend to be housed in temporary camps, which frequently suffer from crowding, insufficient food, water, and shelter, as well as unsanitary waste disposal systems. These conditions predispose refugees to the development of communicable diseases and malnutrition. Particularly vulnerable groups include unaccompanied children, households headed by women, and minority ethnic or religious groups.

Internally Displaced Persons (IDPs)

Internally Displaced Persons (IDPs) are caught in similar situations as refugees in that they are forced to flee their home communities and seek refuge elsewhere. The primary difference is that they remain within their country of origin and therefore have a different administrative status with regard to international laws governing treatment of refugees. As such, their numbers are more difficult to measure and may be larger than official counts suggest. Significant populations of IDPs in 2004 were found around the world in countries on many continents, including: Columbia, Azerbaijan, Liberia, Sri Lanka, the Russian Federation, Bosnia and Herzegovina, Georgia, Serbia and Montenegro, Afghanistan, and Côte d'Ivoire. Many come from rural areas that have been destroyed or severely disrupted by conflict and migrate to larger cities. In contrast to refugees, IDPs may blend into the local population or form their own urban tent settlements or shantytowns. Like refugees, many may have endured periods of inadequate food, water, and shelter during flight from the region of conflict and suffer from malnourishment, illness, and/or injury. IDPs may be at continued risk of persecution or may be intentionally deprived of access to assistance through internal sources by their governments if they are viewed as sympathetic to rebel forces.

Locally Entrapped Populations

Locally Entrapped Populations represent civilian groups trapped in their home communities by ongoing local conflict, putting them at risk for illness or injury. They may be unable to flee due to geographic isolation, damage to transportation infrastructure, or risk of injury during flight due to ongoing surrounding hostilities. During the war in Sarajevo from 1991 to 1993, death rates among the local population rose fourfold due to direct violence, food shortages, and destruction of public sanitation and utilities and health services.

EMERGENCY HEALTH NEEDS OF DISPLACED POPULATIONS

Morbidity and mortality rates among refugee populations are often significantly elevated when compared to surrounding non-refugee populations in countries offering asylum. Mortality rates ranged from 8 to 45 times baseline in Thailand (1979), Somalia (1980), and the Sudan (1985). Among Rwandan refugees in Goma, Zaire, the death rates were 60 times that of the surrounding population in 1994. Children less than 5 years old are at particularly high risk for increased mortality.

Waterborne disease epidemics result from contamination of drinking water supplies. Common organisms responsible for these epidemics are those transmitted by the fecal–oral route, such as *Vibrio cholerae* and Shigella species. Cholera causes a toxin-mediated profuse watery diarrhea, leading to rapid dehydration. Shigella is an infectious enteritis resulting in bloody diarrhea and systemic illness.

Food shortages or poor-quality food can lead to protein-calorie malnutrition or micronutrient malnutrition. An important indicator of malnutrition in refugee populations is the prevalence of acute malnutrition (low weight for height) among children less than 5 years old. Vitamin A deficiency is a common micronutrient deficiency seen in refugee populations that causes blindness and increases the risk of severe illness and death from diarrheal diseases and measles. Recent epidemics of micronutrient deficiency-related diseases seen in refugee populations include scurvy, beriberi, and pellagra.

Sixty to ninety five percent of all deaths among refugees and IDPs are due to the following preventable illnesses: measles, malnutrition, diarrheal diseases (cholera, shigella), acute respiratory infections (pneumonia), and malaria. Measles epidemics are common among unvaccinated refugee populations. The disease spreads rapidly via respiratory microdroplets among the crowded conditions often seen in refugee camps. Measles may also be complicated by pneumonia, diarrhea, and malnutrition.

The psychological trauma of disasters on displaced populations is a vital health concern that can result in devastating long-term complications if not adequately addressed. Refugees are often victims of rape, torture, and other human rights abuses. They suffer tremendous personal and community loss as a result of their dislocation. Children are often orphaned or separated from their families. Mental health issues should be addressed as a part of the overall healthcare strategy for refugee populations.

HUMANITARIAN AID PRIORITIES FOR RELIEF EFFORTS

Effective humanitarian relief efforts begin with rapid initial assessments to accurately determine population size, composition, mortality rates, nutritional status and healthcare needs using reliable epidemiological strategies. The goal of initial assessments is to determine which problems are likely to pose the greatest threat to the population so that interventions can be planned strategically to accomplish the greatest good for the greatest number. Health needs assessments and planning must be coordinated with other sector assessments (environmental, sanitation, security, etc.) because problems in one sector affect every other sector. Ongoing assessment of the health status of the refugee population are essential for determining the effectiveness of relief efforts and for refocusing interventions as conditions on the ground change.

The initial public health priorities for disaster-affected populations are to ensure provision of adequate clean water, food, shelter, sanitation, and protection from conflict-related trauma. The UNHCR recommendations for meeting these basic needs of refugees and IDP include: at least 15 liters of clean water per person per day, an average of 2,100 kilocalories of energy per person per day (as well as basic requirements of protein and essential micronutrients), one latrine per 20 persons, and adequate shelter, particularly in cold climates.

The critical components of a comprehensive public health intervention for refugee populations in austere environments include: environmental health issues (clean water, sanitation, disease vector management); communicable disease control and epidemic management (preventative measures including immunization, and curative medical services); nutrition (adequate caloric intake and essential micronutrients); and emergency health information systems.

REFERENCES

UNHCR: the refugee agency [internet website]. (Geneva). Available at http://www.unhcr.ch/cgi-bin/texis/vtx/home. Accessed on 28 January 2005.

Leaning J, Briggs SM, Chen LC, eds. 1999. *Humanitarian crises: the medical and public health response*. Cambridge: Harvard UP.

Hollifield M, Warner TD, Lian N, Krakow B, Jenkins JH, Kesler J, Stevenson J, Westermeyer J. 2002. Measuring trauma and health status in refugees: a critical review. *JAMA* **288**(5): 611–21.

Toole MJ, Waldman RJ. 1997. The public health aspects of complex emergencies and refugee situations. *Annu Rev Public Health* **18**:283–312.

80

CHILD SOLDIERS

Sophie Skarbek-Borowska* and
George W. Skarbek-Borowski, MD**

OVERVIEW

In 1997 the United Nations (UN) defined a child soldier as "anyone under the age of 18 who serves in any kind of armed force in any capacity, thereby including those too small to bear arms and girls taken as wives." There are currently over 300,000 active child soldiers, in addition to uncertain numbers of former child soldiers left to fend for themselves once peace has been established. These children can be found across the world's poorest regions, but primarily in Southeast Asia and Africa. Kidnapping, forced acts of violence (often against family members or other children), torture, and drugs are all used to induct children into an armed force and prevent their escape.

PHYSICAL, PSYCHOLOGICAL AND SOCIOECONOMIC SEQUELAE

The main difficulties faced by former child soldiers and those trying to help them are limited healthcare access and social stigma. Local hospitals do not have the equipment or the medications to provide adequate treatment, and as a result many child soldiers go without medical attention for long periods of time. Common combat-related injuries include hearing loss, blindness, and limb amputations, usually from landmines or grenades. Prostheses are in high demand because so many amputees are still growing and need frequent replacements. Sexually transmitted diseases (STDs), malaria, skin and respiratory diseases, malnutrition, bone deformation from carrying heavy loads, as well as drug and alcohol addiction are widespread.

*Verso Publishing, London

**Department of Emergency Medicine, Brown University, Memorial Hospital, Providence, Rhode Island

Apart from the physical injuries sustained by child soldiers, another area of concern for aid agencies and healthcare workers is the psychological health of these children. A recent Belgian study revealed the extent of this problem in a voluntary survey of former child soldiers of Uganda's notorious Lord's Resistance Army. Of the 301 children interviewed, 77% had witnessed at least one killing, 39% had been forced to kill, 39% had abducted other children, 63% had looted and burned civilian homes, and 52% had been seriously beaten. A secondary survey was conducted on a randomly selected subgroup of 75 children, of whom 71 agreed to participate. They completed a questionnaire designed to evaluate the extent of posttraumatic stress disorder (PTSD). A score of greater than 24 on the impact of event scale-revised (IES-R), which is a self-report scale akin to the DSM-IV criteria for PTSD, indicates clinically significant symptoms. The mean IES-R score was 53.5, with 97% of participants falling into the clinically significant category. Symptoms reported by respondents included nightmares, memory problems, drug and alcohol abuse, and an inability to function in social life. Similar findings have been reported in Sri Lankan child soldiers, including somatization, depression, PTSD, and a more severe reactive psychosis termed malignant PTSD.

Growing up in a culture of war, particularly during a child's vulnerable and impressionable formative years, only reinforces the role of violence as the primary means of conflict resolution. These psychological and emotional problems have as much a debilitating effect as their physical handicaps, seriously impeding a child's ability to work productively and interact normally in society.

The issue of social stigmatization particularly affects girls, who are often dependent on being accepted into a family in order to support themselves and, in many cases, the children of their military "husbands." As a result, it is extremely difficult for outsiders to make contact with former girl soldiers and address their needs. Interviews and tests for STDs, rape trauma, and other conditions are almost impossible to conduct without identifying girls as former fighters, which may result in their being rejected by the adoptive family. Furthermore, girls, many pregnant or with small children, are greatly underrepresented in demobilization and reintegration programs.

A Human Rights Watch report from December 2002 on the status of former child soldiers in Angola revealed that the vast majority of those interviewed wanted to return to school and find work, but had no means of doing so. Scarce resources mean that governments have focused on the needs of adults, leaving behind large numbers of hungry, jobless, and homeless youths who return to violence as their only means of survival.

SOLUTIONS

Guidelines for preventing child recruitment and for identifying and providing assistance to former child soldiers are outlined in UNICEF's *Cape Town Principles and Best Practices*. The physical assessment and care of child soldiers is a top priority, but the consensus among aid agencies, governments, and the UN is that helping these children transition into healthy adults requires investment in schooling, vocational training, and family support, not just in short-term medical assistance.

The UN has established a policy of disarmament, demobilization, and reintegration (DDR) that equates the psychological stability of former child soldiers with the well-being of their communities. While emphasizing the reunification of families in order to establish regular emotional links for these children, the DDR principles also require that children be the first soldiers demobilized, a policy that, at least legally, prevents them from being re-recruited. The role of human rights and other workers revolves around identifying and monitoring those children most at risk from recruiters. Such risk is particularly real in places such as refugee camps, where children are displaced, abused, separated from families, and living in extreme poverty.

Interviews to assess the psychosocial needs of the children and their communities should be done as early as possible. Risk-mapping and evaluations of the socioeconomic environment to which children will return are aimed at building local support networks. Military "service," paradoxically, may have provided recruits with certain technical skills (particularly mechanical and electrical), which, coupled with traditional apprenticeships, can aid in the reintegration process. The Spanish Red Cross has set up programs to establish vocational training in several Angolan provinces, and in northern Sri Lanka a Liberation Tigers of Tamil Eelam (LTTE) and UNICEF rehabilitation plan includes health services, vocational training, and the provision of microcredit so that children can afford to buy school and work materials. The Christian Children's Fund, a nongovernmental organization involved in the rehabilitation of child soldiers, has successfully reintegrated 2,153 children into their home communities using such techniques as job skills training, literacy instruction, monetary grants, and "cleansing rituals" designed to mark the end of a child's military "career" and appease the spirits of their victims.

The UN, its constituent nations, and nongovernmental organizations alike must strive to augment their efforts at demobilization and reintegration of child soldiers worldwide. The greatest challenge, apart from physical rehabilitation, will be in providing the requisite socioeconomic and psychological support to transition these unfortunate children into functional adults.

RESOURCES

Amnesty International: www.amnesty.org
Caritas International: www.caritas.org
Coalition to Stop the Use of Child Soldiers: www.child-soldiers.org
Human Rights Watch: www.hrw.org
Medical Association for the Prevention of War: www.mapw.org.au
United Nations Children's Fund: www.unicef.org
United Nations Children and Armed Conflict: www.un.org/special-rep/children-armed conflict/English/index.html
World Vision: www.worldvision.org
Quaker United Nations (New York): www.quno.org/newyork/girlsandwar/default.htm In-depth interviews with girl soldiers from the Philippines, Colombia, Sri Lanka and Angola.
SOS-Kinderdorf International:www.sos-childrensvillages.org (builds reintegration communities for former Ugandan child soldiers)
International Centre for Rights and Democracy: www.ichrdd.ca Focus on girl soldiers.

REFERENCES

Coalition to Stop the Use of Child Soldiers. 2004. *Child soldier use 2003: a briefing for the 4th UN Security Council open debate on children and armed conflict*. Geneva: Human Rights Watch. http://hrw.org/reports/2004/childsoldiers0104/

Derluyn IE, Broekaert G, Schuyten E, De Temmerman E. 2004. PTSD in former Ugandan child soldiers. *Lancet* **363**:861–3.

Haggstrom H. 2004. *Stop the use of child soldiers*. www.mapw.org.au/childsoldiers. Accessed 15 August 2004.

Human Rights Watch. 2003. *Forgotten fighters: child soldiers in Angola*. Geneva: HRW. http://www.eldis.org/static/DOC14020.htm.

Lamberg L. 2004. Reclaiming child soldiers' lost lives. *JAMA* **292**(5):253–254.

McKay S, Mazurawa D. 2004. *Where are the girls? Girls in fighting forces in Northern Uganda, Sierra Leone and Mozambique: their lives during and after war*. Montreal: International Centre for Rights and Democracy, 2004. http://www.ichrdd.ca/english/commdoc/publications/women/Girls/girlsmainEN.html

Somasundaram DJ. 2002. Child soldiers: understanding the context. *BMJ* **324**:1268–1271.

Somasundaram DJ. 1998. *Scarred minds*. New Delhi: Sage.

UNICEF. 1997. *Cape Town principles and best practices*.

81 REPRODUCTIVE HEALTH

Barbara Kilian, MD*

> "Reproductive health is a state of complete physical, mental, and social well-being and not merely the absence of disease or infirmity, in all matters relating to the reproductive system and to its functions and processes. It implies that people are able to have a satisfying and safe sex life and that they have the capability to reproduce and the freedom to decide if, when and how often to do so.
>
> —WHO-DRH brochure on reproductive health.

Although reproductive health, as an issue unto itself, has only been in the spotlight of international emergency aid since the early 1990s, the amount of research and initiatives that have since been created is at times overwhelming. In the context of emergency aid, reproductive health is a broad-spanning term that includes all aspects of sexual health: maternal and newborn care, sexually transmitted diseases (STDs)/HIV, family planning (including abortion issues), female genital mutilation, and gender-based violence (GBV). The importance of incorporating reproductive health as an integral part of humanitarian aid cannot be emphasized enough. Each of these topics is complex and expansive. The goal of this chapter is to contextualize an often-overlooked issue and give a brief overview of these issues.

Maternal and newborn care addresses issues related to pre-, peri-, and postnatal care. Approximately 585,000 women die each year from pregnancy-related causes, with 95% of these deaths occurring in developing countries. Girls aged 15–19 are twice as likely to die from childbirth as those in their twenties, and girls aged less than 15 are five times as likely to die from childbirth. Death from pregnancy-related causes is often the leading cause of death among women. Bleeding, infection, obstructed labor, eclampsia, and unsafe abortions are all significant causes of death among mothers. Aid should attempt to provide medical care for these issues as well as ensuring that comprehensive reproductive health services are offered. There is a wide range of aid that can be offered, from the most basic of clean delivery kits to comprehensive maternal care. In an emergent/unstable environment, the first priority should be provisions for clean/safe delivery either at home or at established centers. It is vital that the

*Department of Emergency Medicine, St. Luke's/Roosevelt Hospital Center, New York

affected population be aware of services offered and that there is an appropriate number of trained staff at service centers. Education regarding breast-feeding can have a dramatic positive impact on the neonate.

STDs and HIV are complex and difficult issues in providing care in emergency settings, and the political environment surrounding them often make individuals shy away from these issues. However, the impact of these issues is astounding. Across the world, greater than 330,000 million new cases of STDs occur every year. In developing countries, the morbidity from these easily curable diseases is staggering. At the end of 2003, approximately 37.8 million people worldwide have HIV/AIDS. It is estimated that in 2003 4.8 million individuals were infected with HIV, worldwide, with more than 95% of these occurring in developing countries. The goals of aid should be to treat individuals affected by these diseases and help educate and prevent further spread of the disease. In regards to HIV, even simple healthcare measures may be beneficial.

In the disaster/emergency setting, the right of couples and individuals to choose when to have children often seems inconsequential. However, family planning can have a pronounced effect on the economical and social circumstances of a woman and her family. Family planning involves the care and treatment of complications from unsafe abortions, offering safe abortions, education regarding birth control options, and increasing the availability of birth control methods. It is estimated that 68,000 women die as a result of complications from unsafe abortions annually. The education and incorporation of birth control options is often a large-scale event that comes once an emergency environment has become stable and more complex issues can be addressed. It is important for healthcare providers to recognize the myriad reasons why family planning needs are not met, including but not limited to: limited access, limited methods, lack of information, safety concerns/side effects, partner disapproval, and religious/social customs.

The partial or complete removal of the external genitalia and/or damage to the genital organs of women for cultural or nonmedical reasons is termed Female Genital Mutilation (FGM). Approximately 130 million women and girls have been subjected to this practice, with another 2 million at risk to undergo FGM each year. The practice is most common in African countries, but it is known to also exist in Asia and other parts of the world. Special care during pregnancy and labor is vital, as there are often serious complications as a result of FGM. Education of girls and women is vital. Many relief organizations are also targeting education campaigns at men and religious leaders, as they are often the decision-makers in households.

Gender-based violence remains an elusive and difficult-to-study aspect of reproductive health. In displaced populations, loss of social structures and the need for exchanging sex for material goods and/or protection are all known to increase GBV. Under normal circumstances, violence against women is underreported secondary to feelings of powerlessness, fear of retribution, embarrassment, and difficulty accessing resources. In refugee environments, these situations are often magnified. In refugee and politically unstable environments, the violence is often sexual. Rape is common, and relief workers should assume this is a problem, unless proven otherwise. It is an extremely frustrating issue but should not be neglected. Efforts should be made to increase security and awareness, distribute foodstuffs and other essential material goods (to decrease the need for sexual trade), and to treat victims of GBV, including emergency contraception.

RESOURCES

Reproductive Health and Research: part of the World Health organization. www.who.int/reproductive-health/index.htm

International Planned Parenthood Federation: www.who.int/reproductive-health/index.htm

CDC's Department of Reproductive Health: www.cdc.gov/reproductivehealth/logistics/global_rrh.htm

Center for Reproductive Rights: www.crlp.org/

United Nations High Commissioner for Refugees: www.unhcr.ch

World Health Organization, Emergency and Humanitarian Action (EHA): www.who.int/disasters

REFERENCES

Reproductive health in refugee situations: an inter-agency field manual. 1999. Geneva: United Nations High Commissioner for Refugees. http://www.unfpa.org/emergencies/manual/.

UNAIDS. 2004. *Report on global aids epidemic.* http://www.unaids.org/bangkok2004/GAR2004_pdf/UNAIDSGlobalReport2004_en.pdf (July). http://www.unaids.org/wad2004/EPIupdate2004_html_en/epi04_00_en.htm (December 2004 update). Geneva: UNAIDS.

WHO. 1998. *World health day—safe motherhood,* 7 April 1998. WHD 98.11 (Pamphlet).

WHO. 2000. *Unsafe abortion: Global and regional estimates of the incidence of unsafe abortion and associated mortality in 2000,* 4th ed. Geneva: Department of Reproductive Health and Research, World Health Organization. http://www.who.int/reproductive-health/publications/MSM_97_16/MSM_97_16_abstract.en.html

PART VII

EDUCATION, HEALTH ISSUES, AND RESOURCES

82 EMERGENCY PREPAREDNESS

Dan Wiener, MD*

The Joint Commission on Accreditation of Healthcare Organizations (JCAHO) has created clear standards for the creation and implementation of an emergency management plan. This chapter will focus on the operational aspects of implementing a response to an external disaster in a hospital setting.

NOTIFICATION

A hospital may learn of an external disaster through the media, notification by governmental agencies, EMS, or simply by the arrival of a number of injured patients at its emergency department. Every plan must have a clear mechanism for declaring a disaster and activating its emergency management plan (EMP). This requires a clear channel of communication between clinical leadership and senior administration. Once the determination is made that a disaster exists, the extent of mobilization of resources and personnel needs to be determined. Disasters can and should be categorized by the level of resources needed to meet demands. A hospital that has defined these levels in advance will be prepared to mobilize an appropriate and proportional response. Planners need to be aware that in many disasters most victims will arrive on foot or by personal vehicles within 1.5 hours of the disaster. Often it is the less injured that arrive first, with a second wave of more critically injured patients arriving later via EMS.

SECURITY

Security is essential to the successful implementation of an EMP. In any disaster there is a significant potential for disruption of ongoing care and interference with implementation of the EMP. Security needs to have and implement plans for crowd control, communication with local police, and locking down of the emergency department and facility. Issues of biological and chemical terrorism pose unique problems of quarantine and decontamination.

*Department of Emergency Medicine, St. Luke's/Roosevelt Hospital Center, New York

COMMAND CENTER: HEICS

As soon as the EMP is activated, the incident command structure needs to be activated and the incident command center established. The command staff is responsible for overall leadership and management of the incident. The HEICS structure calls for the command center to be staffed by the Incident Commander, Public Information Officer, Safety and Security Officer, and a Liaison Officer. The Incident Commander is in charge of the overall emergency operation. The Safety and Security Officer has authority over the safety of internal disaster operations and hazardous conditions. This includes security and traffic control. The Public Information Officer represents the facility to the news media. The Liaison Officer coordinates external communications with outside agencies and facilities. Incident command supervises the five major functions: operations, logistics, planning, and finance/administration.

- Operations — organizes all activities related to clinical care.
- Logistics — organizes and directs maintenance of the physical plant as well as food and shelter. The major subcategories are facilities, communications, transportation, materials, and nutrition.
- Planning consolidates management and distribution of information. It also manages the collection and inventory of medical, nursing, and staff in separate labor pools.
- Finance monitors and documents the utilization of financial assets in support of the disaster operation.

The location of the command center should be identified in the emergency preparedness plan. An alternative should be identified as well in case the primary site is part of an internal disaster.

As hospital leadership responds to the disaster notification, they will assume the roles defined in the HEICS table of organization. Staff will have been trained in the role they will assume but can also rely on printed job action sheets to guide them.

COMMUNICATION

The command center must be able to communicate throughout the organization and with outside agencies (police, fire, EMS, public health). Mobilization of staff should be facilitated by preexisting phone and paging list of key personnel. Lists to notify key hospital leadership as well as outside agencies should be kept in the command center and with telecommunications. Individual departments should also keep lists of key personnel. Redundant systems must be created to ensure that at least one system continue to be functional. The choices are varied and include beepers (numeric and text messaging), telephones (land-based, fax lines, wireless, bypass, and satellite), Internet access (telephone, cable and wireless), handheld two-way communication devices, access to television and radio, radios (800 mHz, short wave), and individuals to serve as "runners." Some states and municipalities are now utilizing web-based communication during disasters to disseminate information and to obtain from hospitals an ongoing assessment of their bed and resource availability as well as their needs. The Public Information Officer should handle communications from the hospital to the media. Ideally, these communications will convey information that will permit the public to optimize their contribution to the emergency response.

SURGE CAPACITY

The surge of patients during a disaster will require increasing the availability of outpatient and inpatient beds. The Emergency Department needs to identify in advance areas of the hospital it could utilize for acute care if space became an issue. The plan should move the ambulatory, non-acute patients and keep the emergent patients in the ED. Other areas should be surveyed for the adequacy of electricity, water, and medical gases. If these resources are not available, plans should be in place to bring them to the area from a central location.

Patients currently under treatment in the ED should receive a disposition as soon as possible. Admitted patients and those likely to be admitted should be moved to inpatient beds. The remainder of patients should either be treated and released or moved to other patient care areas as soon as possible. Inpatient services should have a system in place to assess and immediately discharge those patients who do not need to be in the hospital. Consideration should be given to canceling elective surgical cases, clinic appointments, and diagnostic procedures. Hospitals should have plans to treat patients in areas of the hospital that are not usually used for patient care (lounges, auditoriums, hallways, cafeterias). Mutual aid agreements should be in place with other hospitals and healthcare facilities to transfer patients if they exceed their own capacity.

For every physical casualty of a disaster there will be a significant number of "worried well" and psychological victims. It is estimated for every casualty there will be 4 to 20 psychological victims. This can include not only those patients at the scene of the event but those in proximity or even watching on television. Hospitals need to be prepared to set up a treatment and counseling area for these patients; however, this area should be separate from the acute care areas.

SUPPLIES

The hospital must ensure that there are adequate supplies to stabilize, decontaminate, and treat patients. Hospitals will need to have enough food, resources, and medical supplies, including pharmaceuticals, to be self-sufficient for 48–72 hours. Hospitals need to inventory their supplies, maintain internal stockpiles, and have agreements with outside vendors to deliver additional supplies in the event of an emergency. There should be a stockpile of supplies that can be immediately moved to the ED and designated treatment areas from central supply. Hospitals can utilize their hazard vulnerability analysis to identify the most likely emergencies and create caches of supplies to cope with those emergencies. The potential need for mortuary space should also be considered. Additional resources can be expected as the federal government mobilizes and FEMA (Federal Emergency Management Agency), NDMS (The National Medical System), USAR (Urban Search and Rescue), and the CDC (Centers for Disease Control and Prevention) respond. The Strategic National Stockpile (SNS) may take up to 48 hours to deliver antibiotics to areas were they are needed. The Department of Health and Human Services suggests that hospitals maintain enough antibiotics on hand for the first 48 hours of an emergency. Which agency responds and the exact nature of the response will depend on the specifics of the emergency.

STAFF NEEDS

Hospitals must have a reliable method to mobilize personnel. Disruptions in communication and transportation should be anticipated. Staff will expect to have the needs of their families addressed. It should be anticipated that staff will only come to work if they know that their families are safe and that their children and elderly dependents are cared for. In some instances arrangements will need to be made to feed and house staff. Transportation into the hospital may also need to be arranged. It is important to keep staff apprised of what is going on within the organization and across organizations so they can gain a sense of control. Personnel who are reporting to the hospital for duty when it is not their regular shift should report to the labor pool. From there they can be assigned to other areas of the hospital at the direction of the command center.

TRIAGE

Most emergency department triage systems are designed to deliver as much care as needed to each patient. In a disaster situation this may be harmful, as medical resources, personnel, supplies, and facilities must be allocated to provide the greatest good for the greatest number. Most field EMS triage systems use color-coded tags to identify patients by level of severity. "Red" is for patients who require immediate intervention; "yellow" is for those who are seriously injured but whose care can be delayed in order to treat category red patients; "green" includes patients who are ambulatory and those with psychological reactions; "black" is for those who are dead or near-dead. Once in the ED, patients can be triaged using the modified START system.

PATIENT TRACKING

Hospitals will also need to have in place a system to track all patients brought to the hospital during the disaster. This should include the patient's name or a description of the patient, location, type of injuries, initial care, and disposition. There should be a system to take calls from concerned family members and accurately report who is being treated in the hospital. Hospitals need to be able to accurately identify if a person is currently in the hospital receiving care.

DECONTAMINATION: CHEMICAL AND RADIATION

During some emergencies, decontamination will need to be performed at triage. Triage staff must be able to recognize the signs and symptoms of patients exposed to hazardous materials. If these patients are not recognized, they have the potential to contaminate the hospital. For this reason public health officials are now advocating an all-hazards approach to victims. In this approach it is assumed that all victims are contaminated until public health officials declare that there is no evidence of radioactive or chemical contamination. Decontamination equipment and personnel protective equipment need to be readily available and staff trained in their use. Issues of securing the decontamination facility, water supply, drainage, lighting, ventilation, and storage of contaminated runoff all need to be considered. Some facilities have built permanent decontamination structures, while others have temporary showers, which can be erected at the time they are needed. The training of staff in the use of the appropriate personnel protective equipment (PPE) is an essential element of preparedness. OSHA has developed guidelines for use of this equipment in hospitals where staff will be the "first receivers" of contaminated patients.

BIOLOGIC: ISOLATION

Communicable diseases, which occur naturally, such as SARS, and potential bioterrorism agents, such as smallpox and pneumonic plague, make it essential that hospitals rapidly identify and isolate these patients. All medical staff should be educated in the recognition and immediate isolation and treatment of these patients. Triage should have appropriate signage instructing patients to identify themselves if they have a fever and a rash or if they have a fever and a cough and have traveled to area of the world known to be endemic for SARS. Once a patient has been identified they should be placed in an isolation room. Healthcare workers should use appropriate precautions and don an N-95 respirator (employees should be fit tested), gown, gloves, and eye protection. Procedures should be in place for safely moving the patient from triage to the treatment area, quarantining the waiting room, notifying public health officials, and providing educational materials to quarantined patients, staff, and others anxious about their possible exposure. An inventory of all airborne isolation rooms should be kept in the command center and a floor identified as a potential isolation floor if necessary. The ventilation system of the ED and proposed isolation floors should be tested in advance to assure they will not contaminate other areas of the hospital. Hospitals should also have a plan to provide prophylaxis and/or vaccination to the staff and community as directed by the local department of health.

FAMILIES

Family members of victims will need to have an area set aside. Services provided should include counseling, stress debriefing and interactions with physicians, social services, relief agencies, and clergy. Basic needs for food, bathrooms, and access to phones need to be provided. Informational packets should be prepared in advance for scenarios identified as likely in the HVA.

VOLUNTEERS

Hospitals should expect a large volume of volunteers during an emergency. Some volunteers will be known to the hospital and can report to the labor pool with other hospital employees. A system should be created to direct nonaffiliated volunteers to a separate area where the needs for their services can be ascertained and individuals can be appropriately vetted. Volunteering physicians and nurses present a unique problem in terms of verification of identity and credentials. Hospitals need to work with the state to determine the level of verification that is required in an emergency. JCAHO has advocated for a credentialing database to support a national emergency volunteer system for healthcare professionals. Hospitals that are part of a healthcare network should put in place a mechanism for physicians and nurses at one hospital to work at another during an emergency. Transferring patients within a hospital system has the advantages of allowing physicians and nurses to work in the familiar environment of their own hospital and decompressing the hospital most affected by the emergency. However, during a disaster transportation is often difficult, as ambulances are occupied with acute care. Hospitals must be aware that the EMTALA laws remain in effect during an emergency.

POST-DISASTER RECOVERY PERIOD

During this period the focus of the hospital will shift back to the everyday needs of the population. All departments should assess their specific needs, including destroyed or used equipment, including computers and telephones. Needs for medical supplies, food, water, linen, and other patient care products should be assessed. An assessment of adequacy of staffing should also be made. The results of these surveys are reported to the incident commander. Once the incident commander is certain that the staff, equipment, and supplies necessary for operation are secured, the order can be given to reopen the facility or reestablish normal operations. Consideration should be given to the psychological needs of the medical personnel who responded. Most will recover from the initial trauma, but some will manifest symptoms of post-traumatic stress disorder.

REFERENCES

Bisell RA, Becker BM, Burkle FM. 1996. Healthcare personnel in disaster response: reversible roles or territorial imperatives? *Emerg Med Clin North Am* **14**:267-289.

Garner A, Lee A, Harrison K, Schultz CH. 2001. Comparative analysis of multiple-casualty incident triage algorithms. *Ann Emerg Med* **38**:541–548.

Guide to emergency management planning in healthcare. 2002. Chicago: JCAHO.

Health care at the crossroads. 2003. Chicago: JCAHO. http://www.jcaho.org/about+us/public+policy+initiatives/emergency.htm.

Kaji AH, Waeckerie JF. 2003. Disaster medicine and the emergency medicine resident. *Ann Emerg Med* **41**:865–870.

San Mateo County Emergency Medical Services Agency. 1998. *Healthcare facility emergency incident command system III—January*. http://www.emsa.cahnet.gov/dms2/heics3.htm.

Tintinalli J, Kelen G, Stapczynski J, eds. 2000. *Emergency medicine: a comprehensive study guide*, pp. 2631–2640. New York: McGraw-Hill.

Ursano RJ. 2002. Post-Traumatic Stress Disorder [editorial]. *New Engl J Med* **2**:130–131.

Waeckerle J. 1991. Disaster planning and response *N Eng J Med* **324**:815–821.

83 SYNDROMIC SURVEILLANCE

Dan Wiener, MD*

OVERVIEW

Early recognition of a BT attack presents a significant challenge to healthcare providers and public health officials. Although there was some recognition of the risk of biological attack prior to the World Trade Center attack of September 11th and the anthrax attacks later in the fall of 2001, these events provided impetus to the efforts to develop, standardize, and validate syndromic surveillance across the country. Surveillance activities in the United States until then had been focused on traditional surveillance.

The goal of syndromic surveillance is to identify a bioterrorist attack at the earliest possible moment, before microbiologic confirmation. Early identification can lead to early treatment and prophylaxis with antibiotics and a reduction in morbidity and mortality. Developers of these systems have struggled with a number of challenging issues: What syndromes should be examined? How should those syndromes be defined? How can the early nonspecific symptoms of bioterrorism agents be distinguished from other infectious diseases? How can data be collected in a timely manner? What data should be collected? What is the best format for the data? How should the data be transmitted efficiently in accordance with current privacy laws? What are the sensitivity and specificity of the systems being developed? How can the seasonal variation in infectious disease be distinguished from a bioterrorist attack? What should be the standards for development and evaluation? Will these systems successfully identify a biologic attack?

DEFINITION

The CDC defines surveillance as "the ongoing, systemic collection, analysis, interpretation, and dissemination of data about a health-related event for use in public health action to reduce morbidity and mortality and to improve health".

*Department of Emergency Medicine, St. Luke's/Roosevelt Hospital Center

Traditionally, the primary method for collecting surveillance data was manual reporting of suspicious and notifiable clinical and laboratory data from clinicians, hospitals, and laboratories to public health officials. These systems provide information that can be utilized to estimate the magnitude of a public health problem, detect outbreaks, and determine the distribution of illness. This information is used to evaluate public health practice, stimulate research, and facilitate planning. However, these passive systems that rely on disease recognition and manual reporting are inadequate for rapidly identifying emerging patterns of illnesses.

Unlike traditional systems, syndromic surveillance is a system of data collection and analysis in which a clinical syndrome (signs and symptoms) or incident disease clusters are the focus of investigation rather than a specific disease. Systems are designed to collect data during the earliest manifestations of a disease, before a diagnosis is made. By identifying abnormally high visit rates for a specific syndrome, an early signal of BT attack may be detected. For example, in an anthrax attack the initial clinical presentation of patients with respiratory complaints would proceed a laboratory diagnosis by a few days. Early identification would allow public health officials to limit the scope of the outbreak. Ideally, these systems would not only identify disease outbreaks early but would do so with 100% sensitivity and a high degree of specificity. Systems may be designed for one or more of the following purposes: (1) to identify early cases of disease caused by terrorism, (2) to find aberrant patterns of disease in the context of a widespread exposure, (3) to track proxy syndromes by geographic and temporal distribution to identify possible cases, and (4) to provide reassurance that terrorism has not been found.

HISTORY

Immediately after the terrorist attacks on the World Trade Center in New York, the NYC Department of Health and Mental Hygiene became concerned about the possibility of a secondary attack with a biological agent. Fifteen city hospitals participated in a manual system that involved coding each ED visit into one of twelve syndromes. Based on this coding, patients could be classified as having symptoms that might result from exposure to a BT agent or as a sequela of the WTC attacks. Both geographic and hospital alarms prompted further investigation. Although no syndrome of bioterrorism was identified, a number of important lessons were learned: (1) significant technical and staff resources at the DOHMH as well as in individual EDs was required and limited the effort to 30 days, (2) manual data entry resulted in coding errors, (3) although 7 patients in the city had cutaneous anthrax during this period they were not picked up by this system, as 6 of the 7 did not seek care in the ED, and (4) due to the heterogeneity of symptoms and diagnosis within syndromes, deciding when to pursue and investigate with chart review was difficult. Although this system did not detect the anthrax attack, it did serve to identify a number of the issues that needed to be addressed by those planning syndromic surveillance systems. Electronic collection and analysis, the development of appropriate syndrome categories, and the need to look beyond the ED for data collection would become the focus of work in New York and elsewhere.

BIOLOGICAL WEAPONS: CDC CATEGORIES

The Centers for Disease Control has identified 35 potential BT agents that have can be utilized as biologic weapons. Three categories have been created to set priorities for public health preparedness. Category A agents are those that are easily disseminated or transmitted from person to person, result in high mortality, are likely to cause panic and social disruption, and present the greatest risk to national safety. These include: anthrax, smallpox, plaque, tularemia, hemorrhagic fever viruses, and botulism. With the exception of botulism, these illnesses present initially as flu-like illnesses with fever and malaise. The presence of GI symptoms, rash, and hemorrhagic syndromes may also aid in the diagnosis. The challenge is to define syndromes that are broad enough to include all likely presentations but narrow enough to exclude patients with common illnesses.

DATA COLLECTION

Fortunately the need for this type of surveillance has occurred at the same time computerized records have become more prevalent in hospitals, pharmacies, Emergency Departments, and EMS systems across the country. This allows for automated collection, transfer, and processing of information. The challenge is to develop a system that recognizes an abnormal event in a timely manner in order to reduce morbidity and mortality. The developers of these systems must deal with issues of privacy, archiving, issuing alerts, sensitivity, validity, and cost.

The Emergency Department has been the primary focus of syndromic surveillance implementation. Other data sources that have been reported include clinical impressions of ambulance log sheets, over-the-counter drug sales, consumer health hotline telephone calls, ambulatory visit care record, and school or work absenteeism.

ED Logs: Chief Complaints

In 1999 Wayne State University developed and tested the feasibility of a web-based surveillance program based on patients' chief complaints in the Emergency Department. Triage data was sorted into five chief complaint groups. Separate chief complaint groups were identified for all Category A threats. For example, the anthrax group consists of cough, dyspnea, fever, lethargy, pleuritic chest pain, headache, upper respiratory infection, weakness or fatigue, vomiting, and generalized abdominal pain. Historical data was used as a control. Using the anthrax criteria, they were able to successfully identify the influenza outbreak within the first week. They emphasize, as do other public agencies, that syndromic surveillance can only detect potential threat exposures. Once an aberrant signal is detected it is essential that public heath officials follow-up with field investigations.

Traditionally, the nurses at triage record chief complaints in free-text format. This results in a large degree of variability. Patients express their symptoms in different terminology, which is then recorded by the triage nurse. Aronsky demonstrated that all chief complaints to the ED could be categorized into 57 categories. Day utilized computer algorithms to recognize a combination of words, word fragments, and word patterns to link free-text-compliant fields to 20 reason-for-visit categories. They suggest that reason-for-visit taxonomy is well suited for syndromic surveillance, as patients who look similar on presentation will be grouped together for analysis.

ICD-9 Codes

ICD-9 codes are universally used in the United States and are considered diagnostically more accurate than chief complaints. There is a great deal of latitude that the coder can exercise when picking a particular code. As a result, an increase in incidence of a disease may not be recognized as cases are distributed across a number of related codes. For example, an asthmatic with a chief complaint of difficulty breathing might be labeled with a number of ICD-9 codes: wheezing (786.07), acute asthma (493), acute bronchiolitis (466.1), and viral infection (480). Additional disadvantages of ICD-9 codes are the delay from the time care is provided to the time a code is assigned as well as the biases of physicians and coders as they seek to enhance revenues.

The Department of Defense's ESSENCE program has developed broad syndrome groups using ICD-9 codes that approximate natural infectious disease outbreaks or bioterrorism. Syndrome groups were created using all possible codes. These syndrome groups are now being used for routine surveillance at all military medical treatment facilities. These syndrome definitions and associated ICD-9 coded syndrome groups can be used in syndromic surveillance systems to allow for comparability and evaluation among programs.

Correlation Between Chief Complain and ICD-9

Beitel and colleagues at Children's Hospital in Boston compared the sensitivity and specificity of ED chief complaints and ICD-9 codes. Both chief complaints and ICD-9 codes demonstrated excellent specificity and moderate specificity for all respiratory infections. They were also able to demonstrate that adding the chief complaint codes of fever and earache could raise the sensitivity but lower the specificity. Although ICD-9 codes are superior to chief complaints, the timeliness of chief complaints and the possibility of improving the accuracy and/or sensitivity of chief complaint codes make them an attractive alternative.

Issues of Sensitivity and Specificity

A challenge for all systems is to establish the correct balance between sensitivity and specificity. Systems that are too sensitive will result in frequent false alarms. This will tax the resources of public health officials as well as EDs and other clinicians. Frequent expenditures of resources investigating false alarms could potentially erode the confidence of the medical professionals utilizing the system. From a practical point of view, no public health system will be able to sustain a system that identifies more alarms than it can muster the resources to investigate. However, a system that is too specific and lacks sensitivity risks missing a significant event. The degree of sensitivity needs to be flexible and allow for a decrease in threshold levels during periods of high concern. To date no system has provided an early warning of a bioterrorist event. However, the sensitivity of these systems can be tested using naturally occurring outbreaks such as annual influenza epidemics and through simulation models.

DATA ANALYSIS

Essential to the recognition of an aberrant event is the establishment of the baseline incidence of disease syndromes. In the Emergency Department the baseline for utilization rates for different syndromes must be established and the predictable effects of seasonal and epidemic variability understood. Once the baseline is established, alarm thresholds can be set.

The statistical methodology utilized needs to be able to identify both temporal and geographic clusters of events that may merit additional investigation. The ability to examine small geographic areas is important, as disease outbreaks in a BT event may be confined. Analysis that includes that area in a larger region may be unable to detect the outbreak. Most of the statistical techniques being utilized for syndromic surveillance have been adapted from analytical methods designed for other purposes. The application of advanced space-time analytic methods may detect aberrations in bioterrorism surveillance data with greater sensitivity, specificity, and timeliness.

REGULATORY REQUIREMENTS

The HIPPA Privacy Rule should not limit a state's ability to perform its public health functions. Public health authorities can utilize the surveillance to determine the existence of cases of an illness and disseminate that information to benefit the community. These efforts should be made with respect for individual's privacy rights. Strategies to lessen the risk of privacy violations include: collecting the minimum amount of identifiable data necessary, assigning collection and storage to agencies with a legal mandate and tradition of maintaining confidentiality, collecting aggregated data rather than individual data, de-identifying aggregated data, and using decentralized data. It is assumed that public health agencies have systems to keep confidential the large amount of data they receive. In some systems encrypted identifiers are utilized and individuals are identified and contacted only in the event of an aberrant signal. This increases the burden on primary-care providers to provide timely information in the event of an outbreak. Most public health functions occur at a state level. Local disease reporting laws should be consulted before the establishment of a syndromic surveillance system.

SYSTEM EXAMPLE: NEW YORK CITY

Since November 2001, the NYC Department of Health and Mental Hygiene has operated a syndromic surveillance system using ED visit data supplied in an electronic format. All ED visits from 40 hospitals in the city are logged for date and time of visit, age, sex, home zip code, and free-text chief complaint. An algorithm scans chief complaints for character strings and places these complaints into a single syndrome category. The two syndromes of interest for bioterrorism are acute respiratory and fever syndromes in persons greater than 13 years of age. Citywide daily temporal analysis and spatial clustering analysis are both used to identify significant signals. A signal is investigated by reviewing the data provided by the ED. This is followed by a phone call to the ED to alert them to the unusual disease pattern and ask if they have noted an increase in the frequency of syndrome visits or admission of seriously ill patients. If there is concern a field investigation is done with chart review, patient interviews, and on-site discussions with clinicians. In the first year of operation the system did not identify any BT-related illness but was able to identify community increases in gastrointestinal illness, respiratory illness, and fever associated with the peak of influenza activity.

CDC VALIDITY: HOW ARE SYSTEMS EVALUATED?

The CDC has created a framework for evaluating public health surveillance systems for early detection of outbreaks. A comprehensive evaluation will address four categories: system description, outbreak detection, experience, and conclusions and recommendations. Further details can be obtained online at http://www.cdc.gov/mmwr.

CONCLUSIONS

The ability of an ED-based surveillance system to provide early detection of a BT event remains unproved, and the optimal method of surveillance is a matter of ongoing debate and research. What is clear is that these systems ideally must be timely and provide a high level of sensitivity and specificity.

REFERENCES

Aronsky D, Kendall D, Merkley, K, James BC, Haug PJ. 2001. A comprehensive set of coded chief complaints for the emergency department. *Acad Emerg Med* **8**:980–989.

Beitel A, Olson KL, Reis BY, Mandl KD. 2004. Use of emergency department chief complaint and diagnostic codes for identifying respiratory illness in a pediatric population. *Pediatr Emerg Care* **6**:355–360.

Begier EM, Sockwell D, Branch LM, Davies-Cole JO, Jones LH, Edwards L, Casani JA, Blythe D. 2003. The national capital region's emergency department syndromic surveillance system: do chief complaint and discharge diagnosis yield different results? *Emerg Infect Dis* **9**: 393–396.

Bravata DM, McDonald KM, Dmith WM. 2004. Systemic review: surveillance systems for early detection of bioterrorism-related diseases. *Ann Intern Med.* **140**:910–922.

Buehler JW, Hopkins RS, Overhage JM, Sosin DM, Tong V. 2004. Framework for evaluating public health surveillance systems for early detection of outbreaks. *MMWR* **7**(53):1–11.

Day FC, Schriger DL, La M. 2004. Automated linking of free-text complaints to reason-for-visit categories and international classification of diseases diagnoses in emergency department patient record databases. *Ann Emerg Med* **43**:401–409.

Department of Defense. 2001. *Global emerging infections system. ESSENCE: electronic surveillance system for the early notification of community-base epidemics.* http://www.geis.ha.osd.mil/geis/surveillanceactivities/essence/essence.asp.

Heffernan R, Mostashari F, Das D, Karpati A, Kulldorff M, Weiss D. 2004. Syndromic surveillance in public health practice, New York City. *Emerg Infect Dis* **10**:858–864.

Irvin CB, Nauhan PP, Rice R. 2003. Syndromic analysis of computerized emergency department patients' chief complaints: an opportunity for bioterrorism and influenza surveillance. *Ann Emerg Med* **41**:447–445.

Kaufman AF, Meltzer MI, Schmid GP. 1997. The economic impact of a bioterrorist attack: are prevention and post-attack intervention programs justifiable? *Emerg Infect Dis* **3**:83–94.

Moran GJ, Talan DA. 2003. Update on emerging infections: News from the Centers for Disease Control and Prevention. *Ann Emerg Med* **41**:414–418.

Mostashari F, Hartman J. 2003. Syndromic surveillance: a local perspective. *J Urban Health* **80**: 11–17.

Reis BY, Mandl KD. 2003. Time-series modeling for syndromic surveillance. *BMC Med Inform Decis Mak* **3**(1):2.

84

JCAHO EMERGENCY MANAGEMENT STANDARDS

Dan Wiener, MD*

JCAHO

The mission of the Joint Commission on the Accreditation of Hospitals (JCAHO) is to continuously improve the safety and quality of care provided to the public through the provision of healthcare accreditation and related services that support performance improvement in healthcare organizations. JCAHO accomplishes this mission by setting standards for performance in specific areas affecting the quality of patient care and emergency management.

In January 2001, the Joint Commission's disaster preparedness standards were modified to introduce the concepts of emergency management and community involvement in the management process. These modifications call for accredited organizations to take an "all-hazards" approach to disaster planning—reviewing, analyzing and addressing all hazards that are determined to be credible and serious threats to the community. JCAHO defines an emergency as a natural or manmade event that significantly disrupts the environment of care, that significantly disrupts care and treatment, or that results in sudden and significantly changed or increased demands for the organization's services.

The JCAHO 2004 Environment of Care Standards contains two elements that are relevant to emergency management:

— The Hospital Addresses Emergency Management (EC 4.1)
— The Hospital Conducts drills regularly to test emergency management (EC 4.20)

*Department of Emergency Medicine, St. Luke's/Roosevelt Hospital Center

THE HOSPITAL ADDRESSES EMERGENCY MANAGEMENT (EC 4.1)

The plan needs to address the four phases on an emergency: mitigation, preparedness, response and recovery, and hazard vulnerability analysis. The plan must be flexible and allow response to different situations involving both internal (institution-based) and external (community-based) disasters. The plan must also be scalable: it must have the ability to respond to emergencies as diverse as a heat wave or a terrorist attack. Plans must clearly describe areas of responsibility, circumstances under which the plan is to be activated, who is in charge, and who is authorized to activate the plan. It is required that the organization have an incident command structure for emergency management that is consistent with that used by the local community.

JCAHO advocates taking an all-hazards approach to emergency preparedness. Hazard Vulnerability Analysis (HVA) is an essential first step in the planning process. HVA is defined as the identification of potential emergencies and the direct and indirect effects these emergencies have on the healthcare organization's operations and the demand for its services. HVA is a formal assessment of hazards that might affect the organization or the surrounding community. External threats could involve hazardous weather, power outages, civil disturbances, terrorism, hazardous material release, or transportation accidents. Internal threats could involve fire or explosion, fumes, loss of environmental services (heat, water, power), loss of medical gases, or a hazardous material release. Once an organization has identified the potential threats, an attempt should be made to assess the likelihood of each of these possibilities occurring. Preparatory sessions, which involve brainstorming and a review of historical data, will assist in this process. The local community planning board may be able to provide the needed historical information. Once a list of vulnerabilities is established, it should be rank-ordered in terms of probability and severity. Finally, the organization must determine its level of preparedness and that of community for each of these possibilities. Performing a "gap analysis" will help organizations understand toward what areas it needs to direct future resources. Sample HVA tools are available from Joint Commission Resources.

Once the HVA analysis is complete, the issues of mitigation, preparedness, response, and recovery can be addressed. Mitigation is defined as the activities undertaken to lessen the severity and impact of a disaster or emergency. Some mitigation activities involve improving structural elements of the hospital, such as fireproofing or providing uninterrupted power through standby generators. A number of hospitals have recently built or purchased decontamination facilities in response to the threat of biologic and chemical terrorism. Other activities may involve a series of steps to respond to and lessen the impact to the institution or community of an unpreventable event (i.e., sandbags during a flood). One approach to mitigation is to utilize a cost-benefit analysis. In this way, scarce resources can be allocated to areas most likely to provide the greatest protection.

Preparedness is defined as activities an organization undertakes to build capacity and identify resources that may be used should a disaster or emergency occur. Organizations must plan to be self-sufficient for a period of 72 to 96 hours. Some activities that will assure preparedness include an inventory of resources and creating a system for procuring additional resources. This can be accomplished through prearranged agreements with vendors and other healthcare organizations. A system should also be in place for credentialing of licensed personnel who may assist during an emergency. Plans should also be in place for utilization of hospital volunteers during an emergency. Mutual aid agreements with other organizations should be in place. Preparedness is an ongoing process, and the organization must have a system in place to constantly assess its state of preparedness and needs.

Response is the actual emergency management. It defines how an organization treats victims as well as how it reduces the secondary impact on the organization.

Recovery is the process by which an organization deescalates after an emergency. It is essential that an organization have a plan to get back to normal functioning. This plan should include specific steps and stages. Financial, staffing, and service needs all should be incorporated into this portion of the plan.

STAFF EDUCATION AND TRAINING

An emergency preparedness plan can only be successfully implemented if all staff are appropriately oriented and educated. This education must take place before an emergency occurs and on an ongoing basis. Education needs to address issues appropriate to the individual: specific roles and responsibilities during emergencies; how to recognize specific types of emergencies; the information and skills required to perform assigned duties during emergencies; the backup communication system used during emergencies; and how supplies and equipment are obtained during emergencies. These educational goals should be part of employee orientation programs as well as core competency programs. The competencies required will vary throughout areas of the organization and by job category. Although the Joint Commission expects staff to possess competency, there is no specific recommendation on the frequency of training. It does recognize that annual training is one way to meet the competency goals it has established. The plan should specifically address who is responsible for training and how frequently it is conducted.

ANNUAL REVIEW

The plan must provide for procedures for an annual evaluation of the organization's HVA and of the emergency management plan, including objectives, scope, functionality, and effectiveness. Annual reviews should assess what aspects of the plan did and did not function well in the previous year as well as anticipated and identify issues for the upcoming year. Discussing specific scenarios will reveal gaps in the plan and allow for the greatest number of issues to be addressed. How this evaluation occurs must be specifically stated. It is recommended that this work be done by an interdisciplinary and interdepartmental committee. Representatives from administration, risk management, safety and security, public relations, materials management, pharmacy, and clinical staff should all be included. It is essential that planning be done in cooperation with outside organizations, including volunteer agencies and community contacts.

THE HOSPITAL CONDUCTS DRILLS REGULARLY TO TEST EMERGENCY MANAGEMENT (EC 4.20)

The response phase of the emergency management plan should be tested twice a year, either in response to an actual emergency or in planned drills. Drills are conducted at least four months apart, and no more than eight months apart. At least one drill a year must include an influx of volunteer or simulated individuals (a tabletop drill cannot be substituted). The organization must participate in at least one community-wide (local geographic area, town, city, or region) practice drill annually relevant to the priority emergencies identified by the organization's HVA, which assesses the communication, coordination, and effectiveness of the organization's and community command structures.

Drills are an essential part of the planning process. They are the best way to identify problems with the plan and areas that need improvement. In advance of the drill, leadership and staff have the opportunity to review the training they have received in emergency preparedness. Each drill should be critiqued to identify the strengths and weaknesses in the emergency management plan. This critique should include an assessment of the adequacy of staff training. Strategies for improving the response should be identified. This should be a multidisciplinary process and involve licensed and non-licensed staff as well as participants from other organizations.

COMMAND STRUCTURE

One of the tasks of the planning team is to determine the most effective command structure for the organization. The healthcare organization and community must use similar terminology to facilitate integration. Although no specific system is required, the most common model being utilized is the Hospital Emergency Incident Command System (HEICS). It defines responsibilities (job action sheets), reporting channels, and common terminology for hospitals, fire departments, local governments, and other agencies. The HEICS template can be found at www.emsa.cahwnet.gov. The key members of the command structure include: Incident Commander, Public Information Officer, Safety and Security Officer, and a Liaison Officer. Certain types of disasters may require representation from community organizations in the hospitals command structure.

COMMUNICATION

The plan needs to clearly define how and under what circumstances the organization will communicate with outside agencies and staff. Creation of redundant systems will be a key element of this preparation. In the HEICS structure the Public Information Officer will be responsible for communication with the media, and the Liaison Officer will coordinate communication with outside agencies.

OPERATIONS

The plan needs to address a number of operational contingencies that would be needed to operate during the events identified in the HVA. This could include mass casualty events, biologic events, chemical events, or events that require evacuation or establishment of alternative care sites. The logistics of ongoing patient care activities, staff support, critical supplies (pharmaceuticals, medical, food), transportation, and security all need to be specified. The plan should also address the means of preserving essential building services such as electricity, water, ventilation, fuel, and medical gases.

INTERACTION WITH THE COMMUNITY

The emergency management plan and HVA should be integrated with local and regional emergency management agencies. Integration of the organization's role in relation to community-wide emergency response agencies, including identification of the command structure in the community, must be defined. It is essential that the organization and local agencies integrate planning activities and agree on the levels of responsibility that reside with each. The plan should be specific about how the relationship between external facilities and agencies will be initiated, continued, and ended. Information must be shared on a timely bases regarding: essential elements of the command structures and specifics regarding the names, roles, and telephone numbers of individuals in the command structures. Resources and assets that could potentially be shared or pooled will need to be shared. Hospitals must maintain accurate lists of the names of care recipients and deceased individuals brought to the organization, so as to facilitate identification and location of victims of a disaster.

RESOURCES

JCAHO. *Healthfinder*. http://www.jcaho.org/general+public/who+jc/index.htm.

REFERENCES

JCAHO. 2002. *Guide to emergency management planning in healthcare*. http://www.jcrinc.com/publications.asp?durki=1022&site=4&return=78.

JCAHO. 2004. *Accreditation manual for hospitals*. http://www.jcrinc.com/subscribers/perspectives.asp?durki=2815&site=10&return=27.

85 HEALTH AND THE HUMANITARIAN/ DISASTER WORKER

John D. Cahill, MD*

OVERVIEW

As long as disasters continue to occur, there will be a need for individuals with certain expertise to respond to these events. To meet this need, there are workers who dedicate their lives to this cause. The nature of disasters places responders in unfamiliar and unstable events and locations. These workers are at risk for a multitude of occupational injuries and disease. Ideally, a prescreening medical/psychiatric process should occur before sending individuals out into the field.

CHALLENGES

Location

Often the environment is unpredictable due to the nature of the event or disaster. There may be damage or destruction to infrastructure (water, sanitation, roads, buildings, communication). Environmental hazards may be a direct cause of the disaster, or the worker may not have been exposed to them before. Regions afflicted with war and conflict pose a threat. Unfamiliar diseases and lack of proper medical care, supplies, and personnel may also exist.

Self-Neglect

Although these workers are concerned about the well-being and safety of those they are assisting, they often neglect their own health. There are endless tragic stories of workers being killed from lack of personal safety equipment, entering a dangerous environment (unsafe buildings, crossfire, landmines), not wearing seatbelts, and not using common sense.

*Department of Emergency Medicine and Division of Infectious Diseases, St. Luke's/Roosevelt Hospital Center, New York

Vaccination

All workers should have appropriate up-to-date vaccinations prior to embarking on a disaster response. These recommendations will vary depending on the affected region. However, basic vaccines would include: MMR (measles, mumps, rubella), dT (diphtheria tetanus), IPV (injectable polio vaccine), Hepatitis B, and Hepatitis A. Depending on the situation/region/age the following vaccines may be considered: yellow fever, Japanese encephalitis, rabies, typhoid, cholera, meningococcal, influenza, and pneumococcal.

Insect-Borne Disease

Malaria, dengue fever, and tick-borne illnesses are only a few of the potential diseases that one can become infected with. Appropriate measures should be taken to avoid insect-borne disease, and these recommendations will vary depending upon location. In general, an insect repellant that contains 25 to 50% DEET should be applied to exposed skin surfaces. Permethrin can be used to treat mosquito nets and clothing. A mosquito net should also be used in malarious regions. The importance of proper compliance with antimalarials cannot be understated. Humanitarian and disaster workers are notorious for refusing to take antimalarials or having a high level of noncompliance. Emergency self-treatment for malaria has no role as an option for chemoprophylaxis in the initial phases of a disaster response.

Food- and Water-Borne Illnesses

A multitude of illnesses can be acquired from food and water. As a rule of thumb, all water should be bottled, boiled, and filtered, or be known to come from a safe source. Ice cubes are generally not an option. Beverages that are generally considered safe include: boiled teas and coffees, bottled soda, wine, and beer. Milk has to be pasteurized. All meats and seafood should be thoroughly cooked. Vegetables need to be cooked or thoroughly cleaned. Fruits need to be washed and peeled. It should be remembered that schistosomiasis is acquired from standing or swimming in freshwater lakes and rivers and is endemic throughout a large part of the tropics.

Traveler's diarrhea is commonplace and usually responds well to fluids (avoid dairy products) and loperamide. An antibiotic (ciprofloxacin) may be considered in those cases where the diarrhea is not responding to loperamide, there is fever and diarrhea, and where the diarrhea is going on for more than 2 to 3 days.

Mental Health

Mental health is a topic that is often neglected and overlooked. The scene of disaster response is often chaotic, unstructured, and stressful. Individuals are placed in dangerous situations and are faced with the anguish, suffering, and death of other humans. Often the numbers can be unimaginable and difficult to accept. Sleep patterns can be altered, placing more stress on the individual. Often there is the feeling that there is no time to rest. Alcohol and drugs can often seem appealing in these circumstances. This is all compounded by the fact that the individual's usual environment and support system is not available (significant other, family, and friends).

Sexually Transmitted Diseases

STDs are not uncommon in workers who spend any significant time in the field. The reason for this is multifactorial: they are away from their significant other, they experience feelings of isolation and loneliness, they use drugs and alcohol, they are outside of cultural norms, they experience a feeling of anonymity, there is a lack of reliable birth control available, and the problem of prostitution as a means to receive money or other goods.

EVALUATION OF THE RETURNED WORKER

Although there is limited data on humanitarian/disaster workers and patterns of disease and injury, some data from travel medicine studies can be extrapolated. It should be remembered that common accidents (car accidents, drowning) and illnesses (coronary artery disease, upper respiratory tract infections, bronchitis, pneumonia, urinary tract infections) still happen abroad. Fever, diarrhea, and skin conditions are common complaints. A detailed discussion of the febrile traveler is beyond the scope of this chapter. However, initial evaluation entails a careful history and physical exam. Laboratory results can help limit the differential diagnosis and should include a complete blood count with differential, thick and thin blood film for malaria (where endemic), blood cultures, urinalysis, and liver function tests. Chest x-ray and serological studies may be obtained depending on the history. Patients with diarrhea should have three sets of stool examined for fecal leukocytes, ova, and parasites, and sent for culture. Screening for sexually transmitted diseases, including HIV, should be performed where appropriate.

It is important to remember that eosinophilia can be caused by infectious sources, allergic disease states, and hematological and neoplastic processes. The physician should always think of noninfectious causes before engaging in the million-dollar workup. Helminths are the most common infectious cause of eosinophilia. Protozoan infections such as malaria do not typically cause eosinophilia. One must remember that multiple infections may be present and that the absence of eosinophilia does not exclude parasitic infection.

Several key points to remember in the evaluation of these patients:

1. Fever after travel may be unrelated to exposures during travel.
2. Always think of malaria.
3. Exposure to many widely distributed infections is more common during travel than during life at home.
4. Reexamine the febrile patient if the initial evaluation does not suggest a specific diagnosis.
5. Keep in mind the public health implications.

86 IMMUNIZATION SCHEDULES AND RECOMMENDATIONS

Arathi Rao, MD, Maria Mileno MD*

Maintaining an adequate defense against infections is an important aspect of public health, and the use of vaccines has been one of the greatest achievements in this regard. Immunization is the act of artificially inducing immunity or protection from disease. There are two types of immunization: active and passive. Active immunization is achieved by administrating a vaccine or toxoid that stimulates the body's immune system to produce antibodies, cell-mediated immunity, or both. Passive immunization is temporary protection through the administration of exogenously produced antibodies. Examples of the latter are either transplacental transfer of antibodies to the fetus or through administration of immunoglobulins. In this chapter we have summarized vaccine schedules in several tables for easy reference.

Table 1 refers to recommended childhood and adolescent immunization schedules. It represents the standard of care for immunizations beginning with newborn individuals. The range of ages considered for those who are "on schedule" are depicted with an extended arrow. Catchup immunization schedules are marked with a "cui." Preadolescent assessment should be done ideally between ages 11 and 12, and recommended vaccines for this age group are depicted with an "X." If a vaccine series is not completed during this age range, they can be administered at the next opportunity. Certain populations may also require Hepatitis A vaccine. Examples include travelers to endemic regions, healthcare workers, and HIV-, Hepatitis B-, and Hepatitis C-infected individuals. Table 2 refers to recommended immunizations for adults.

Advising travelers has become a specialist's task, and advising persons with underlying medical problems can get complicated. Travelers decide best about appropriate vaccinations in the setting of a consultation with a dedicated travel medicine specialist. These practitioners will review the traveler's medications and immune status to determine a safe strategy for their individual itinerary, and address other risks beyond vaccination, such as insect avoidance, malaria prophylaxis, and self-treatment strategies for common infectious disease problems such as travelers diarrhea. Table 3 refers to immunizations recommended for adults with underlying medical conditions. See Table 4 for immunizations recommended or contraindicated in the pregnant wo-

*Division of Infectious Disease, Brown University, Providence, Rhode Island

Table 1. Recommended Childhood and Adolescent Immunization Schedule—United States, 2004

Vaccine	Birth	1 mo	2 mo	4 mo	6 mo	12 mo	15 mo	18 mo	24 mo	4–6 yr	11–12 yr	13–18 yr
		←		→	←			→				
Hepatitis B	HepB #1	Only if mom HbsAg (−)					←	→		HepB series (cui)	X	
Hepatitis B			HepB #2			←	HepB #3	→			X	
Diphtheria, tetanus, pertussis			Dtap	Dtap	Dtap ←		Dtap	→		Dtap	Td X	Td (cui)
Haemophilus influenza type B			Hib	Hib	Hib	←	Hib →				X ←	→
Inactivated poliovirus (IPV)			IPV	IPV		←	IPV	→	←	IPV	X	→
Measles, mumps, rubella (MMR)						←	MMR #1	→	←	MMR #2 →	X	MMR #2
Varicella (Var)					←		Var		←	Var (cui)	X →	→
Pneumococcal (PCV) (PPV)			PCV	PCV	PCV		PCV		PCV (cui)		PPV X	
Influenza (Inf)							Inf (yearly)		←	Inf (yearly)	X	→
			vaccines below this line are for selected people									
HepA										HepA series	X	

X = preadolescent assessment (11–12 yr); cui = catchup immunization; PCV = pneumococcal conjugate vaccine; PPV = pneumococcal polysaccharide vaccine; arrows = range of recommended ages.

Approved by the Advisory Committee on Immunization Practice (ACIP), the American Academy of Pediatrics (AAP), and the American Academy of Family Physicians (AAFP). Table adapted from the CDC.

Table 2. Recommended Adult Immunization Schedule—United States, 2003–2004

Vaccine	19–49 yr	50–64 yr	65 yr and older
Tetanus/diphtheria	1 dose, booster every 10 year ↔		
Influenza	1 dose annually ↔		
Pneumococcal (polysaccharide)	1 dose ↔		1 dose ↔
Hepatitis A	2 doses (0, 6–12 months) ↔		
Hepatitis B	3 doses (0, 1–2, 4–6 months) ↔		
Measles, mumps, rubella (MMR)	1 dose if MMR vaccination history is unreliable; 2 doses for persons with occupational or other indications		
Varicella	2 doses (0, 4–8 wk) for persons who are susceptible ↔		
Meningococcal (polysaccharide)	(1 dose)* ↔		

*Special attention should be placed on vaccinating college-age students with the meningococcal vaccine due to added risks of close living quarters. Other adults who may require this vaccine are military personnel and those traveling to endemic countries of high risk.

This schedule indicates the recommended age groups for routine administration of currently licensed vaccine for person 19 years of age and older. Licensed combination vaccines may be used whenever any components of the combination are indicated and the other vaccine components are not contraindicated. Approved by the Advisory Committee on Immunization Practice (ACIP) and accepted by the American College of Obstetricians and Gynecologists (ACOG) and American Academy of Family Physicians (AAFP). This table is adapted from the CDC.

Table 3. Recommended Immunizations for Adults with Medical Conditions—2003–2004

Vaccine	Diabetes, COPD, heart disease	HIV	Severe immuno-sup-pression	Renal failure	Asplenia	Alcoholism chronic liver disease
Hepatitis A	UI	UI	UI	UI	UI	UI
Hepatitis B	R	R	R	R	R	R
Influenza	R	R	R	R	R	R
Measles, mumps, rubella	R	R**	C	R	R	R
Pneumo-coccal	R	R	R	R	R	R
Polio-myelitis (IPV)	UI	UI	UI	UI	UI	UI
Tetanus/ diphtheria	R	R	R	R	R	R
Varicella	R	C	C	R	R	R
BCG*	UI	C	C	UI	UI	UI
Meningo-coccal	UI	UI	UI	UI	R	UI
Typhoid						
(Vi)	UI	UI	UI	UI	UI	UI
(TY21a)	UI	C	C	UI	UI	UI
Vaccinia*	UI	C	C	UI	UI	UI

R = Recommended, UI = use if indicated, C = contraindicated.
*BCG and vaccinia vaccines are not available in the United States at this time.
**Administer only if CD4 count is >200.
Table adapted from CDC and *Educational Review Manual for Infectious Disease.*

Table 4. Vaccinations During Pregnancy

Vaccine	Recom-mended	Use if Indicated	Contra-indicated	Comment
Routine				
Hepatitis A		UI		Safety data not available; Theoretical risk of vaccination must be outweighed with risk of disease
Hepatitis B	R			
Influenza				
(inactivated)		R		
(live attenuated)			C	
Measles, mumps, rubella			C	
Pneumococcal		UI		? Safety data in 1st trimester
Poliomyelitis (IPV)		UI		For unimmunized women who need immediate protection IPV may be used
Tetanus/ diptheria	R			
Varicella			C	
Travel				
BCG			C	Not available in US
Japanese encephalitis				No data on safety
Meningo-coccal		UI		
Rabies		UI		If substantial risk of exposure
Typhoid				
(Vi)		UI		No data on any the three vaccines
(TY21a)		UI		
Vaccinia			C	Only administer if definite exposure to smallpox virus; not available in US
Yellow fever			C	Only administer if exposure to virus is unavoidable

R = recommended, UI= use if indicated, C = contraindicated.
Table adapted from CDC and *Educational Review Manual in Infectious Disease*.

Table 5. Recommended Dosing Schedules of Commonly Used Vaccines for Travel

Vaccine	Primary series	Booster	Indications
Hepatitis	1 dose for adults/children older than 2 yr	1 dose 6–12mo after 1st dose, Lifelong immunity after two doses	Travel to developing countries, Eastern Europe and Russia
Hepatitis B	3 doses, 1 each at 0, 1, 6 mo, and at 0, 7, 21 or 28 days	Fourth dose is needed at 12 mo for accelerated schedules for life-long immunity	Travelers to developing countries; healthcare workers, sexually active adolescents/adults not previously vaccinated
Hepatitis A and B (combined)	3 doses 0, 1 mo, 6 mo		as above
Immune globulin (IG)	One 2-ml dose IM, gluteus muscle, for 3 mo protction, 5 ml dose for 5 mo; pediatric dose, 0.02 ml/kg for 3-mo trip, 0.06 ml/kg for 5-mo	At 3–5 mo intervals	Exposure or anticipated unavoidable exposure to Hepatitis A. This is suboptimal to protection from Hepatitis A vaccine. May offer some protection for Rabies, Measles, Hepatitis B and Tetanus
Japanese encephalitis	3 doses, 1 each on days 0, 7, 30; 0, 7, 30; 1 ml SC for children >3 yr; 0.5 ml SC for <3 yr	After 3 yr	Travel to endemic countries: Malaysia, Myanmar, Cambodia, Laos, Nepal, Taiwan, Phillippines, Vietnam, Sri Lanka, North Thailand (at least 1-mo stay) Rarely required for short-term travelers
Meningococcus (A/C/Y/W-135)	1 dose subcutaneous	After 3 yr	Travelers to Sub-Saharan Africa during dry season (Dec–June); countries include: Kenya, Tanzania, Burundi, Mongolia. Also required for pilgrims to Mecca for the Hajj
Plague*	Risk to travelers, even those traveling to areas where disease has been reported, is low. Vaccination recommended only for those who have direct contact with diseased rodents or infected animals. This vaccine is not available in the US.		Chemoprophylaxis available to those traveling to high-risk areas
Poliomyeltis (IPV, inactivated)	1 dose at ages 2, 4, 6–18 mo and 4–6 yr	Once before travel	Travel to developing countries
Rabies	3 doses (1 ml IM, deltoid area) on days 0, 7, and 21 or 28	Boost after 2 yr or test serum for antibody level	Travel to developing countries; Endemic areas: Mexico, India, Nepal, Sri Lanka, Thailand, Vietman, and parts of S. Am.

Table 5, cont'd

Vaccine	Primary series	Booster	Indications
Tetanus/diphtheria (for unvaccinated individuals > 7yr of age)	3 doses (0.5 ml SC or IM) 1st and 2nd dose given 4–8 wk apart; 3rd dose at 6–12 mo after	Routinely every 10 yr	Ensure up-to-date on vaccination prior to travel
Typhoid, oral	I capsule orally every other day for 4 doses (> 6 yr old)	5 yr	Travelers anticipating prolonged exposure to potentially contaminated food/water; endemic areas
Typhoid, Vi capsular polysaccharide	single dose (0.5 ml IM) (> 2 yr old)	2 yr	include Indian subcontinent, parts of South, West, North Africa, Mexico, Haiti, Iran
Yellow fever	1 dose (0.5 ml SC) for those over 9 mo of age	10 yr	Required for travel to equatorial South America and Africa
Cholera, parenteral*	2 doses 1 wk or more apart (0.5 ml SC or IM); pediatric dose)0.3 ml for 5–10 yr, 0.2 ml for 6 mo to 4 yr	6 mo	Risk of cholera infection is very low; licensed vaccine in US is only 50% effective; only indicated for high-risk people working/living in endemic areas (S. and C. America, Africa, Asia) and poor sanitation
Cholera, live oral*	1 dose PO on an empty stomach for those 2 yr and older	6 mo (optimal booster not yet not yet determined)	

*Plague vaccine and Cholera vaccines are currently not available in the United States.
Tables adapted from *Infectious Disease Clinics of North America, Current Diagnosis and Treatment in Infectious Diseases, Educational Review Manual in Infectious Disease.*

man. Table 5 refers to dosing schedules and indications for administering travel vaccines. Note that BCG and vaccinia vaccines are not available in the United States at this time.

RESOURCES

CDC: http://www.cdc.gov/travel/htm

REFERENCES

American Academy of Family Physicians. 2005. *Age charts for periodic health examinations.* Available at http://www.aafp.org/exam/table2.html and http://www.aafp.org/exam/table4.html.

CDC. 2004. Recommended childhood and adolescent immunization schedule—United States, July–December 2004. *MMWR* **53**(16). http://www.cdc.gov/mmwr/pdf/ wk/mm5301-Immunization.pdf.

CDC. 2004. Recommended adult immunization schedule—United States, 2003–2004. MMWR **52**(40):965–969. http://www.cdc.gov/mmwr/preview/mmwrhtml/mm5240a6.htm.

CDC. 2004. Recommended immunizations for adults with medical conditions—United States, 2003–2004.

Hale D, Milne C. 2001. Infections in travelers. In *Current diagnosis and treatment in infectious diseases.* Ed W Wilson, M Sande.

Jong E. 1998. Immunizations for international travel. *Infect Dis Clin North Am* **12**(2):249–266.

Mileno M. 2004. Immunizations. In *Educational Review Manual in Infectious Disease*. Ed B Cunha. New York: Castle Connolly Graduate Medical Publishing.

Mileno M. 2004. Preparation of immunocompromised travelers. In *Travel medicine*, pp. 249–255. Ed JS Keystone, PE Korasrsky, DO Freedman, HD Nothdurff, BA Connor. Edinburgh: Mosby.

Pickering LK, Baker C, Overtuff G, Prober C. 2003. Active and passive immunization. In: *Red Book: 2003 report of the committee on infectious diseases*, 26th ed. Ed LK Pickering. Elk Grove Village: American Academy of Pediatrics.

Suk K, Mileno M. 2005. Challenging scenarios in a travel clinic: advising the complex traveler. *Infect Dis Clin North Am*. In press.

87 HEALTHCARE WORKER EXPOSURES TO BLOOD AND BODY FLUIDS

Roland Merchant, MD*

INTRODUCTION

Healthcare workers frequently come in contact with blood or body fluids from patients harboring communicable diseases. Respiratory droplets, weeping skin lesions, needlesticks, human bites, contaminated instruments, etc., provide means of exposure to these diseases. Although most contacts do not result in infections, some can lead to disastrous consequences. It is fortunate that consequent serious infections are rare and the vast majority of concerning exposures are preventable. When accidental exposures or breaches to infection control procedures do occur, post-exposure prophylaxis (PEP) might help reduce the chances of acquiring selected diseases.

TRANSMISSION RISK

Transmission necessarily depends on the type and means of exposure, the body fluids involved, the disease and health status of the source and exposed person, and the inoculum, pathogenicity, and transmissibility of the organism in question. Knowing these factors for a particular organism and exposure type helps in assessing the risk and in most cases can immediately reduce a healthcare worker's concern. For example, if an exposure cannot result in infection, e.g., a urine splash from an HIV-infected source, then further anxiety-provoking evaluation and treatment can be avoided.

Herpes, influenza, meningococcus, pertussis, syphilis, tuberculosis, and varicella are some of the many infections healthcare workers can acquire from their patients (see Resources section). Transmission risk is not estimable for most of these organisms

*Department of Emergency Medicine, Brown University, Providence, Rhode Island

since only case reports or series exist describing healthcare worker infections. Given that many of these diseases are common, patient visits to healthcare workers for them are innumerable, and the case reports are few, the transmission risk for the majority of these pathogens must be quite small. In general, exposures involving percutaneous injuries, mucosae, and non-intact skin are of higher transmission risk than to other body surfaces.

INITIAL POST-EXPOSURE MANAGEMENT

Healthcare workers sustaining blood or body fluid exposures should enact basic first aid practices to prevent infection. For percutaneous injuries, the sharp object should be removed and the injured body part washed with clean or sterile water. Hydrogen peroxide, povidone/iodine, bleach, or alcohol solutions are generally harmful in wound management so should not be used. Soap solutions may be of benefit in cleaning the wound but likely do not mitigate the risk of transmission. Apply direct pressure to bleeding wounds with sterile bandages. A topical antibiotic may help reduce bacterial contamination and speed wound healing. Cutting wounds or expressing blood from wounds is not advised, as it will likely not reduce the risk of infection and will only cause further damage and risk of another percutaneous injury. Although there are no data on this subject for HIV- and hepatitis-contaminated wounds, closure of lacerations after proper irrigation should not increase the risk of HIV or hepatitis and in most cases helps reduce the risk of bacterial infections. Mucocutaneous injured surfaces should be promptly washed with clean or sterile water with or without soap. Contact lenses should be removed and not worn again. Eyes should be flushed with copious amounts of clean or sterile water. The immediate source of exposure, e.g., needle or sharp object, should be disposed of in accordance with proper biohazard procedures. Contaminated needles or sharp objects should not be sent to a laboratory for testing since injury to laboratory workers or others may occur from handling these objects.

POST-EXPOSURE PROPHYLAXIS

HIV PEP

Several public health groups recommend PEP with antiretroviral medications for healthcare workers potentially exposed to HIV. Table 1 summarizes the CDC recommendations. PEP may be more efficacious if administered within an hour of the exposure and may not be helpful (although not contraindicated) 72 hours post-exposure. PEP should be taken for 28 days; shorter periods may not confer adequate protection against HIV. Pregnant women may take HIV PEP, but should be aware of the unknown effects of HIV PEP on their fetus. PEP should only be taken voluntarily, and recipients should be aware that it may not be effective for them. It is preferable for PEP recipients to be under the care of a healthcare provider experienced in monitoring HIV PEP. Baseline and follow-up for hematologic, electrolyte, renal, and liver profile testing is necessary depending upon the PEP regimen prescribed. PEP recipients should undergo HIV testing at the time of their exposure as well as at least 3 months post-exposure, but testing should not delay receipt of HIV PEP. HIV PEP is unnecessary if

Table 1. HIV PEP Recommendations from the CDC

Exposure type	Source's HIV status HIV infected sources	Unknown HIV status sources
Percutaneous sharp exposures		
Higher-risk events (e.g., solid bore needlesticks)	3 PEP drug regimen	Consider a 2 PEP drug regimen when likelihood of source HIV infection is high
Lower-risk events (e.g., hollow bore needlesticks)	2–3 PEP drug regimen depending upon severity of source's HIV illness and viral load	Consider a 2 PEP drug regimen when likelihood of source HIV infection is high
Mucous membrane exposures		
Higher-risk events (e.g., large volume exposures)	2–3 PEP drug regimen depending upon severity of source's HIV illness and viral load	Consider a 2 PEP drug regimen when likelihood of source HIV infection is high
Lower-risk events (e.g., small volume exposures)	Consider a 2 PEP drug regimen	Consider a 2 PEP drug regimen when likelihood of source HIV infection is high

PEP regimens
2 PEP drug regimen: zidovudine 150 mg BID + lamivudine 150 mg BID p.o. for 28 days
3 PEP drug regimen: zidovudine 300 mg BID + lamivudine 150 mg BID + nelfinavir 1250 mg BID OR indinavir 800 mg TID p.o.

the source is not HIV infected or if the healthcare worker sustaining the exposure is known to be HIV infected.

The CDC advocates a hierarchical approach to HIV PEP: the greater the perceived risk, the more medications prescribed. Other groups support using two nucleoside reverse transcriptase inhibitors and a protease inhibitor or tenfovir for any significant HIV exposure. The CDC believes the expense and added potential for adverse side effects for additional medications is usually not warranted. The effectiveness of either method is not known. In general, availability of medications, expense, belief in the likelihood of transmission, compliance concerns, etc., will determine which approach to take. Other PEP regimens are possible and might be more, the same, or less effective.

Hepatitis B PEP

The preferred prophylaxis for hepatitis B is vaccination prior to being exposed. Unless otherwise contraindicated, all healthcare workers who will may come in contact with blood or body fluids should be vaccinated against hepatitis B. A small proportion of those vaccinated may require a second round of shots, and a smaller pro-

Table 2. HBV PEP Recommendations from the CDC

HBV vaccination status of exposed healthcare worker	Recommended treatment Source is $HBsAg^+$	Source is $HBsAg^-$	Unknown HBsAg status
Never vaccinated	HBIG and HBV vaccination	HBV vaccination	HBV vaccination
Previously vaccinated			
Known responder	No treatment	No treatment	No treatment
Known non-responder	HBIG x 1 and HBV if only vaccinated once, otherwise HBIG x 2	No treatment	If perceived source's HBV risk is high, proceed if source is
HBsAg+			
Unknown response	Test healthcare worker's HBV status first, then proceed based upon their antibody response	No treatment	Test healthcare worker's HBV status first, then proceed based upon their antibody response

portion may never develop a detectable immune response. The CDC recommends a hierarchical approach to hepatitis B PEP (summarized in Table 2). The greater the transmission risk, the stronger the recommendation to provide either post-exposure vaccination, immunoglobulin, or both. It is likely the source's HBeAg status will not be known initially for most exposures. If the status can be determined rapidly (i.e., within the 72-hour recommended window period for PEP), then immunoglobulin administration can be delayed. The exposed healthcare worker should be vaccinated prior to receiving the HBeAg results. The CDC does not currently recommend a hepatitis B booster for those successfully vaccinated previously or are known to be immune.

Hepatitis C PEP

Although there are antiviral medications and immunoglobulin agents available for hepatitis C treatment, none are yet proven effective for PEP. The CDC does not currently recommend any regimen for hepatitis C PEP, and there are no large sample randomized controlled trials evaluating hepatitis C PEP. Furthermore, there are no putative regimens for hepatitis C PEP. However, recent trials support the early use of antiviral medications for acute hepatitis C infections.

RESOURCES

University of Iowa Department of Public Health: http://www.idph.state.ia.us/adper/cade_content/epifacts/epifactcontents.htm (healthcare worker exposure transmission risk information)

PEP Intranet Resources:

Centers for Disease Control and Prevention: http://www.cdc.gov/mmwr/PDF/rr/rr5011.pdf
European Commission: http://www.eurosurveillance.org/em/v09n06/0906-222.asp
UCSF Center for HIV Information: http://hivinsite.ucsf.edu/InSite?page=kb-07-02-06#S2.4X
UK Department of Health: http://www.advisorybodies.doh.gov.uk/eaga/PDFS/prophylaxisguidancefeb04.pdf
WHO Post Exposure Prophylaxis: http://www.who.int/hiv/topics/prophylaxis/en/index.html

REFERENCES

Cardo DM, Culver DH, Ciesielski CA, Srivastava PU, Marcus R, Abiteboul D, Heptonstall J, Ippolito G, Lot F, McKibben PS, Bell DM. 1997. A case-control study of HIV seroconversion in health care workers after percutaneous exposure. *New Engl J Med* **337**(21):1485–90.

Gerberding JL. 1994. Incidence and prevalence of human immunodeficiency virus, hepatitis B virus, hepatitis C virus, and cytomegalovirus among health care personnel at risk for blood exposure: final report from a longitudinal study. *J Infect Dis* **170**(6):1410–1417.

Kato-Maeda M, Ponce-de-Leon S, Sifuentes-Osornio J, Rangel-Frausto MS, Calva-Mercado J, Infante-Surez L, Villareal FM, Ponce-de-Leon S. 2000. Bloodborne viral infections in patients attending an emergency room in Mexico City: estimate of seroconversion probability in healthcare workers after an occupational exposure. *Infect Control Hosp Epidemiol* **21**(9):600–602.

Merchant RC, Becker BM, Mayer KH, Fuerch J, Schreck B. 2003. Emergency department blood or body fluid exposure evaluations and HIV post-exposure prophylaxis usage. *Acad Emerg Med* **10**(12):1345–1353.

New York State Department of Health. 2004. *HIV prophylaxis following occupational exposure*. New York: New York State Department of Health.

Petrosillo N., Puro V, Jagger J, Ippolito G. 1995. The risks of occupational exposure and infection by human immunodeficiency virus, hepatitis B virus, and hepatitis C virus in the dialysis setting: Italian multicenter study on nosocomial and occupational risk of infections in dialysis. *Am J Infect Control* **23**(5):278–285.

Puro V, Cicalini S, De Carli G, Soldani F, Ippolito G. 2004. Towards a standard HIV post exposure prophylaxis for healthcare workers in Europe. *Euro Surveill* **9**(6). Epub ahead of text.

United Kingdom Health Department. 2004. HIV post-exposure prophylaxis: guidance from the UK chief medical officer's expert advisory group on AIDS. London: Department of Health.

Updated US public health service guidelines for the management of occupational exposure to HBV, HCV, and HIV and recommendations for postexposure prophylaxis. 2001. *MMWR Recomm Rep* **50**(RR-11):1–52.

Werner BG, Grady GF. 1982. Accidental hepatitis-B-surface-antigen-positive inoculations: use of E antigen to estimate infectivity. *Ann Intern Med* **97**(3):367–369.

World Health Organization. 2005. *Post-exposure prophylaxis*. http://www.who.int/hiv/topics/prophylaxis/en/index.html.

88 POST-TRAUMATIC STRESS DISORDER

Brian Wolfson, MD*

OVERVIEW

Posttraumatic stress disorder (PTSD) develops in persons who have experienced a traumatic event that has involved experiencing, witnessing, or being confronted with actual or threatened death, serious injury, or a threat to one's physical integrity. Examples include combat, physical assault, rape, and disasters. The three major elements of PTSD include:

1. Reexperiencing the trauma through dreams or recurrent and intrusive thoughts
2. Emotional numbing such as feeling detached from others
3. Symptoms of autonomic arousal such as irritability and exaggerated startle response

These symptoms must last for longer than one month
Two subtypes are specified:

1. Acute: duration of the symptoms is less than 3 months
2. Chronic: symptoms last 3 months or longer

If onset is delayed more than 6 months after the stressor, that delay is specified.

HISTORICAL SIGNIFICANCE

The term posttraumatic stress disorder was introduced in 1980 in the DSM-III, although the concept of this disturbance has a long history. In the past, it the syndrome was recognized in wartime as shell shock or war neurosis, because it was seen most commonly in wartime situations. Many of its typical symptoms, however, such as

*Department of Emergency Medicine, Allegheny General Hospital, Pittsburgh

intrusive thoughts and autonomic arousal, were also recognized in victims of other traumatic events, such as natural disasters.

EPIDEMIOLOGY

The prevalence of PTSD in the general population has been estimated to be 0.5% among men and 1.2% among women. Most men with the disorder have experienced combat. For women, the most frequent precipitating stressor is a physical assault or rape. The disorder can occur at any age, and children have been reported to develop the disorder.

CLINICAL FINDINGS

The disorder can be chronic and has been reported to last in some cases for 30 or 40 years (see Table 1). Symptoms tend to fluctuate and worsen during periods of stress. Predictors of good outcome include rapid onset of symptoms, adequate premorbid functioning, strong social supports, and an absence of psychiatric or medical comorbidity.

PATHOPHYSIOLOGY

While much of the pathophysiology of PTSD is unclear, interesting findings are accruing from research being done in the area. Studies using PET scans have shown that there is decreased hippocampal volume in patients with PTSD compared with matched controls. Other reports have demonstrated increased central norepinephrine levels with downregulated central adrenergic receptors, chronically decreased glucocorticoid levels, and decreased serotonin activity.

ETIOLOGY

The major etiological event leading to PTSD is the stressor. Because not all persons who experience a major stressor develop the disorder, other variables such as underlying personality and biological vulnerability are undoubtedly important. Stressors of all types may contribute to the development of PTSD, but they must be severe enough to be outside the range of normal human experience. Certain experiences are highly linked to the development of PTSD: witnessing a friend being killed in action, witnessing wartime atrocities, and, especially, participating in atrocities.

Individual differences that can predispose to the development of PTSD include age, history of emotional disturbance, social support, and proximity to the stressor. Eighty percent of young children who sustain a burn injury, for example, show symptoms of posttraumatic stress 1–2 years after the initial injury, but only 30% of adults who sustain this injury have symptoms after 1 year. Persons with a prior history of psychiatric treatment have a greater likelihood of developing the syndrome, presumable because the previous illness reflects a greater sensitivity to stress; and persons with adequate social support are less likely to develop the disorder than persons with poor support.

Table 1. DSM-IV Criteria for Posttraumatic Stress Disorder

A. The person has been exposed to a traumatic event in which both of the following were present:
 1. The person experienced, witnessed, or was confronted with an event or events that involve actual or threatened death or serious injury, or a threat to the physical integrity of self or others.
 2. The person's response involved intense fear, helplessness, or horror. In children, it may be expressed instead by disorganized or agitated behavior.

B. The traumatic event is persistently reexperienced in one (or more) of the following ways:
 3. Recurrent and intrusive distressing recollections of the event, including images, thoughts or perceptions. In young children, there may be frightening dreams without recognizable content.
 4. Recurrent distressing dreams of the event. Note: In children, there may be frightening dreams without recognizable content.
 5. Acting or feeling as if the traumatic event were recurring (including a sense of reliving the experience, illusions, hallucinations, and dissociative flashback episodes, including these that occur on awakening or when intoxicated). In young children, traumatic specific reenactment may occur.
 6. Intense psychological distress at exposure to internal or external cues that symbolize or resemble an aspect of the traumatic event.
 7. Physiological reactivity on exposure to internal or external cues that symbolize or resemble as aspect of the traumatic event.

C. Persistent avoidance of stimuli associated with the trauma and numbing of general responsiveness (not present before the trauma), as indicated by three (or more) of the following:
 8. Efforts to avoid thoughts, feelings, or conversations associated with the trauma.
 9. Efforts to avoid activities, places, or people that arouse recollections of the trauma.
 10. Inability to recall an important aspect of the trauma.
 11. Markedly diminished interest or participation in significant activities.
 12. Feeling of detachment or estrangement from others.
 13. Restricted range of affect (e.g., unable to have loving feelings).
 14. Sense of foreshortened future (e.g., does not expect to have a career, marriage, or children, or a normal life span).

D. Persistent symptoms of increased arousal (no present before the trauma), as indicated by two (or more of the following:
 15. Difficulty falling or staying asleep.
 16. Irritability or outbursts of anger.
 17. Difficulty concentrating.
 18. Hypervigilance.
 19. Exaggerated startle response.

E. Duration of the disturbance symptoms in criteria B, C, and D is more than 1 month.

F. The disturbance causes clinically significant distress or impairment in social, occupational, or other important areas of functioning.

Specify if:
Acute: if duration of symptoms is less than 3 months
Chronic: if duration of symptoms is 3 months or more

Specify if:
With delayed onset: if onset of symptoms is at least 6 months after the stressor.

COMPLICATIONS

Complications of PTSD may include violence and aggression, alcohol and drug abuse, and poor impulse control. Although many war veterans have claimed that PTSD has led them to commit criminal offenses, one study found that felonious behavior in combat veterans occurred only in those who had had similar behavior before military service.

DIFFERENTIAL DIAGNOSIS

The differential diagnosis for PTSD includes major depression, adjustment disorder, panic disorder, generalized anxiety disorder, acute stress disorder, obsessive compulsive disorder, depersonalization disorder, factitious disorder, or malingering. Occasionally, a physical injury may have occurred during the stressor so that a mental disorder secondary to brain injury must be considered as well. Many patients with PTSD meet criteria for another Axis I disorder (e.g., major depression, panic disorder), in which case both disorders should be diagnosed.

TREATMENT

There are few controlled studies of the pharmacological and psychotherapeutic strategies for the treatment of PTSD. Medication helps to decrease depression, to reduce intrusive symptoms such as nightmares and flashbacks, and to normalize sleep.

Serotonin Reuptake Inhibitors

Selective serotonin reuptake inhibitors (SSRIs) reduce flashbacks, arousal, and avoidance in patients with PTSD. The efficacy of the SSRIs was demonstrated in a randomized double-blind placebo-controlled trial of 53 civilians with PTSD who received fluoxetine (median dose 30 mg daily) or placebo. Compared with the placebo group, the group treated with fluoxetine showed better global improvement and less disability at 12 weeks.

Anxiolytics

Anxiolytics are generally ineffective in PTSD, which is surprising considering the constellation of anxiety, jitteriness, hyperarousal, and autonomic instability commonly observed in these patients. One study comparing alprazolam and placebo found a modest reduction of anxiety in patients with PTSD, although symptoms specific to PTSD were not changed. Given the prevalence of comorbid substance abuse in patients with PTSD and the lack of efficacy, benzodiazepines should generally be avoided.

Psychotherapy

Psychotherapy can be enormously helpful. Behavioral techniques involving direct therapeutic exposure (i.e., flooding), are particularly helpful in reducing the intrusive symptoms of PTSD. Cognitive therapies may also help to reduce anxiety by providing patients with the skills to control anxiety. More psychodynamic approaches may help persons to integrate the traumatic event into their understanding of the meaning of life and their self-concept. Group and family therapy have been advocated.

REFERENCES

Braun P, Greenberg D, Dasberg H, Lerer B. 1990. Core symptoms of posttraumatic stress disorder improved by alprazolam treatment. *J Clin Psychiatry* 51:236–238.

Bremner JD, Randall P, Scott TM, Bronen RA, Seibyl JP, Southwick SM, Delaney RC, McCarthy G, Charney DS, Innis RB. 1995. MRI-based measure of hippocampal volume in patients with PTSD. *Am J Psychiatry* **152**(7):973–81.

Connor KM, Sutherland SM, Tupler LA, Malik ML, Davidson JR. 1999. Fluoxetine in post-traumatic stress disorder: randomised, double-blind study. *Br J Psychiatry* **175**:17–22.

Geracioti TD Jr, Baker DG, Ekhator NN, West SA, Hill KK, Bruce AB, Schmidt D, Rounds-Kugler B, Yehuda R, Keck PE Jr, Kasckow JW. 2001. CSF norepinephrine concentrations in posttraumatic stress disorder. *Am J Psychiatry* **158**:1227–1230.

Van der Kolk BA. 1997. The psychobiology of posttraumatic stress disorder. *J Clin Psychiatry* **58**(suppl 9):16–24.

89

INTERNATIONAL LAW: A PRIMER FOR HEALTHCARE PROFESSIONALS

Michael H. Hoffman*

INTRODUCTION

This chapter presents (1) basic concepts and principles from international law relevant to the work of healthcare professionals responding to peacetime emergencies and armed conflict, and (2) selective field notes that illustrate some of the more challenging implications of these principles.

This is introductory text for readers who are not lawyers. This chapter does not provide legal advice of any sort and should not be used for that purpose. Readers should consult qualified attorneys to resolve legal issues that arise in connection with their work.

INTERNATIONAL LAW

International law traditionally addressed the relationship between nations (referred to as states in international law and through the remainder of this chapter). Generally speaking, individuals and organizations did not have a role to play in the international legal system. Only states could officially speak, act on, or complain about implementation or violation of international rules. Since the late nineteenth century, international law has been changing in respect to the participants who are authorized to get involved in these events.

Since that time, international organizations established by treaty (e.g., the World Health Organization) have also played a role in developing and implementing the law. However, individuals could say little or nothing on their own behalf in the international legal system until more recently. Though the antislavery movement achieved major progress in the development of an international law to protect human beings in

*Office of International Humanitarian Law and Policy, American Red Cross, Washington, DC

earlier generations, and rules for protection during wartime have existed for centuries, it took the horrors of the Second World War to bring about the development of a modern law of human rights. In our time states have legal obligations to individual human beings as well as each other.

These still-evolving historical trends are important to healthcare professionals in several respects. (1) States and selected international organizations established or recognized by treaty play the lead role in developing and implementing international law. (2) Private nongovernmental organizations (NGOs) such as those involved in healthcare delivery can be influential and informative in the international legal system. However, they do not have the authority to create or enforce the law. (3) There are established international legal standards for the protection of human beings, and sometimes, but not always, these standards take into account the specific role of healthcare professionals (e.g., the Geneva Conventions).

For purposes of this chapter, contemporary international law is narrowly defined as the rules and principles adopted by states and (sometimes) international organizations that (1) set standards and obligations for protection of the vulnerable; and (2) regulate the status, rights, responsibilities, and protection of healthcare professionals performing services abroad, especially in response to armed conflict and peacetime emergencies.[1]

RELATIONSHIP OF INTERNATIONAL AND DOMESTIC LAW

Modern international law imposes certain humanitarian and human rights obligations on states. In most other respects, however, states retain full sovereign control over law-making. In most cases domestic (national) law is not superseded by international law. States hold the authority to determine who may enter their territory, and whether and to what extent humanitarian organizations and their staff will be exempt from local laws and regulations. Healthcare professionals performing services in a foreign state are bound to follow national laws (e.g., professional licensing requirements where this is an issue, traffic rules, customs and tax obligations).

There are exceptional circumstances where the application, interpretation, manipulation, or misuse of domestic law may put the state in breach of international legal obligations: (1) where the state fails to honor treaty commitments (e.g., on reciprocal privileges for visiting workers), (2) where the state fails to honor commitments made to a humanitarian organization, (3) where national law, policy, or conduct conflicts with, or violates, international humanitarian, human rights or refugee law.

REFUGEE LAW

There is one universally recognized legal definition of refugees. It is found in the UN Convention relating to the Status of Refugees of 1951 and its Protocol of 1967. Taken together, these define a refugee as one who "owing to well-founded fear of being persecuted for reasons of race, religion, nationality, membership of a particular social group, or political opinion, is outside the country of his nationality and is unable or, owing to such fear, is unwilling to avail himself of the protection of that country." Individuals who meet this legal test are entitled to the assistance and protection of the UN High Commissioner for Refugees (UNHCR).

More expansive definitions have been regionally adopted by treaty in Africa (OAU Convention Governing the Specific Aspects of Refugee Problems in Africa), and by way of a legally nonbinding resolution passed by states in the Americas (Cartagena Declaration on Refugees), that encompass situations such as those where individuals cross international borders to escape from generalized violence, armed conflict, and other circumstances seriously disturbing public order. The popular notion of a refugee as someone fleeing from any conceivable form of crisis or chaos (e.g., economic collapse) is not supported by international law.

Additionally, those who flee from danger or upheaval but remain within their home country are known as internally displaced persons (IDPs). Refugee law does not address the well-being of IDPs, but they do benefit from the protections of international humanitarian and human rights law. In some circumstances UNHCR extends assistance to IDPs as well as refugees. The International Committee of the Red Cross takes the lead in assisting IDPs during armed conflict.

States have an obligation (1) to make a fair determination of whether someone is entitled to refugee status, (2) not to send refugees back home while they are in danger (sometimes referred to as the principle of non-refoulement), and (3) to assist them in securing public services where such are otherwise available and let them earn a livelihood.

Field note: Within one refugee camp, whose residents seem legally indistinguishable from one another, it may be possible that some will qualify as refugees and others as internally displaced persons, while yet others have no claim to belong in either of these groups. In such circumstances the legal status, protection, and options available to individuals within such communities may vary significantly.

INTERNATIONAL HUMANITARIAN LAW

International humanitarian law (IHL) is comprised of the laws and principles that are used to save lives and alleviate suffering during armed conflict. Armed forces sometimes prefer to use "the law of war" or "the law of armed conflict" as terminology that identifies these rules.[2] IHL has roots going back many centuries in customary, non-treaty-based practices such as the use of white flags to request a suspension of hostilities. Its systematic development in the form of treaties began in the nineteenth century.

The core treaties of modern IHL are the four Geneva Conventions of 1949, which establish humanitarian standards and obligations for protection of wounded, sick, and shipwrecked members of armed forces, prisoners of war, and civilians detained by the other side or living in war zones or occupied areas. (These treaties are the primary focus of this section.) The Geneva Conventions of 1949 are supplemented by two Protocols that were adopted in 1977.[3] Under the Geneva Conventions, the International Committee of the Red Cross (ICRC) is accorded special status and responsibility for the protection of prisoners of war and civilians.

It should also be noted that some IHL treaties have a different focus. Some regulate tactics and targeting in combat (Hague Conventions IV and IX of 1907 and some sections in the Protocols to the Geneva Conventions of 1977), and others the kinds of weapons that can be used (e.g., the Convention on the Prohibition of the Use, Stockpiling, Production, and Transfer of Anti-Personnel Mines and on their

Destruction). A recent treaty established an international court to try defendants for alleged war crimes (Rome Statute of the International Criminal Court).

Most rules of IHL apply during international armed conflict (meaning between states). A subset of these rules also applies during internal armed conflict (meaning within one state). States have never agreed to apply the full rules of IHL to internal armed conflicts. The rules described below therefore apply in full during international armed conflict only. However, many of the rules along with the broad principles of humane treatment for the wounded, sick, civilians, and captives, and for protection of those rendering them assistance, apply during internal armed conflict as well.[4] IHL only applies during armed conflict and not in other circumstances involving use of force.[5]

Field note: There is another branch of international law (not IHL) that deals with the legal standards justifying or prohibiting the initiation of armed conflict: (1) such rules are not immediately relevant to humanitarian work in the field, (2) such rules are separate from those that actually regulate behavior during armed conflict and therefore not part of IHL, and (3) once armed conflict actually begins, all parties are expected to apply IHL whether or not their cause is legally or morally justifiable. A cause worthy of support may be marred by war crimes. Combatants serving a cause lacking international sympathy might, on the other hand, be highly creditable for their diligent application of IHL.

The wounded, sick, and shipwrecked are to be spared from attack, rescued from the field, and protected. Wounded and sick must receive medical treatment regardless of which side they are on. Only urgent medical reasons authorize priority in the order of treatment. There are strict prohibitions against violence, torture, or biological experiments on the wounded and sick, prisoners of war, and civilians.

Prisoners of war and civilians detained for security reasons must be humanely treated and protected, given proper medical care, food, and shelter, and must be accorded protective visits from the ICRC to ensure that they are being humanely treated and allowed to communicate with their families.

Civilians, civilian communities, and civilian infrastructure are protected from attack. Protection of women from rape, enforced prostitution, and other crimes of violence is an increasingly emphasized facet of IHL. A pattern of systematic, brutal crimes instigated or abetted by the authorities sometimes collectively constitutes an additional and separate category of offenses known as Crimes Against Humanity. Crimes Against Humanity could be committed during armed conflict or peacetime but most often occur in the former circumstances. Genocide is also a crime that could occur either during armed conflict or peacetime (see International Human Rights Law below).

IHL protects military medical units, transport, and personnel from attack. IHL also protects civilian hospitals and personnel from attack.[6] In turn, using language from the Geneva Conventions, military and civilian medical facilities and transport are not to be used "to commit, outside their humanitarian duties, acts harmful to the enemy" (e.g., using a hospital to disguise a military command center). To do so risks loss of protection.[7]

Certain humanitarian emblems can be used to mark such medical units, transport and facilities. When used for that purpose, the emblems signal the medical character of these sites and staff, and protect them from attack. The Red Cross and Red Crescent are the two humanitarian emblems recognized in the Geneva Conventions that are presently in use. They are used to mark military medical units and facilities and civilian hospitals, and to identify personnel who are engaged in medical and supporting administrative duties at those sites.

The International Committee of the Red Cross and the International Federation of Red Cross and Red Crescent Societies are also authorized similar emblem use. Civilian hospitals cannot use these emblems without prior authorization from the authorities. Use of protective emblems is optional for those organizations and facilities that are authorized to employ them. Even if not so identified by a protective emblem, IHL still protects these personnel, medical units, hospitals, and staff from attack.

Field note: Use of protective emblems is highly regulated. No one is permitted to wear or utilize them unless they are performing humanitarian duties with an organization or facility that is clearly authorized their use under the terms of the Geneva Conventions.

To the fullest extent of the means available to it, a military occupation force is responsible for ensuring food, medical supplies, medical facilities, and public health in occupied areas if local resources are inadequate. If resources are inadequate and the occupation forces cannot meet needs, then they are obligated to allow and cooperate in relief schemes that bring in outside sources of humanitarian assistance. Local and outside organizations may continue to provide assistance and relief so long as they operate in a manner compatible with humanitarian status and obligations.

Field note: Healthcare providers serving in humanitarian organizations are present to provide services and not to support an occupation force. They should maintain an independent view on whether the authorities are properly implementing IHL. In other respects, the occupation force stands in a similar relationship to humanitarian organizations as do the civil authorities in peacetime. Occupation authorities can impose temporary and exceptional measures for urgent reasons of security. These cannot be ignored, just as the laws and regulations implemented by civil authorities cannot be ignored in peacetime.

INTERNATIONAL HUMAN RIGHTS LAW

International human rights law encompasses the rules that protect human beings from state oppression and abuse, and ensure their political, social, and religious freedoms. It also addresses (sometimes with debate on the state of the law and its application to such issues) individual economic and social rights and well-being, and group rights such as self-determination. All human rights law applies in peacetime.

However, it only applies to a more limited extent during armed conflict, as IHL is the body of law that has been specifically adopted for use in those circumstances. The Convention on the Prevention and Punishment of the Crime of Genocide of 1948 offers the starkest example of a crime prohibited by international law that could take place either in peacetime or during armed conflict. This treaty prohibits and criminalizes certain acts committed "with intent to destroy, in whole or in part, a national, ethnic, racial, or religious group."

Human rights emerged as a major component of international law with adoption, by the UN General Assembly, of the Genocide Convention and the Universal Declaration of Human Rights in 1948. Other landmark sources of human rights law include the International Covenant on Economic, Social, and Cultural Rights, the International Covenant on Civil and Political Rights, and the Convention Against Torture and Other Cruel Inhuman or Degrading Treatment or Punishment. The latter defines torture, in part, as "any act by which severe pain or suffering, whether physical or mental, is intentionally inflicted on a person ... by or at the instigation of or with the consent or acquiescence of a public official or other person acting in an official capacity."

Core human rights protections prohibit slavery, genocide, torture, and denial of religious and political freedom. One influential line of thought suggests that human rights law advances in generations, with the first ensuring political rights, the second economic and social rights, and the third collective or group rights.

Protections for women have recently emerged as a key focus of human rights law. The concept of rights-based programming draws upon international human rights law as well. However, international law does not recognize or incorporate a principle of rights-based programming.

Where rules of IHL are often specific, and almost all designed for application in unstable or turbulent circumstances, the rules found in human rights law are broad and sometimes more a statement of principles than a source of specific guidance. Also, human rights law is principally designed for application in stable settings rather than emergencies. It is thus more difficult to identify human rights rules that apply specifically to healthcare professionals and services during emergency response. However, broad principles of human rights law barring discrimination and mistreatment are sufficiently developed to bar states from discrimination against disfavored segments of the population in delivery of emergency relief or healthcare services.

Human rights law is important to the work of healthcare professionals in emergency settings: (1) Any indication that the authorities are attempting a favored or malicious allocation of healthcare services or resources should put healthcare professionals on alert for possible human rights violations. (2) Healthcare professionals will sometimes be the first to find evidence of serious human rights law violations such as torture or discriminatory relief distribution. (3) Local laws and customs may be in conflict with human rights law standards that your organization looks to apply in its field work (e.g., rules on gender discrimination).

Field note: Care should be taken to avoid inadvertent facilitation of human rights violations. For example, a reasonable impulse to inform the police about property theft might be weighed against the reputation, record, and professionalism of local law enforcement. If they take a heavy-handed approach the result could be a human rights disaster for all concerned.

EMERGING ISSUES

International law is a dynamic field that's undergoing rapid change. Several notable examples of other, newly emerging issues that may impact the work of healthcare professionals include the international law of terrorism and international disaster response law.

Several legal problems contribute to the ongoing debate on terrorism and state response: (1) no treaty provides a comprehensive definition of terrorism, and (2) it is sometimes unclear whether threats posed by terrorism are more military or criminal in their characteristics. This can make it difficult to determine whether IHL (military response) or human rights law (police response) applies. This problem will not be fully resolved any time soon.

In another field, peacetime disasters and emergencies have received surprisingly little legal attention. Some treaties that focus primarily on other subjects also contain provisions for peacetime humanitarian response, and a handful of specialized treaties have been specifically adopted to address peacetime emergency response (e.g., Tampere Convention on the Provision of Telecommunication Resources for Disaster Mitigation and Relief Operations).

However, until recently such sources were never systematically examined or applied. The International Federation of Red Cross and Red Crescent Societies is leading collaborative efforts (with states, the United Nations, and others actively participating) to remedy this gap by collecting, publishing, and analyzing relevant treaties, laws, and regulations, which are sometimes known as International Disaster Response Laws (IDRLs). Over time these efforts should help to improve the efficiency of peacetime disaster response.

PROFESSIONAL STATUS, STANDARDS AND ETHICS

International law has not fully caught up with the globalization of healthcare delivery in emergency settings. The standards of international humanitarian and human rights law apply in this work, but in other respects licensing and professional standards remain fully in the purview of domestic law. There is no international licensing authority or board of professional responsibility that oversees the work of healthcare professionals.

Healthcare professionals should nonetheless remain alert to evolving international standards and expectations against which their work may be measured. Best practices (e.g., Sphere Standards) may eventually acquire sufficient standing to be accepted as a prospective legal standard. Resolutions passed by international professional societies (e.g., the World Medical Association) are also influential in determining the ethical standards and responsibilities of healthcare professionals who provide international emergency assistance. The impact and influence of such standards will likely grow in the twenty-first century.

IMPLEMENTATION OF INTERNATIONAL LAW

International law is formally implemented through a variety of mechanisms, including, among others, diplomatic negotiation and persuasion, sanctions, international and domestic courts, humanitarian fieldwork by organizations officially mandated to perform these tasks by treaty, and training programs for armed forces. Important sources of unofficial persuasion in the implementation of international law include media coverage, human rights monitoring activities, NGO field work, advocacy, legal scholarship, and public opinion.

Field note: Extreme care should be used by healthcare professionals in deciding how they might or might not contribute to implementation of international law in the field. Missteps might endanger staff or beneficiaries. Silence or inaction, on the other hand, might contribute to further breaches of the law. Depending on the specific circumstances, careful consideration might be given to appropriate response methods including among others dialogue, negotiation, evacuation, and reporting. On the brighter side, there may sometimes be opportunities for proactive improvement in the situation via friendly persuasion and education efforts.

RESOURCES

There are numerous websites dedicated to issues covered by this chapter. Care should be used in utilizing such sites to distinguish between actual legal sources (e.g., statutes and treaties), interpretation and explanation of the law (which may or may not be professional and insightful), and polemics, which sometimes add nothing to the readers' understanding of international law. A few helpful professionally sponsored sites are identified here.

For treaties, resolutions, and specialized discussion of international humanitarian law see the following sites:

www.icrc.org/eng

www.ihlresearch.org/ihl/portalhome.php

For treaties and resolutions on international human rights and refugee law see the following site:

www1.umn.edu/humanrts/

For background on international disaster response laws and links to other relevant IDRL sources, see the following site:

www.ifrc.org/what/disasters/idrl

NOTES

1. Topics covered here fall within the much wider field known as public international law, which covers numerous other important subjects as well (e.g., international environmental law, the law of the sea, the law of treaty interpretation).

2. War, in the legal sense, is a term used to describe armed hostilities initiated by states via formal declaration. The Geneva Conventions apply during armed conflict, meaning almost any form of armed interstate (and sometimes intrastate) hostilities whether or not formally declared.

3. Convention I for the Amelioration of the Condition of the Wounded and Sick in Armed Forces in the Field; Convention II for the Amelioration of the Condition of Wounded, Sick, and Shipwrecked Members of Armed Forces at Sea; Convention III relative to the Treatment of Prisoners of War; Convention IV relative to the Protection of Civilian Persons in Time of War; the Protocol Additional to the Geneva Conventions of 12 August 1949, and relating to the Protection of Victims of International Armed Conflicts (Protocol I); the Protocol Additional to the Geneva Conventions of 12 August 1949, and relating to the Protection of Victims of Non-International Armed Conflicts (Protocol II).

4. Article 3, common to all four Geneva Conventions of 1949, provides the core rules applicable during internal armed conflict, and these are bolstered by the rules in Protocol II to the Geneva Conventions.

5. IHL protections do not apply in peacetime. Use of force in response to riots, violent demonstrations, and other turbulent or unstable situations falling short of armed conflict (sometimes referred to as internal disturbances and tensions) is, however, addressed by international human rights law.

6. Hospital, safety, and neutralized areas can also be set up in some circumstances to protect the wounded and sick as well as civilians.

7. Geneva Convention I provides "Protection may, however, cease only after a due warning has been given, naming, in all appropriate cases, a reasonable time limit, and after such warning has remained unheeded."

90

A GUIDE TO THE WORLDWIDE WEB

Barbara Kilian, MD*

The scope of the Internet can make doing research a frustrating task. Before listing resources, a primer of web-based research is offered. The first step in web-based research is to find a search engine/directory you are comfortable using. A search engine/directory is a website tool that allows users to find information on the World Wide Web (WWW).

The primary problem that most people encounter when searching the web is encountering too much information, as there are millions upon millions of websites. There are several types of search engines/directories that can be utilized. Search directories are databases arranged in a hierarchical database that reference websites. The websites that are listed are chosen by individuals and classified according to the rules of that particular search directory. The Yahoo! Directory is the classic example of a search directory. These are good when you only have a general idea of what you are looking for, as subjects are divided into broad categories and then subdivided when you choose the topic. You can often utilize a search within the directory. When you utilize this function, you are not actually searching the text of actual webpages, but are instead searching the text in the title and site description (composed by the site owner themselves).

Search engines are "robots" that crawl the WWW and look for new websites. They take the information in the websites and put the text into a large database that you access when you search. The largest search engines are Google and Yahoo!Search. Search engines should be the first choice when you know exactly what you are looking for.

Once you have decided on a search engine/directory, you can begin your search. The best way to make your search effective is to use the BOOLEAN method. This is a code that allows the search engine to better narrow down your search. When you are using multiple words in your search, you can tell the search engine what to include and what to exclude. Using "AND" will tell the computer to find only web pages with

*Department of Emergency Medicine, St. Luke's/Roosevelt Hospital Center, New York

both words. By utilizing "AND NOT," the computer will exclude the word following the command. "OR" will tell the search engine to include either of the words.

You can also use phrases with your search by utilizing "double quotation marks." This will tell the computer to look for those words together and does not look for each individual word. Most search engines also have an advanced search option that will guide you through more advanced questions to help refine your search. Keep in mind that there is no librarian or card catalogue to go with the web, which can be frustrating. Think about the question you want answered and search effectively. It may take several refinements before finding exactly what you need. The more you search, the easier it becomes.

HELPFUL SITES

http://www.cdc.gov: home site for the Center for Disease Control and Prevention. It has a search engine in the top right hand corner for specific searches. It covers information from birth defects, diseases, emergency preparedness, vaccinations, etc.

http://www.fema.gov: home site for the Federal Emergency Management Agency. FEMA is responsible for "responding to, planning for, recovering from, and mitigating against disasters." Site includes general information, a library, maps, and regional updates. Site is for United States ONLY. It does not include information on international disasters.

http://www.epa.gov: home site for the Environmental Protection Agency. Under "Quick Links," select "More Links" for an alphabetical listing. Under "Emergencies," there are subheadings for Emergency Preparedness and Emergency Responses.

http://www.nih.org: home site for the National Institutes of Health. Search engine includes the National Library of Medicine.

http://www.who.int: the World Health Organization is a United Nations agency specialized in health. Their goals are to pursue the best available health care for all people, including physical, mental, and social well-being. There is a search function in the upper right-hand corner.

http://www.redcross.org: the American Red Cross is a nonprofit volunteer organization that works to provide relief services to victims of disasters and to help prevent, prepare for, and respond to emergencies.

http://www.emergencyjournal.com/pn06001.html: home site for the *Journal of Emergency Management*, a quarterly journal whose goal is "to better equip all those responsible for emergency preparedness and response to deal effectively with everything from acts of terror, fires, floods, and weather emergencies to gas explosions and catastrophic accidents on land, in the air, or at sea."

INDEX

Note: Page numbers followed by *t* indicate tables.

B

C

D

F

I

N

O

P

Q

R

S

T

W

X

Y

Z

DATE DUE

Printed in the United States of America